SURGICAL ANATOMY

of the

HEART

SECOND EDITION

Benson R. Wilcox, MD
Professor of Surgery
Chief, Division of Cardiothoracic Surgery
University of North Carolina
Chapel Hill, North Carolina, USA

Robert H. Anderson,
BSc, MD, MRCPath
Joseph Levy Professor of
Paediatric Cardiac Morphology
Cardiothoracic Institute
University of London
Honorary Consultant
The Brompton Hospital
London, UK

foreword by

David C. Sabiston, Jr. MD
James Buchanan Duke Professor of Surgery
and Chairman of the Department
Duke University Medical Center
Durham, North Carolina

Gower Medical Publishing · London · New York

Distributed in the USA and Canada by:
J B Lippincott Company
East Washington Square
Philadelphia
PA 19105
USA

Distributed in the UK and Continental Europe by:
Gower Medical Publishing
Middlesex House
34–42 Cleveland Street
London W1P 5FB
UK

Distributed in Australia and New Zealand by:
Harper Educational (Australia) Pty Ltd
PO Box 226
Artamon
NSW 2064
AUSTRALIA

Distributed in Southeast Asia, Hong Kong and Taiwan by:
APAC Publishers Services
30 Jalan Bahasa
Singapore 1129

Distributed in Japan by:
Nankodo Co Ltd
42–6 Hongo 3-chome
Bunkyo-ku
Tokyo 113
JAPAN

Distributed in South America by:
Harper Collins Publishers Latin America
701 Brickell Avenue
Suite 1750
Miami, Florida 33131
USA

Project Managers:	Sally Paviour
	Zak Knowles
Designer:	Mark Willey
Illustration:	Sue Tyler
Paste-up:	Nancy Chase
	Alan Wood
Index:	Nina Boyd
Production:	Susan Bishop
Publisher:	Fiona Foley

British Library Cataloguing in Publication Data:
Wilcox, Benson R.
Surgical anatomy of the heart – 2nd Ed.
I. Title   II. Anderson, Robert H.
616.1

Library of Congress Cataloging in Publication Data:
available on request

ISBN 0–397–44842–2

Text set in Bembo and Helvetica

Typesetting by M to N Typesetting, London

Originated by Chroma Graphics, Singapore

Produced by Imago, Singapore

Printed and bound in Singapore

A Slide Atlas of Surgical Anatomy of the Heart Second Edition, based on the contents of this book, is available. In the slide atlas format, the material is split into volumes, each of which is presented in a binder together with numbered 35mm slides of each illustration. Further information can be obtained from:

Gower Medical Publishing
101 Fifth Avenue
New York
NY 10003
USA

Gower Medical Publishing
Middlesex House
34–42 Cleveland Street
London W1P 5FB
UK

PREFACE TO THE FIRST EDITION

The books and articles devoted to technique in cardiac surgery are legion. This is most appropriate, since the success of cardiac surgery is greatly dependent upon excellent operative technique. But excellence of technique can be dissipated without a firm knowledge of the underlying cardiac morphology. This is as true of the 'normal heart' as for those hearts with complex congenital lesions. It is the feasibility of operating upon such complex malformations which has highlighted the need for a more detailed understanding of the basic anatomy in itself. thus, in recent years surgeons have come to appreciate the necessity of avoiding damage to the coronary vessels, often invisible when working within the cardiac chambers, and particularly to the vital conduction tissues, invisible at all times. Although detailed and available since the time of their discovery, only rarely have their positions been described with the cardiac surgeon in mind. Indeed, to the best of our knowledge there are no books which specifically display the anatomy of normal and abnormal hearts as perceived at the time of operation.

In writing this book we have tried to satisfy this need by combining the experience of a practising cardiac surgeon with that of a professional cardiac anatomist. We have emphasized the significant advances made in the last decade in appreciating the value of a detailed knowledge of cardiac anatomy. It is also our hope that the book will be of interest not only to the surgeon, but also the cardiologist, anaesthesiologist and surgical pathologist who ideally should have some knowledge of cardiac structures and its exquisite intricacies. Where appropriate, we have displayed our illustrations as seen by the surgeon, in many cases using material obtained in the operating room. To clarify the various orientations of each illustration, we have included a set of axes showing the directions of superior (S), inferior (I) anterior (A), posterior (P), left (L) and right (R). All our accounts are based on the anatomy as it is observed and, except in the case of aortic arch malformations, owe nothing to speculative embryology.

PREFACE TO THE SECOND EDITION

The books and articles devoted to technique in cardiac surgery are legion. This is most appropriate, since the success of cardiac surgery is greatly dependent upon excellent operative technique. But excellence of technique can be dissipated without a firm knowledge of the underlying cardiac morphology. This is as true for the 'normal heart' as for those hearts with complex congenital lesions. It is the feasibility of operating upon such complex malformations that has highlighted the need for a more detailed understanding of the basic anatomy in itself. Thus, in recent years, surgeons have come to appreciate the necessity of avoiding damage to the coronary vessels, often invisible when working within the cardiac chambers, and particularly to the vital conduction tissues, invisible at all times. Although detailed and accurate descriptions of the conduction system have been available since the time of this discovery, only rarely has its position been described with the cardiac surgeon in mind. At the time our first edition was published, to the best of our knowledge, there were no other books that specifically displayed the anatomy of normal and abnormal hearts as perceived at the time of operation. We tried in our first edition to satisfy this need by combining the experience of a practising cardiac surgeon with that of a professional cardiac anatomist.

This second edition expands and, we believe, improves upon this approach. It contains an entirely new chapter on valvar anatomy and a greatly expanded treatment of coronary arterial anatomy. The format has been altered to allow the reader to find a particular subject more easily. This edition contains more than 200 new illustrations. As in our first edition, we have endeavoured, where appropriate, to illustrate the anatomy as seen by the surgeon, using, in many cases, material obtained in the operating room. To clarify the orientation of the various illustrations, we have included a set of axes showing the directions of superior (S), inferior (I), anterior (A), posterior (P), left (L), right (R), apex (a) and base (b). All our accounts are based on the anatomy as it is observed and, except in the case of malformation of the aortic arch, owe nothing to speculative embryology.

It is our hope that the second edition of this book, like the first, will be of interest not only to the surgeon, but also to the cardiologist, anaesthesiologist and surgical pathologist, all of whom should have some knowledge of cardiac structures and their exquisite ideally, intricacies.

ACKNOWLEDGMENTS

As with our first edition, our many friends and collaborators deserve credit both for our illustrative material and for many of the concepts we espouse within these pages. From the stance of the anatomy, the many changes made from the first edition would not have been possible without the tremendous support and hospitality provided over the period between editions by Dr Bob Zuberbuhler, Chief of Pediatric Cardiology at Children's Hospital of Pittsburgh. We remain indebted to Professor Becker, University of Amsterdam, Dr Siew Yen Ho of the National Heart and Lung Institute, London, and Dr Audrey Smith of the Institute of Child Health, University of Liverpool, for their continuing support. The help of Dr. Ho was also invaluable in preparing artwork and photographs, as was that of Charles Wright and his staff in the Department of Medical Illustrations and Photography, University of North Carolina. We are equally indebted to Christine Anderson and Betsy Mann for their help during the preparation of the manuscript.

In all ventures of this kind, a debt is due to colleagues who shoulder the burden when our minds are on writing rather than on other responsibilities. In this respect, we thank Peter Starek, Blair Keagy, Michael Mill, and Thomas Egan of the University of North Carolina. The experience gained in studying the malformed hearts would have been impossible without the support of Christopher Lincoln, Darryl Shore, Elliot Shinebourne, Jane Somerville, Michael Rigby, and Andrew Redington of the Royal Brompton National Heart and Lung Hospital in London. It is again our pleasure finally to acknowledge the support and encouragement provided by Fiona Foley and her colleagues in the London office of Gower Medical Publishing, who transcended all the impediments placed in our way to ensure that the quality of this second edition surpasses that of the first.

B.R.W. & R.H.A

Introduction

In the normal individual the heart lies in the mediastinum with two-thirds of its bulk to the left of the midline (Fig. 1.1). Therefore, the heart and great vessels can be approached either through the thoracic cavity or anteriorly directly through the midline. To make such approaches safely, it is necessary to know the salient anatomical features of the chest wall, as well as the vessels and nerves that course through the mediastinum.

Median Sternotomy

The approach used most frequently is a median sternotomy, where a soft tissue incision is made in the midline and extends from the suprasternal notch to below the xiphoid process. Inferiorly, the linea alba is incised between the two rectus sheaths, taking care to avoid entering the peritoneal cavity or damaging an enlarged liver. Folding back the origin of the rectus muscles in this area reveals the xiphoid process, which is then incised to provide

access to the anterior mediastinum. Superiorly, a vertical incision is made between the sternal insertions of the sternocleidomastoid muscles, exposing the relatively bloodless midline raphe between the right and left sternohyoid and sterno-thyroid muscles. An incision through this raphe gives access to the superior aspect of the anterior mediastinum. The anterior mediastinum is immediately behind the sternum and is devoid of vital structures, so that these two incisions can safely be joined by a blunt dissection in the retro-

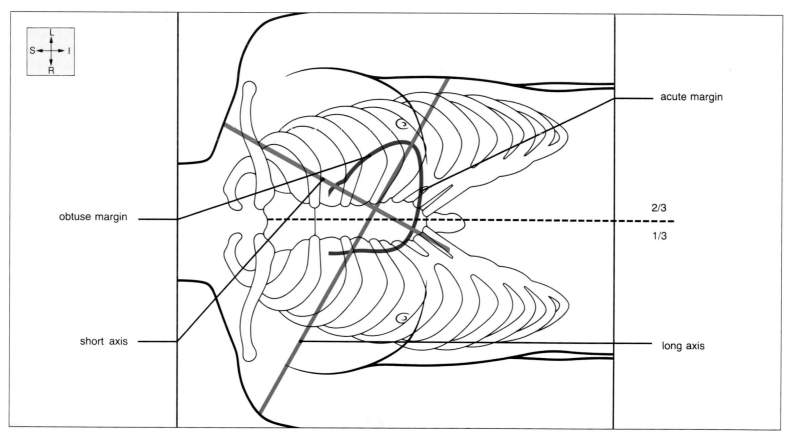

Fig. 1.1 *Diagram showing the usual position of the heart within the thorax showing vital landmarks and areas seen with the patient supine on the operating table.*

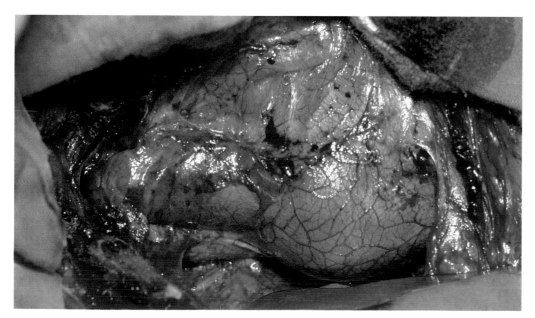

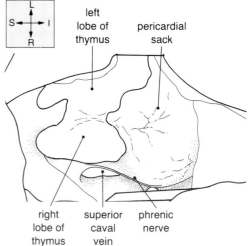

Fig. 1.2 *Operative view through a median sternotomy showing the extent of the thymus gland in an infant.*

sternal space. When the sternum has been split, retraction will reveal the pericardial sack lying between the pleural cavities.

Thymus Gland

Superiorly, the thymus gland wraps itself over the anterior and lateral aspects of the pericardium in the area of exit of the great arteries, the gland being a particularly prominent structure in the infant (Fig. 1.2).

It has two lateral lobes joined more or less in the midline, which sometimes must be divided, or partially excised, to provide adequate exposure. The arterial supply to the thymus is from the internal thoracic (mammary) and inferior thyroid arteries. If divided, these arteries tend to retract beneath the sternum and can produce troublesome bleeding. The veins are fragile, often emptying into the left brachiocephalic (innominate) vein via a common trunk (Fig. 1.3). Undue traction

on the gland may lead to damage to this major vessel.

When the pericardial sack is exposed within the mediastinum, gaining access to the heart should not pose any problem. Although the vagus and phrenic nerves traverse the length of the pericardium, they are lateral to the operative field (Fig. 1.4). On each side the phrenic nerve passes anteriorly and the vagus nerve posteriorly to the hilum of the lung.

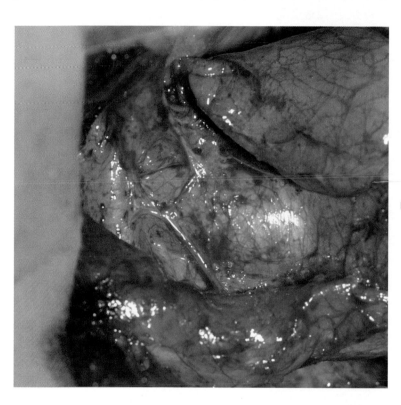

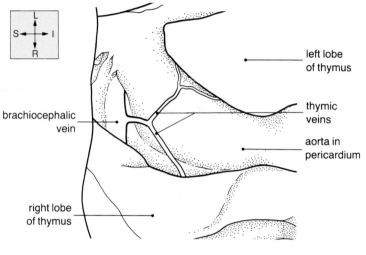

Fig. 1.3 *Operative view through a median sternotomy showing the delicate veins that drain from the thymus to the left brachiocephalic vein.*

left lobe of thymus

thymic veins

aorta in pericardium

brachiocephalic vein

right lobe of thymus

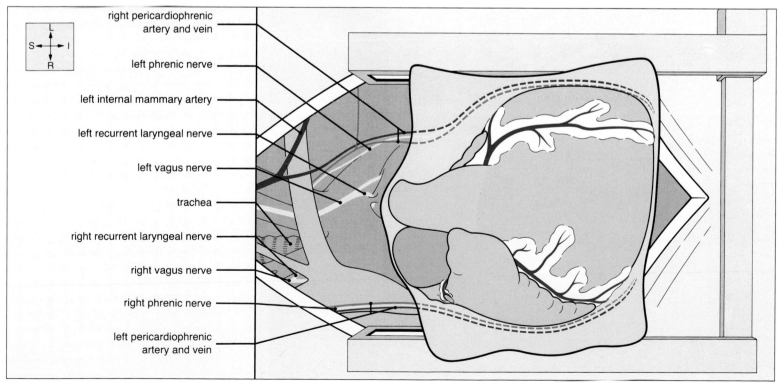

right pericardiophrenic artery and vein

left phrenic nerve

left internal mammary artery

left recurrent laryngeal nerve

left vagus nerve

trachea

right recurrent laryngeal nerve

right vagus nerve

right phrenic nerve

left pericardiophrenic artery and vein

Fig. 1.4 *Diagram of an operative view through a median sternotomy, with the pericardium opened, showing the phrenic and vagus nerves well clear of the operative field.*

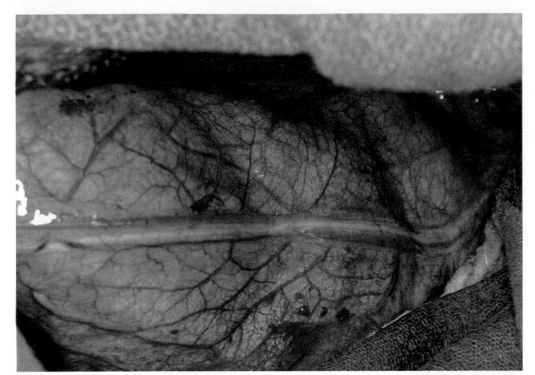

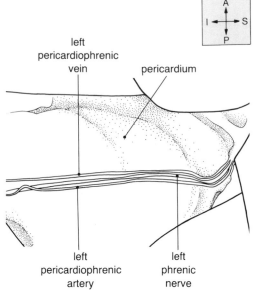

Fig. 1.5 *Operative view through a left lateral thoracotomy showing the left phrenic nerve coursing over the pericardium.*

left
pericardiophrenic
vein

pericardium

left
pericardiophrenic
artery

left
phrenic
nerve

Fig. 1.6 *Operative view through a median sternotomy showing the right phrenic nerve seen (a) through the pericardium and (b) in relationship to the superior caval vein and the right pulmonary veins.*

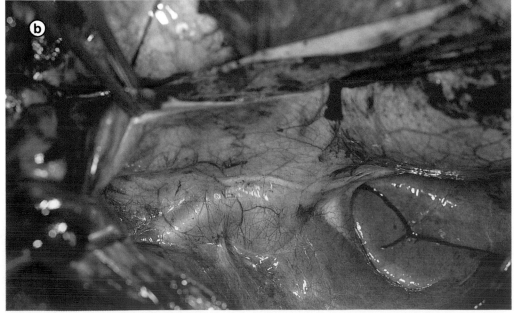

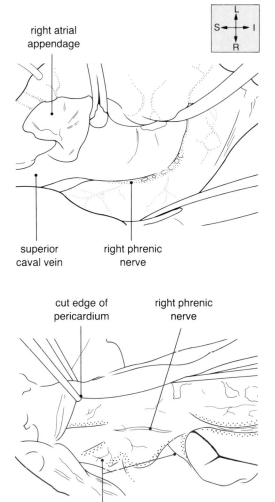

right atrial
appendage

superior
caval vein

right phrenic
nerve

cut edge of
pericardium

right phrenic
nerve

right pulmonary
veins

Phrenic Nerve

The course of the phrenic nerve is seen most readily through a lateral thoracotomy (Fig. 1.5), and so it is in patients undergoing a median sternotomy that this structure is most liable to injury. Although it can sometimes be seen through the pericardium (Fig. 1.6a), its proximity to the caval veins (Figs 1.6b and 1.7) is not always easily appreciated when one dissects these vessels from the anterior approach. Near the thoracic inlet, the phrenic nerve passes close to the internal thoracic artery (Fig. 1.8), exposing it to injury either directly during mobilization of that vessel or by avulsing the pericardiophrenic artery with excessive traction on the chest wall. The internal thoracic arteries are most vulnerable to injury when closing the sternum. The phrenic nerve may be injured when removing the pericardium to use as a cardiac patch or when performing a pericardiectomy. Injudicious use of cooling agents within the pericardial cavity may also lead to phrenic paralysis or paresis.

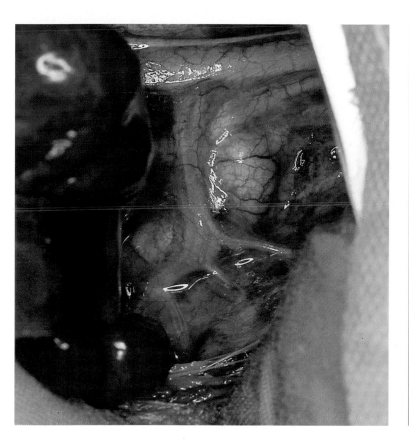

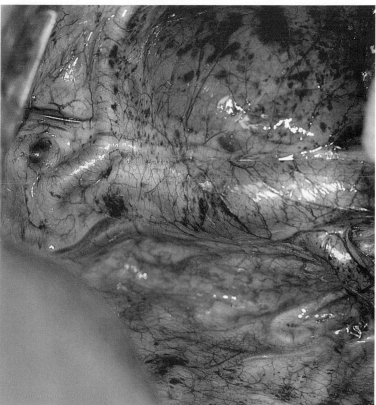

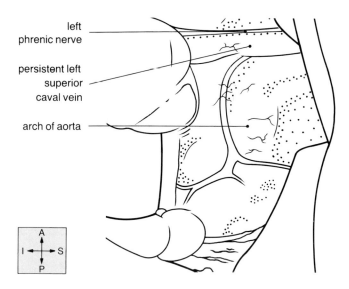

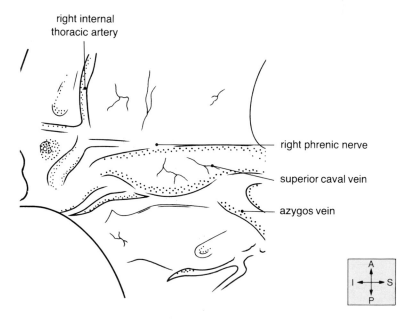

Fig. 1.7 *Operative view through a left thoracotomy showing the relationship of the left phrenic nerve to a persistent left superior caval vein.*

Fig. 1.8 *Operative view through a right thoracotomy showing the relationship of the right phrenic nerve to the right internal thoracic artery and the superior caval vein.*

Lateral Thoracotomy

Left Thoracotomy

Standard lateral thoracotomies provide access to the heart and great vessels via the pleural spaces, with left-sided incisions providing ready access to the great arteries, pulmonary veins and the heart chambers on the left side. Most frequently, the incision is made in the fourth intercostal space. The posterior extent is through the triangular, relatively bloodless, space between the edges of the latissimus dorsi, trapezius, and teres major muscles. The floor of this triangle is the sixth intercostal space. Division of the latissimus dorsi and a portion of the trapezius posteriorly, together with the serratus anteriorly, frees the scapula so that the fourth intercostal space can be identified, although its precise

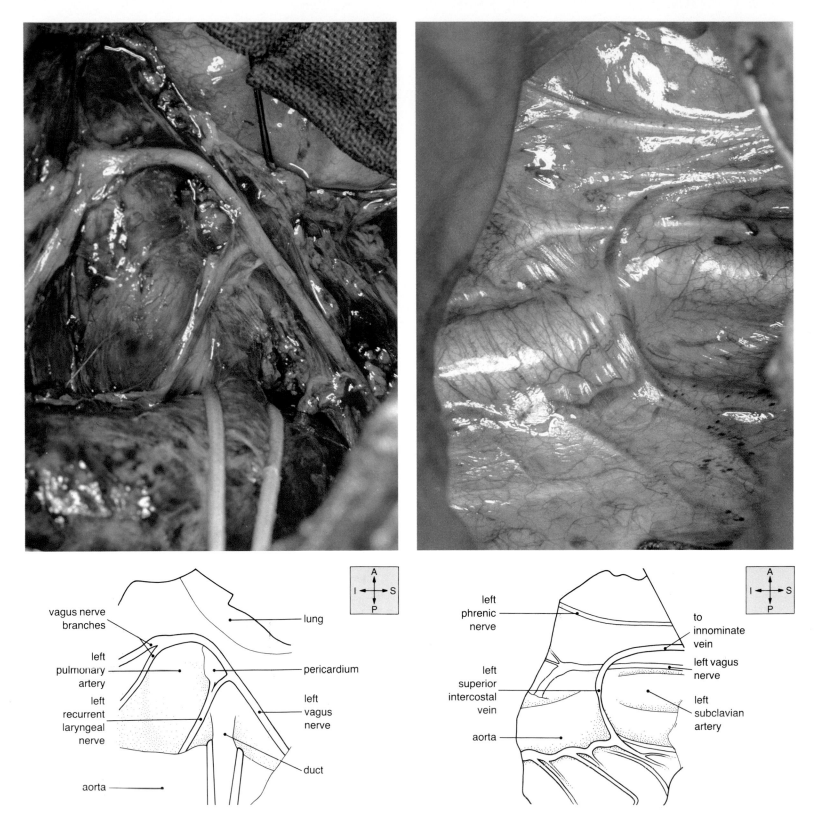

Fig. 1.9 *Operative view through a left lateral thoracotomy in an adult, showing the left recurrent laryngeal nerve passing round the arterial duct.*

Fig. 1.10 *Operative view through a left lateral thoracotomy showing the left superior intercostal vein.*

identity should be confirmed by counting down from above. The intercostal muscles are then divided equidistantly between the fourth and fifth ribs. The incision is carried forward to about the midclavicular line in the submammary position, being careful to avoid damage to the nipple and the tissue of the breast. The intercostal neurovascular bundle is well protected beneath the lower margin of the fourth rib. Having divided the musculature as far as the pleura, the pleural space is entered and the lung permitted to collapse away from the chest wall. Posterior retraction of the lung reveals the middle mediastinum, with the left lateral lobe of the thymus overlying the pericardial sack and the aortic arch with its associated nerves and vessels. Intrapericardial access is usually gained anterior to the phrenic nerve. Occasionally, the thymus may require elevation when the incision is extended superiorly; subsequently, the same precautions should be taken as discussed previously. The lung is retracted anteriorly to approach the aortic isthmus and the descending thoracic aorta; usually the parietal pleura is divided along its mediastinal aspect, posterior to the vagus nerve. In this area, the vagus gives rise to the left recurrent laryngeal nerve, which then passes round the inferior border of the arterial ligament (or duct, if the structure is patent; Fig. 1.9) to ascend towards the larynx on the medial aspect of the posterior aortic wall. Excessive traction on the vagus nerve as it courses into the thorax along the left subclavian artery can cause injury to the recurrent laryngeal nerve just as readily as can direct trauma to the nerve in the environs of the ligament. The superior intercostal vein is seen crossing the aorta and insinuating itself between the phrenic and vagus nerves (Fig. 1.10). This structure, however, is rarely of surgical significance. The thoracic duct ascends through this area (Fig. 1.11) to drain into the junction of the left subclavian and internal jugular veins.

Accessory lymph channels draining into the duct can be troublesome when dissecting the origin of the left subclavian artery.

Right Thoracotomy

A right thoracotomy in either the fourth or fifth interspace is made through an incision similar to that for a left one. The fifth interspace is used when approaching the heart, while use of the fourth permits access to the great vessels on the right side. Access to the pericardium is gained by incising anterior to the phrenic nerve. This approach often necessitates retraction of the right lobe of the thymus. To reach the right pulmonary artery and its adjacent mediastinal structures, it is sometimes useful to divide the azygos vein near its junction with the superior caval vein. Extension of this incision superiorly exposes the origin of the right subclavian branch of the brachiocephalic (innominate)

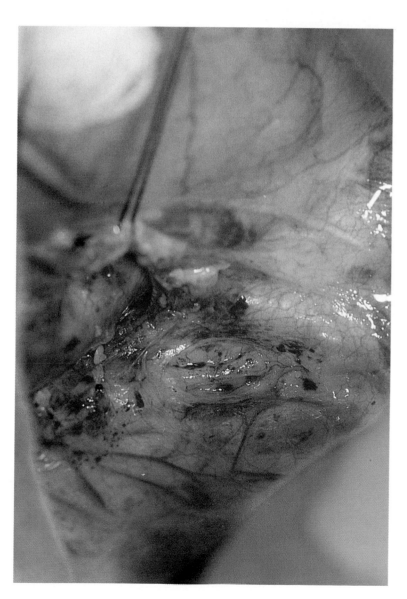

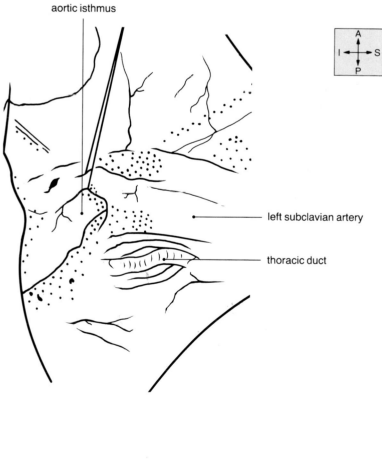

Fig. 1.11 *Operative view through a left thoracotomy showing the thoracic duct coursing below the left subclavian artery to its termination in the brachiocephalic vein.*

aortic isthmus

left subclavian artery

thoracic duct

trunk. Laterally, this artery is crossed by the right vagus nerve, the right recurrent laryngeal nerve originating from the vagus and curling round the posteroinferior wall of the artery before ascending into the neck (Fig. 1.12). Also encircling the subclavian origin on this right side is the subclavian sympathetic loop (ansa subclavia), a branch of the sympathetic trunk that runs up into the neck. Damage to this structure can result in Horner's syndrome.

Congenital Malformations

An anterior right or left thoracotomy is occasionally used in treating congenital malformations. Once the chest is opened, the same basic anatomical rules apply as described above.

Thus far, our account has presumed the presence of normal anatomy. In many instances, the cardiac disposition will be altered by a congenital malformation. These will be described in the appropriate sections.

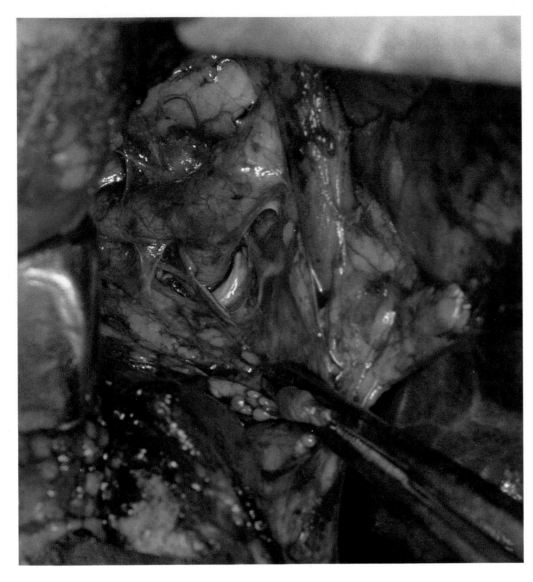

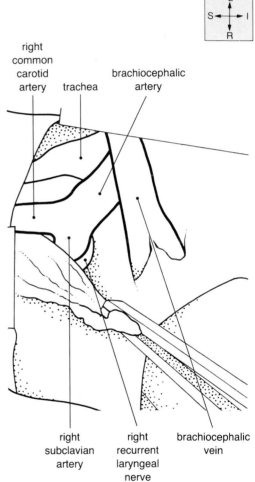

Fig. 1.12 *Operative view through a median sternotomy showing the origin of the right recurrent laryngeal nerve.*

Surgical Anatomy of the Chambers of the Heart and Great Arteries

2

Introduction

When the heart is described in this chapter, and in subsequent chapters, the terms used account for the organ in its anatomical position. Wherever possible, however, the heart is illustrated as it would be viewed by the surgeon during an operative procedure, irrespective of whether the pictures are taken in the operating room or are photographs of autopsied hearts. Where an illustration is in a non-surgical orientation, this is clearly stated.

Pericardium and Pericardial Cavity

Regardless of the approach, the surgeon, having entered the mediastinum, will be confronted by the heart enclosed in its pericardial sack. Although, in the strictest sense, this sack has two layers (fibrous and serous), from a practical point of view it is made up of the tough fibrous pericardium. This fibrous sack encloses the heart's mass, and by virtue of its own attachments to the diaphragm, helps support the heart's position within the mediastinum. The sack is freestanding around the atrial chambers and the ventricles, but becomes adherent to the adventitial coverings of the great arteries and veins at their connexions with the heart, thus closing the pericardial cavity.

The pericardial cavity is contained between two layers of the serous pericardium, this being a thin-walled membrane, folded on itself within the fibrous cavity to produce a double-layered sack. The outer layer of this sack is densely adherent to the fibrous pericardium, while

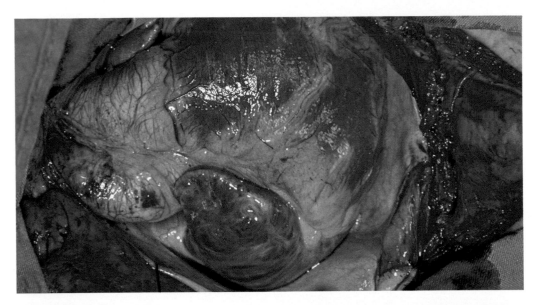

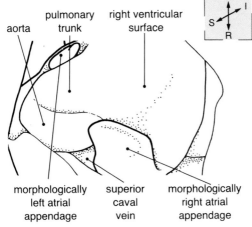

Fig. 2.1 *Operative view through a median sternotomy showing the anterior surface of the heart following a pericardial incision.*

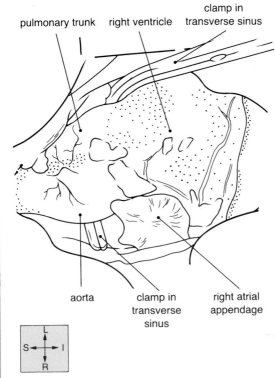

Fig. 2.2 *Operative view through a median sternotomy showing a clamp passed through the transverse sinus.*

the inner layer is firmly attached to the myocardium and is called the epicardium. The pericardial cavity, therefore, is the space between the inner lining of the fibrous pericardium and the surface of the heart (Fig. 2.1).

By virtue of the shape of the cardiac chambers and great arteries, there are two recesses within this cavity that are lined by serous pericardium.

Transverse Sinus

The first is the transverse sinus, which occupies the inner curvature of the heart (Fig. 2.2). Anteriorly, it is bounded by the posterior surface of the great arteries while posteriorly, it is limited by the right pulmonary artery and the left atrial roof. There is also a recess from the transverse sinus that extends between the superior caval and the right upper pulmonary veins.

Its right lateral border is the pericardial fold between these vessels (Fig. 2.3). When exposing the mitral valve through a left atriotomy, incisions through this fold provide good access to the superior aspect of the left atrium and the right pulmonary artery. The fold is also incised when a snare is placed around the superior caval vein. On each side, the ends of the transverse sinus are in free communication with the rest of the pericardial cavity.

Oblique Sinus

The second pericardial recess is the oblique sinus (Fig. 2.4). This is a blind-ending cavity behind the left atrium. The upper boundary of the oblique sinus is formed by the reflection of serous pericardium between the upper pulmonary veins at their entrance to the left atrium. The right border is the reflection of pericardium

around the right pulmonary veins and the inferior caval vein, while to the left is the reflection of pericardium around the left pulmonary veins.

Anterior Surface of the Heart and Great Vessels

With the usual surgical approach through a median sternotomy, the fibrous pericardium is opened more or less in the midline and retracted laterally, exposing the anterior surface of the heart and great vessels (Fig. 2.1). The pulmonary trunk and aorta are then seen to leave the base of the heart and extend in a superior direction, with the aortic root in a posterior and rightward position. Should the aortic root not be in this 'normal' position, then there will almost always be an abnormal ventriculoarterial connexion (see Chapter 7).

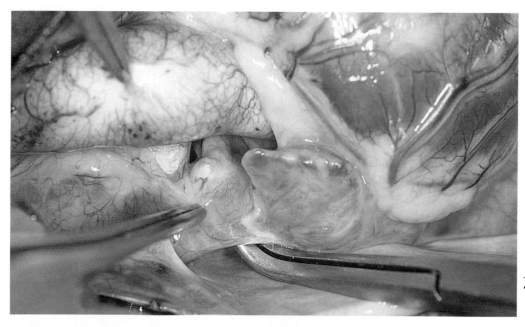

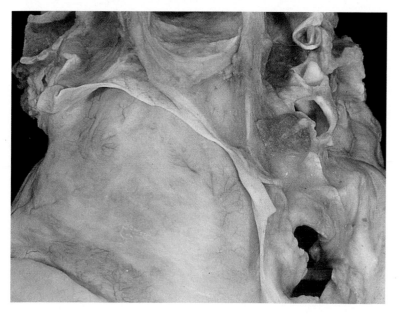

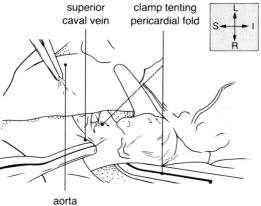

Fig. 2.3 *Operative view through a median sternotomy showing the posterior recess of the transverse sinus limited by a pericardial fold around the superior caval vein. In this picture the fold is being held up by a right-angled clamp passed behind the superior caval vein.*

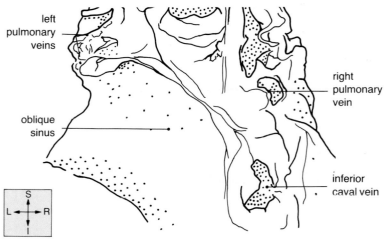

Fig. 2.4 *This heart has been removed and is viewed from behind, showing the recess in the pericardium (the oblique sinus) between the left pulmonary veins and the inferior caval vein.*

Atrial Appendages

Usually the atrial appendages are seen one to either side of the prominent arterial pedicle. The morphologically right appendage is more prominent, having a blunt triangular shape and a broad junction with the atrial cavity (Fig. 2.5). The morphologically left appendage may not be seen immediately. It will be found at the left border of the pulmonary trunk, and is a crennellated structure with a narrow junction with the rest of the atrium (Fig. 2.6). When the two appendages are present on the same side of the arterial pedicle, this is an anomaly called juxtaposition, and is almost always associated with additional malformations within the heart (see Chapter 8).

Inspection of the left border of the heart should always include a search for a persistent left superior caval vein. When present, this venous channel indents the pericardial cavity between the left atrial appendage anteriorly, and the left pulmonary veins posteriorly. Within the cavity, it lies between the left appendage and the left pulmonary artery.

Ventricular Mass

The ventricular mass extends from the base of the heart to the apex; usually its axis extends into the left hemithorax. An anomalous position of either the ventricular mass or of the apex is again highly suggestive of the presence of congenital cardiac malformations (see Chapter 10). The ventricular mass is a three-sided pyramid with diaphragmatic, anterior (sternocostal), and left (pulmonary) surfaces. The margin between the first two surfaces is sharp, the acute (right) margin; while the transition between the latter two surfaces is more gradual, the obtuse margin. The greater part of the anterior surface of the ventricular mass is occupied by the morphologically right ventricle. Its left border, close to the obtuse margin, is marked by the anterior interventricular (descending) branch of the left coronary artery, which curves onto the ventricular surface between the left atrial appendage and the basal origin of the pulmonary trunk. The right border is marked by the right coronary artery which runs obliquely in the atrioventricular groove. Unusually prominent coronary arteries coursing on the ventricular surface should always raise the suspicion of significant cardiac malformations.

Surface Anatomy of the Heart

The surface anatomy of the heart is helpful in determining the most appropriate site for an incision to gain access to a given cardiac chamber. For example, the relatively bloodless outlet region of the

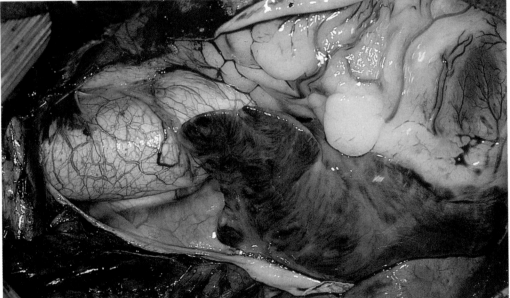

Fig. 2.5 *Operative view through a median sternotomy showing the typical triangular shape of the morphologically right atrial appendage.*

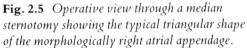

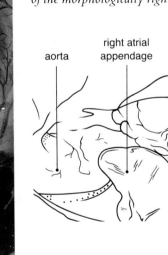

Fig. 2.6 *Operative view through a median sternotomy showing the finger-like morphologically left atrial appendage.*

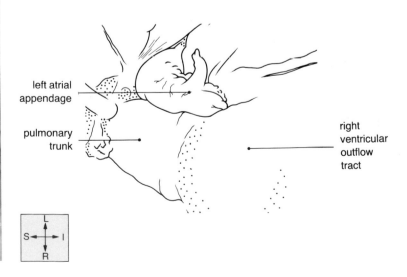

right ventricle, just beneath the origin of the pulmonary trunk, affords ready access to the ventricular cavity.

The important landmark for the right atrium is the terminal groove (sulcus terminalis) between the appendage and the venous component. The sinus node is located within this groove, usually laterally within the superior cavoatrial junction, but occasionally extending over the crest of the appendage (Figs 2.7 and 2.8). The important artery to the sinus node can also be seen occasionally, either as it crosses the crest of the right appendage, or as it courses behind the superior caval vein to enter the terminal groove between the orifices of the caval veins.

Posterior, and parallel, to the terminal groove is a second, deeper, groove between the right atrium and the right pulmonary veins. This interatrial groove (known as Waterston's or Sondergaard's groove) is a guide for surgical incisions into the left atrium (Fig. 2.9).

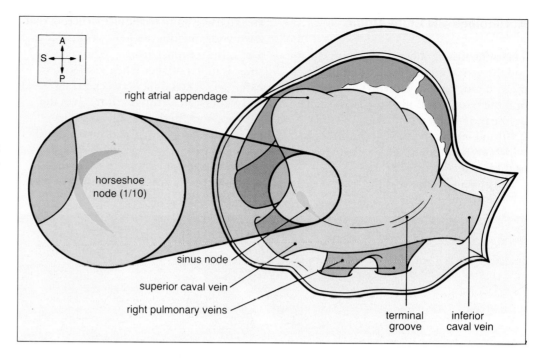

Fig. 2.7 *Drawings showing the usual site of the sinus node within the terminal groove and (inset) the horseshoe arrangement found in about one-tenth of cases.*

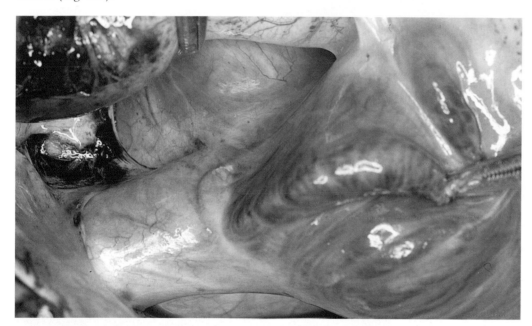

Fig. 2.8 *Operative view through a median sternotomy showing a sinus node arranged in horseshoe fashion across the crest of the right atrial appendage.*

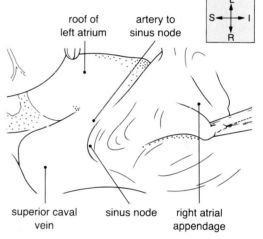

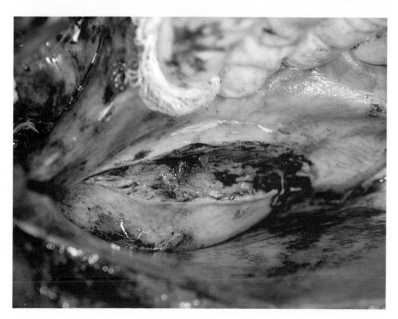

Fig. 2.9 *Operative view through a median sternotomy showing a dissection of the groove between the superior caval and right pulmonary veins (Waterston's groove).*

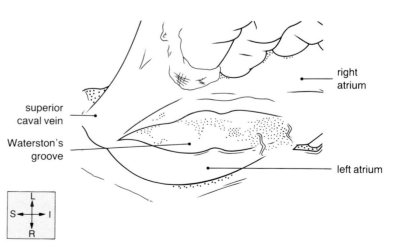

Morphologically Right Atrium

The right atrium consists of the appendage and the venous sinus, the latter receiving the systemic venous return. The junction of these two parts is identified externally by the prominent terminal groove (Fig. 2.10) and internally by the terminal crest, which gives origin to the pectinate muscles of the appendage (Fig. 2.11).

The morphologically right appendage is an extensive blunt triangular structure that has a wide junction with the venous sinus across the terminal groove. The venous sinus is much smaller when viewed externally, extending between the terminal and Waterston's grooves. It receives the superior and inferior caval veins at its extremities. Superiorly and anteriorly, the appendage has an important relationship with the superior caval vein. Here the appendage terminates in a prominent crest, which forms the summit of the terminal groove, and is continuous in the transverse sinus behind the aorta with the interatrial groove (Fig. 2.8).

Sinus Node

As discussed, the sinus node almost always lies within the terminal groove immediately below the epicardium. It is a spindle-shaped structure that usually lies to the

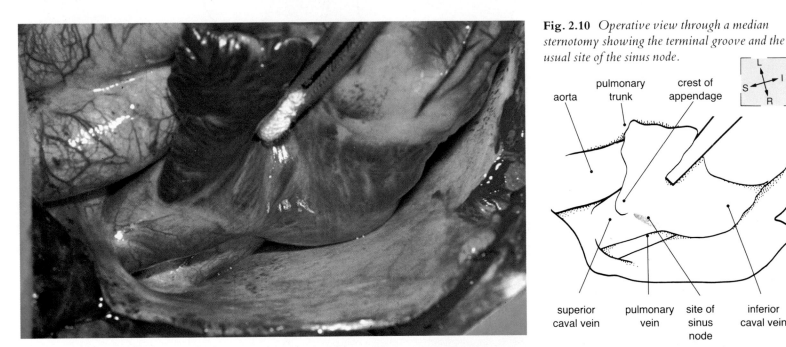

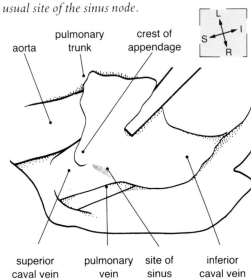

Fig. 2.10 *Operative view through a median sternotomy showing the terminal groove and the usual site of the sinus node.*

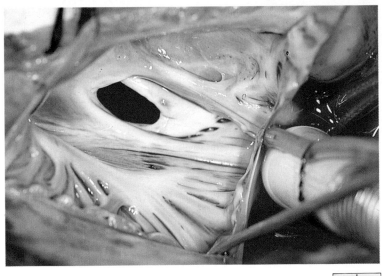

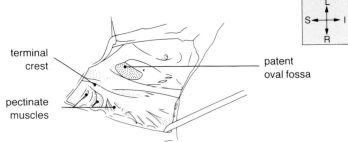

Fig. 2.11 *Operative view through a median sternotomy showing the terminal crest giving rise to the pectinate muscles of the right atrial appendage.*

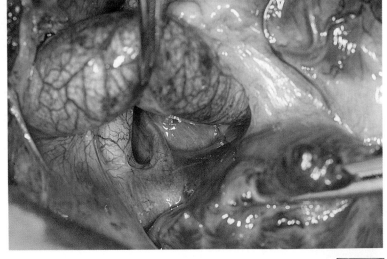

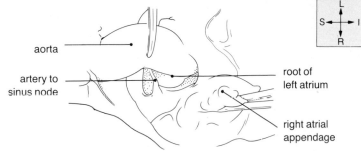

Fig. 2.12 *Operative view through a median sternotomy showing the artery to the sinus node, which originates from the circumflex coronary artery, running within the interatrial groove.*

right of the crest, that is, lateral to the superior cavoatrial junction (Figs 2.7 and 2.10). In about one-tenth of cases, the node extends across the crest into the interatrial groove, draping itself across the cavoatrial junction in horseshoe fashion (Figs 2.7 and 2.8).[1]

Artery to the Sinus Node

Of equal surgical significance is the course of the important artery to the sinus node, which is said to be a branch of the right coronary artery in about 55% of individuals, and a branch of the circumflex artery in the remainder[2]. Irrespective of its origin, it usually courses through the anterior interatrial groove towards the superior cavoatrial junction (Fig. 2.12), frequently running within the atrial myocardium.

The nodal artery usually originates from the proximal segment of its coronary artery (Fig. 2.13), but a significant variant exists when the artery arises from the right or circumflex coronary artery some distance from the aorta. In the case where the nodal artery arises from the right coronary artery, it courses over the lateral surface of the appendage to reach the terminal groove (Fig. 2.14). If it originates from the circumflex artery, however, it crosses the dome of the left atrium (Fig. 2.15). Such a lateral origin is rare in normal hearts[3,4] but more frequent in congenitally malformed hearts[5].

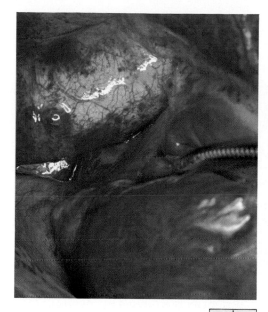

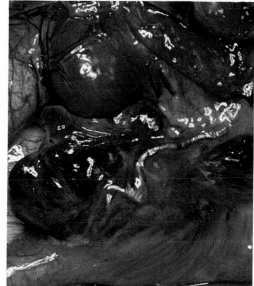

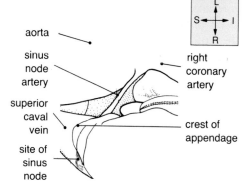

Fig. 2.13 *Operative view through a median sternotomy showing the artery to the sinus node originating proximally from the right coronary artery.*

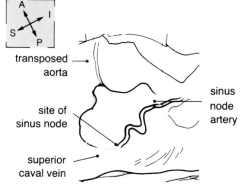

Fig. 2.14 *Operative view through a median sternotomy showing the artery to the sinus node originating distally from the right coronary artery and coursing over the lateral surface of the right atrial appendage.*

Fig. 2.15 *In this specimen, seen in anatomic orientation, the artery to the sinus node originates laterally from the circumflex coronary artery and courses over the dome of the left atrium.*

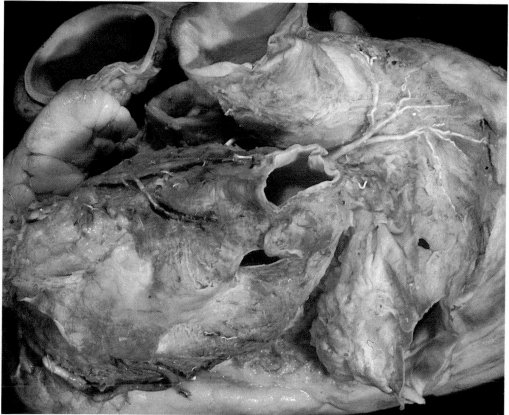

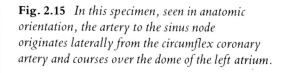

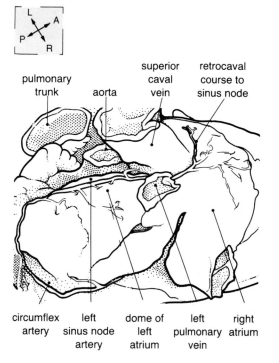

Irrespective of its origin, the artery to the sinus node may cross the crest of the appendage, course retrocavally (Fig. 2.16a), or even divide to form an arterial circle round the junction (Fig. 2.16b). All these variations should be taken into account when planning the safest right atrial incision, particularly when the nodal artery crosses the lateral margin of the right appendage or courses over the dome of the left atrium.

Terminal Crest

Opening the atrium through the most appropriate incision shows that the terminal groove is the external marking of a prominent muscle bundle, the terminal crest. This separates the pectinate muscles of the appendage from the smooth walls of the venous sinus (Fig. 2.11). Anteriorly, the crest curves in front of the orifice of the superior caval vein, and its medial extension forms the border between the appendage and the superior rim of the oval fossa.

The Extent of the Atrial Septum

When first inspecting the right atrium through this incision, there appears to be an extensive septal surface between the orifices of the caval veins and the orifice of the tricuspid valve (Fig. 2.17a). This apparent septal extent is spurious[6,7]. Opening into, and from, this 'septal' surface are the oval fossa and the orifice of the coronary sinus, while the true septum between the right and left atrial chambers is confined to the immediate environs of the oval fossa, as shown by the dissections in Figs 2.17b and 2.18. The extensive superior rim is produced by folding of the interatrial groove between the venous sinus and the pulmonary veins (Fig. 2.18). The inferior rim of the oval fossa is another important muscle bundle, separating the coronary sinus from the orifice of the inferior caval vein (Fig. 2.17a). Only that part of the inferior rim immediately adjacent to the oval fossa is a true inter-atrial septal structure. Similarly, only a small part of the extensive superior rim separates the right from the left atrium. Its larger part is the atrial wall overlying the aortic root (Fig. 2.17a). These limited margins of the true atrial septum are of major surgical importance, since it is easy to pass outside the heart when attempting to gain access to the left atrium through a right atrial approach.

Triangle of Koch

In addition to the position of the sinus node and the extent of the atrial septum, the other major area of surgical significance within the right atrium is the site of the atrioventricular node, which is within the triangle of Koch (Fig. 2.19). This important landmark is bounded by the tendon of Todaro, the attachment of the septal leaflet

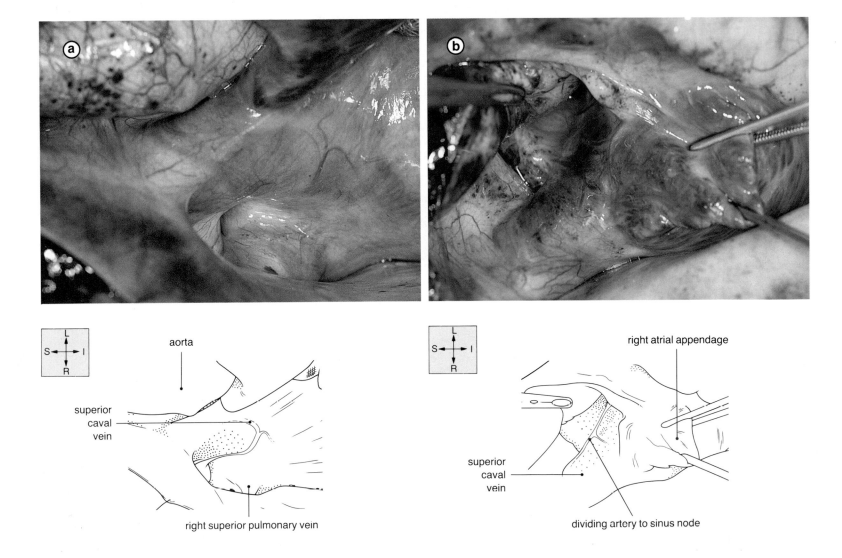

Fig. 2.16 *Operative view through a median sternotomy showing the artery to the sinus node (a) coursing retrocavally and (b) dividing to form an arterial circle around the cavoatrial junction.*

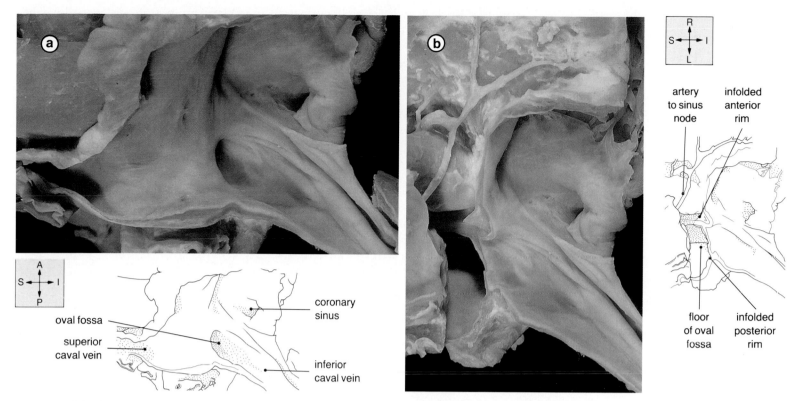

Fig. 2.17 *(a)* *This anatomical specimen viewed in surgical orientation shows an apparently extensive 'septal surface' within the right atrium.* *(b)* *When a cut is made through the oval fossa and the anterior wall is removed the relationships of the aortic root, right coronary artery, and the artery to the sinus node are seen.*

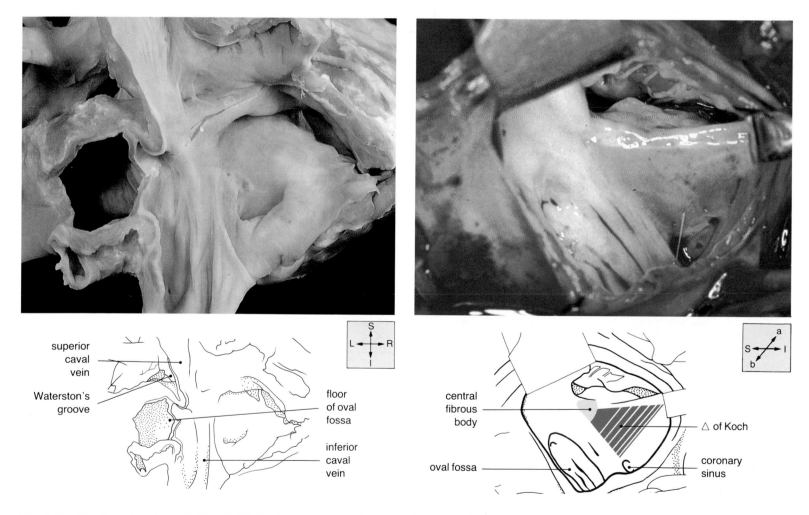

Fig. 2.18 *The dissection shown in Fig. 2.17b has been reconstituted and further dissection has been carried out to show that the superior rim of the oval fossa is the infolded wall of the right and left atrial chambers.*

Fig. 2.19 *Operative view through a right atriotomy showing the triangle of Koch.*

of the tricuspid valve, and the orifice of the coronary sinus. The tendon of Todaro is a fibrous structure formed by the junction (Fig. 2.20a) of the Eustachian valve (the valve of the inferior caval vein) and the Thebesian valve (the valve of the coronary sinus). The tendon of Todaro buries itself in the sinus septum and runs medially to insert into the central fibrous body (Fig. 2.20b). The entire atrial component of the axis of atrioventricular conduction tissues is contained within the confines of the triangle of Koch. If, in hearts with normal segmental connexions, this area is scrupulously avoided during surgical procedures, the atrioventricular conduction tissues will not be damaged. Should the node need to be precisely identified, it should be remembered that the attachment of the tricuspid valve is some way down the surface of the septum relative to that of the mitral valve (Fig. 2.21). The node is located within the atrial musculature on the sloping face of the atrioventricular muscular septum, some distance above the hinge point of the septal leaflet of the tricuspid valve. The atrioventricular bundle, however, penetrates more or less directly at the apex of the triangle of Koch.

Conduction of the Sinus Impulse

Much has been written in recent years concerning the conduction of the sinus impulse to the atrioventricular node by 'specialized' pathways[8-10]. Indeed, it has

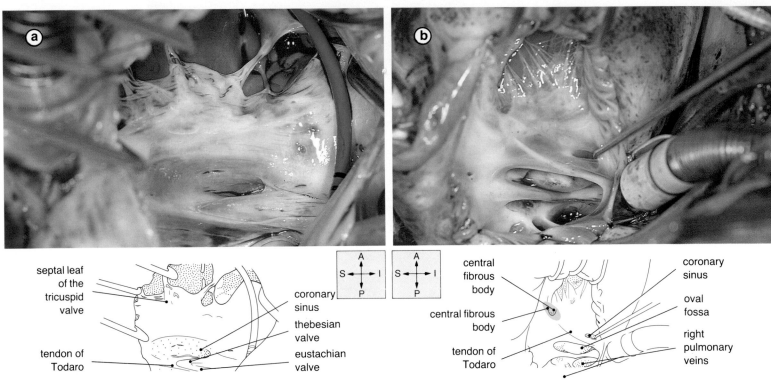

Fig. 2.20 *Operative view through a right atriotomy.* **(a)** *Showing the union of the eustachian and thebesian valves to form the tendon of Todaro.* **(b)** *Showing the tendon of Todaro inserting into the atrioventricular component of the membranous septum.*

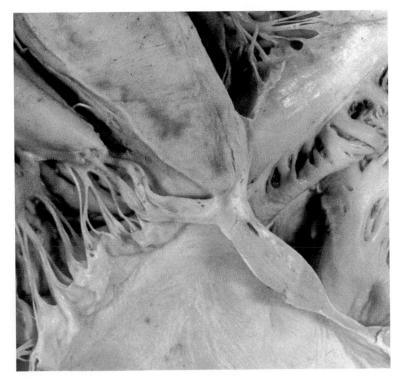

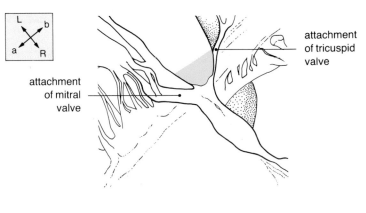

Fig. 2.21 *This four-chamber section of a normal heart is orientated to approximate the surgical view of the heart. It shows how the differential attachments of the atrioventricular valves underscore the existence of the atrioventricular muscular septum.*

been suggested that some surgical operations be specially modified to avoid these presumed tracts[11]. It can now be stated with certainty that there are no insulated or isolated tracts of specialized conduction tissue extending between the nodes that can be avoided in the same way that it is possible to avoid the penetrating and branching atrioventricular bundles[10] The major muscle bundles of the atrial chambers serve as preferential pathways of conduction, but the course of these preferential pathways is dictated by the overall geometry of the chambers. Prominent muscle bundles (such as the terminal crest,

the superior rim of the oval fossa, or the sinus septum) should ideally be preserved during atrial surgery. Even if they cannot be preserved, the surgeon can rest assured that internodal conduction will continue as long as some strand of atrial myocardium connects the nodes, providing that the arterial supply to the nodes, and the nodes themselves, are not traumatized. The key to avoiding post-operative atrial arrhythmias, therefore, is the fastidious preservation of the sinus and atrioventricular nodes and their arteries, rather than concern about non-existent tracts of 'specialized' atrial conduction tissues.

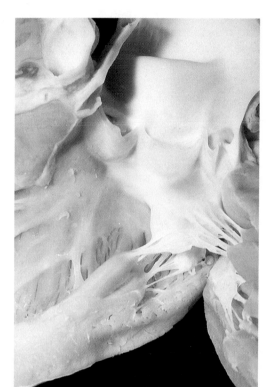

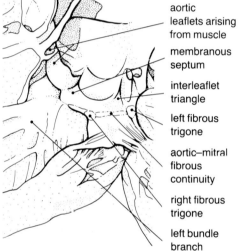

Fig. 2.22 *This specimen, viewed in anatomic orientation, is opened to show how the membranous septum, aortic valve, and the mitral valve all contribute to form the so-called central fibrous body.*

aortic leaflets arising from muscle

membranous septum

interleaflet triangle

left fibrous trigone

aortic–mitral fibrous continuity

right fibrous trigone

left bundle branch

The Central Fibrous Body

The central fibrous body touches on three of the four cardiac chambers, but it is in the right atrium that it becomes first and, perhaps most clearly, evident to the surgeon (Fig. 2.20b). Rather than a specific body, it is as an area within the heart where the membranous septum, the atrioventricular valves, and the aortic valve join in fibrous continuity. Viewed from the left heart (Fig. 2.22), its proximity to the aortic and mitral valves and the left bundle branch of the conduction axis can be seen. Because of this intimate relationship to so many important structures within the heart, the central fibrous body acts as an anatomical focal point for the cardiac surgeon. Operations involving valvar replacement or repair, closure of septal defects, and/or control of arrhythmias all require the surgeon to understand implicitly these anatomical relationships conjoined by the central fibrous body.

The Tricuspid Orifice

The tricuspid orifice, the vestibule to the right ventricle, is continuous with both the venous component and the appendage of the right atrium. The anterior junction of these two parts of the atrium overlies the anteroseptal commissure of the valve and the supraventricular crest of the right ventricle (Fig. 2.23). The posterior junction is at the orifice of the coronary sinus, where there is usually an extensive trabeculated diverticulum found behind

Fig. 2.23 *Operative view through a right atriotomy showing the three leaflets of the tricuspid valve.*

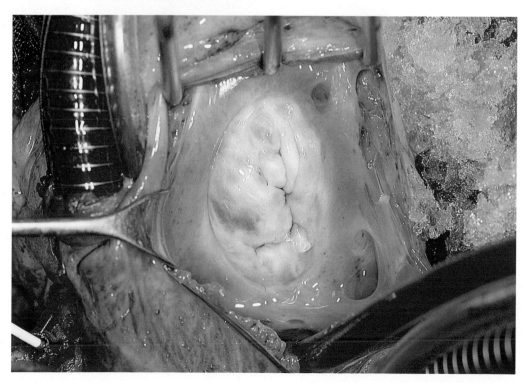

tricuspid valve leaflets (septal, antero-superior and postero-inferior)

coronary sinus

the sinus, the so-called post-Eustachian sinus of Keith (Fig. 2.24).

It is generally possible to distinguish three leaflets in the tricuspid valvar orifice. They lie in anterosuperior, septal, and inferior or mural locations (Fig. 2.23). They are divided from one another by commissures, the apices of which are usually tethered by the fan-shaped commissural cords arising atop the prominent papillary muscles of the valve. The details of valvar and commissural anatomy are discussed in the next chapter.

Morphologically Left Atrium

Owing to its position, only the appendage of the left atrium may be immediately evident to a surgeon on exposing the heart. As with the right atrium, the left has a venous component in addition to its appendage. Unlike the right atrium, however, the venous component of the left atrium is considerably larger than the appendage, and the narrow junction of the two parts is unmarked by either a terminal groove or crest (Fig. 2.25).

Surgical Approaches to the Left Atrium

Because of its posterior position and its firm anchorage by the four pulmonary veins, direct access to the left atrium can be difficult, so the surgeon must use his knowledge of anatomy to gain best exposure of the cavity. Probably the most popular route of access is an incision made just posterior to the interatrial groove (Fig. 2.26). As described above, the extensive infolding between the right pulmonary veins and the venous sinus of the right atrium produces the superior rim of the oval fossa. A posteriorly directed incision along this groove takes the surgeon directly into the left atrium. If necessary, the incision can be extended to the superior aspect of the left atrium by incising the pericardial fold between the superior caval vein and the right superior pulmonary vein (Fig. 2.3). Because the infolding of the interatrial groove also forms the superior border of the oval fossa, much the same access can be gained by approaching through the right atrium and incising just superiorly within the fossa. It must be remembered, nonetheless, that an extensive incision may take the surgeon out of the confines of the atrial chambers and into the pericardial space. Perhaps more importantly, it should be noted that such an incision may damage the artery to the sinus node, either in the interatrial groove or on

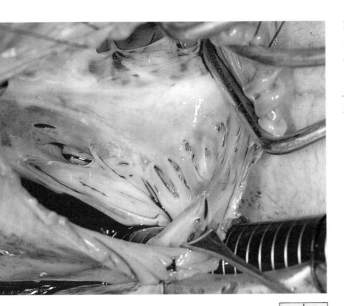

Fig. 2.24 *Operative view through a right atriotomy showing the terminal crest fading out into the post-Eustachian sinus.*

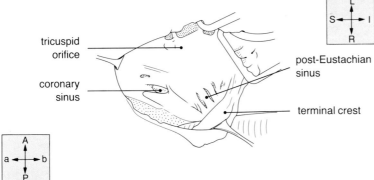

tricuspid orifice

coronary sinus

post-Eustachian sinus

terminal crest

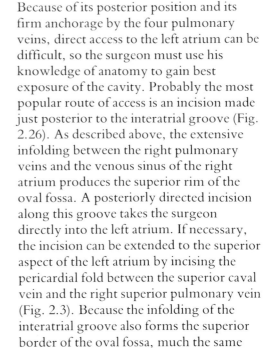

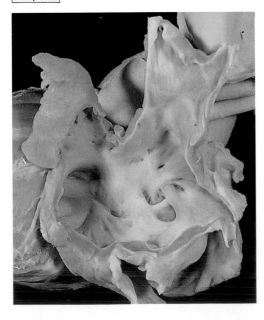

Fig. 2.25 *This dissection of a specimen in anatomic orientation shows the components of the left atrium.*

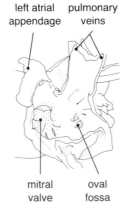

left atrial appendage

pulmonary veins

mitral valve

oval fossa

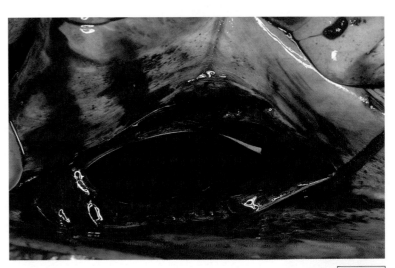

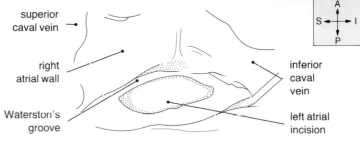

superior caval vein

right atrial wall

Waterston's groove

inferior caval vein

left atrial incision

Fig. 2.26 *Operative view through a median sternotomy showing a subsequent incision to the left atrium after dissection in Waterston's groove.*

the roof of the left atrium.

A further approach to the left atrium is the so-called superior approach, incising directly through the roof. If the aorta is pulled anteriorly and to the left, it can be shown that there is an extensive trough between the two atrial appendages (Fig. 2.27). An incision through the floor of this trough, between the appendages, provides direct access to the left atrium. When making such an incision, it must be remembered that the artery to the sinus node may be coursing through this area if it originates from the circumflex artery (in 45% of cases; Fig. 2.27). Also, in some instances, this artery may pass through the interatrial groove to reach the terminal groove.

Once access is gained to the left atrium, the appendage is seen lying to the left of the mitral orifice and the small size of its opening is apparent. The greater part of the pulmonary venous atrium will usually be located inferiorly, away from the operative field, and the vestibule of the mitral orifice will dominate the picture (Fig. 2.28). The septal aspect will be anterior, in a relatively inferior position, exhibiting the typically roughened flap-valve aspect of its left side. The large sweep of tissue between the flap-valve of the septum and the opening of the appendage is the internal aspect of the deep anterior interatrial groove.

Mitral Valve

Details concerning the mitral valve are given in Chapter 3. The important features are that its two leaflets, supported by two prominent papillary muscles and their commissural cords, have widely differing appearances (Fig. 2.29). The anterosuperior leaflet is short, squat, and relatively square. This leaflet, in fibrous continuity with the aortic valve, is best termed the aortic leaflet, since it is not strictly in either anterior or superior position. The other leaflet is narrower and its junctional attachment more extensive, being connected to the parietal part of the left atrioventricular junction. It is accurately termed the mural leaflet. Detailed descriptions of the relationships of these units are given in Chapter 3.

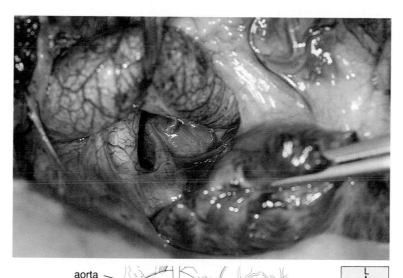

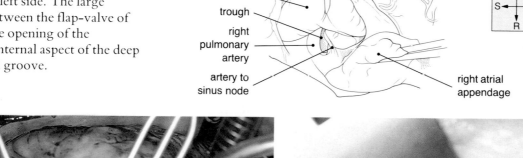

Fig. 2.27 *Operative view through a median sternotomy where the aorta has been retracted to the left to reveal the deep trough inferior to the right pulmonary artery and between the atrial appendages. Note that, in this heart, the artery to the sinus node courses through this trough.*

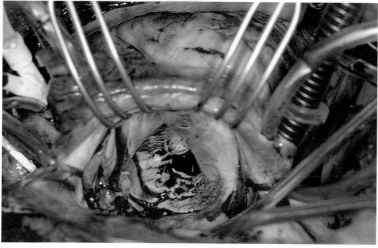

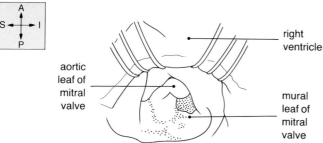

Fig. 2.28 *On gaining access through a right-sided left atriotomy, the vestibule of the mitral orifice dominates the surgical picture.*

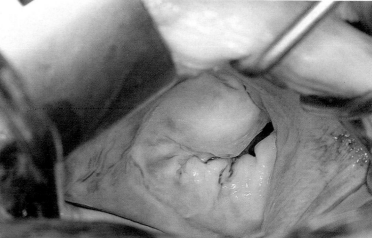

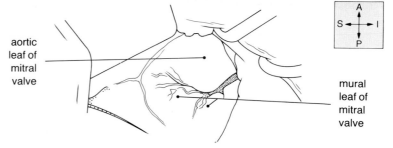

Fig. 2.29 *This operative view through a left atriotomy shows the markedly different appearances of the aortic and mural leaflets of the mitral valve.*

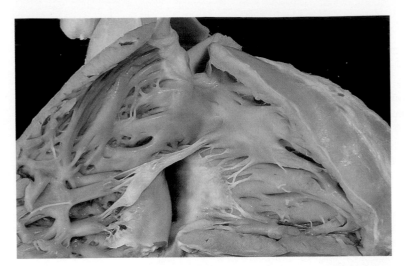

Fig. 2.30 *This specimen, viewed in anatomical orient- ation, shows the three components of the morphologically right ventricle.*

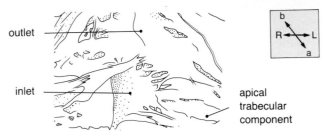

outlet

inlet

apical trabecular component

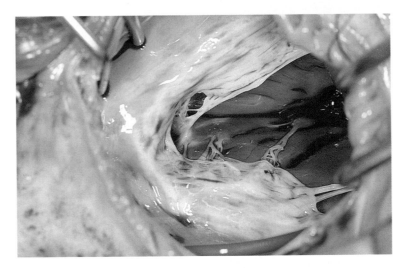

Fig. 2.31 *Operative view through a right atriotomy showing the direct cordal attachments to the septum of the septal leaflet of the tricuspid valve. Note the appearance of the medial papillary muscle.*

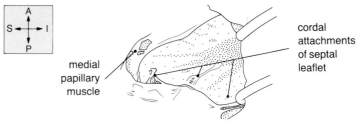

medial papillary muscle

cordal attachments of septal leaflet

Morphologically Right Ventricle

Understanding of ventricular morphology in general is greatly aided by considering the ventricles in terms of three components (Fig. 2.30), rather than the traditional 'sinus' and 'conus' parts. The three components are the inlet, trabecular, and outlet parts[12,13].

The inlet portion of the right ventricle contains, and is limited by, the tricuspid valve and its tension apparatus. The most constant distinguishing feature of the tri- cuspid valve is the direct septal attachments of the cords of its septal leaflet (Fig. 2.31).

The trabecular component of the right ventricle extends out to the apex, where its wall is particularly thin and especially vulnerable to perforation by cardiac catheters and pacemaker electrodes.

The outlet component of the right ventricle is a complete muscular structure, the infundibulum, which supports the pulmonary valve. As described in Chapter 3, the three leaflets of the pulmonary valve do not have a ring or an annulus, being attached to the infundibular musculature in semilunar fashion.

Supraventricular Crest

A distinguishing feature of the right ventricle is the prominent muscular shelf called the supraventricular crest which separates the tricuspid and pulmonary valves. Although it may first appear (Fig. 2.32a) as a large muscle bundle, much of the crest is no more than the infolded inner heart curve (Fig. 2.32b). Incisions or deep sutures through this part run into the transverse sinus and right atrioventricular groove and can jeopardize the right coronary artery[14]. Only the most medial part of the crest is a septal structure, separating the subpulmonary from the subaortic outflow tracts (Fig. 2.32c).

Septomarginal Trabeculation

The supraventricular crest inserts into the septum between the limbs of a prominent and important right ventricular septal landmark. This structure, which we term the septomarginal trabeculation, has anterior and posterior limbs that clasp the crest (Fig. 2.32a). The anterior limb runs up to the attachment of the leaflets of the pulmonary valve, overlying the outlet part of the muscular septum, while the posterior limb extends backwards, inferior to the interventricular component of the membranous septum, to run onto the inlet septum. The medial papillary muscle (Fig. 2.31) usually arises from this posterior limb near its junction with the anterior limb.

The body of the septomarginal trabecu- lation runs to the apex of the ventricle, breaking up into a sheath of smaller trabeculations. Some of these mingle into the trabecular portion and some support the tension apparatus of the tricuspid valve. Two trabeculations may be particu- larly prominent: one becomes the anterior papillary muscle while the other extends from the septomarginal trabeculation to the papillary muscle, the latter being termed the moderator band.

Other significant right ventricular trabeculations are usually found in the transitional zone to the infundibulum. Variable in number, these are the septo- parietal trabeculations (Fig. 2.32a).

Apical Trabeculations

The coarse apical trabeculations serve as the most constant feature of the morpho- logically right ventricle. In the normal

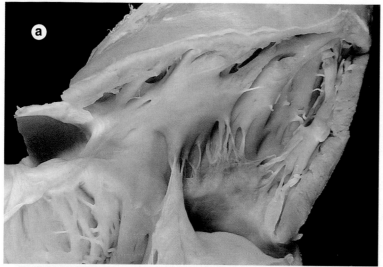

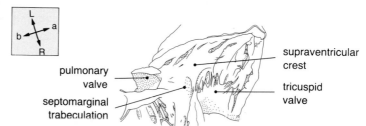

Fig. 2.32 *(a) In this anatomic specimen, viewed in surgical orientation, the prominent supraventricular crest of the right ventricle is seen between the leaflets of the tricuspid and pulmonary valves. (b) Dissection of this heart shows that most of the supraventricular crest is the curvature of the inner heart or ventriculo–infundibular fold. Note the location of the right coronary artery. (c) Further dissection of this heart reveals that part of the crest between the limbs of the septomarginal trabeculation is a true interventricular septal structure.*

supraventricular crest

pulmonary valve

septomarginal trabeculation

tricuspid valve

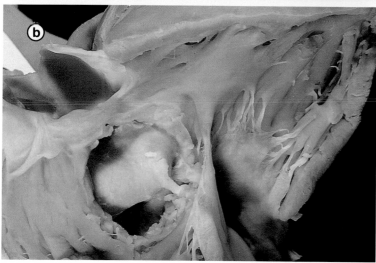

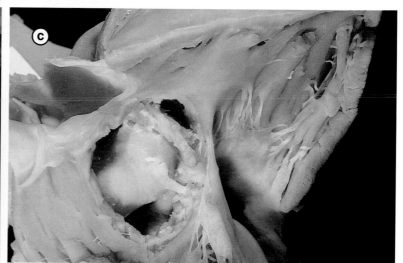

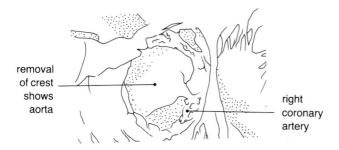

removal of crest shows aorta

right coronary artery

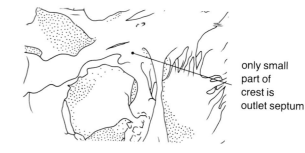

only small part of crest is outlet septum

heart, there are a number of morphological differences between the two ventricles, including the arrangement and attachments of the leaflets of the atrioventricular valves, the shape of the ventricles, the thickness of their walls, and the configuration of the outflow tracts. These features, however, can be altered or lacking in the congenitally abnormal heart, so that, in final arbitration of ventricular morphology, one must rely on the contrast between the coarse trabeculations of the right ventricle and the much finer ones seen in the apical part of the left ventricle (Fig. 2.33).

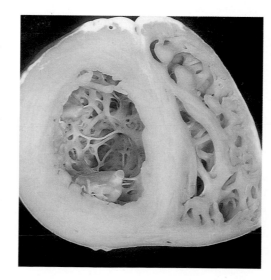

Fig. 2.33 *This apical component of the ventricular mass, viewed from above in anatomical orientation, shows the different patterns of the trabeculations of the left versus the right ventricle.*

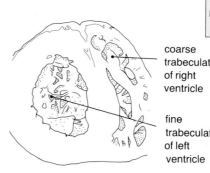

coarse trabeculations of right ventricle

fine trabeculations of left ventricle

Morphologically Left Ventricle

As with the right ventricle, the left ventricle is conveniently considered in terms of inlet, trabecular, and outlet components (Fig. 2.34), although the inlet and outlet components overlap considerably.

The inlet component surrounds, and is limited by, the mitral valve and its tension apparatus. Because the aortic leaf of the mitral valve forms part of the outlet of the left ventricle (Fig. 2.34), the distinction of inlet and outlet is somewhat blurred. The papillary muscles of the valve, although basically located in anterolateral and posteromedial positions, are close to each other at their origin (Fig. 2.35). Unlike the tricuspid valve, the leaflets of the mitral valve have no direct septal attachments (Fig. 2.23). This is because the deep posterior diverticulum of the subaortic outflow tract displaces the aortic leaflet of the valve away from the area of the atrio-ventricular septum (Fig. 2.36).

The trabecular component extends to the ventricular apex and characteristically has fine trabeculations (Fig. 2.33). As in the right ventricle, the apical myocardium is surprisingly thin. This feature is important to the cardiac surgeon who has reason to place catheters and electrodes in the right ventricle or drainage tubes in the left. Immediate perforation, or delayed rupture, may occur. This may be a particular problem with catheters stiffened by hypothermia, which are then pushed against the apical endocardium as the heart is manipulated during surgery on the coronary arteries[15].

The outlet component supports the aortic valve, but, unlike its right ventricular counterpart, it is not a complete muscular structure. The septal wall is largely composed of muscle, but the membranous septum forms part of the subaortic outflow tract. The posterior portion of the outflow tract is composed of the fibrous curtain joining the apparatus of the aortic valve to the aortic leaflet of the mitral valve (Fig. 2.22). The left lateral quadrant, continuing around to the septum, is a muscular structure that is the lateral margin of the inner heart curvature, lined on the outside by the transverse sinus.

Septal Surface

The muscular septal surface of the outflow tract is characteristically smooth, and the

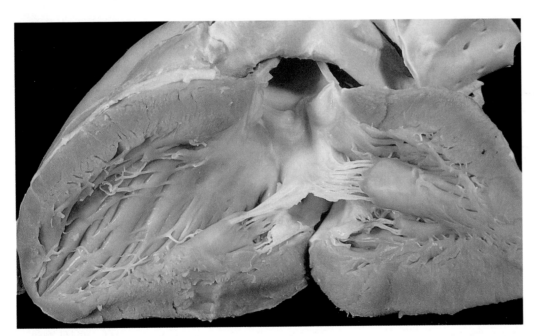

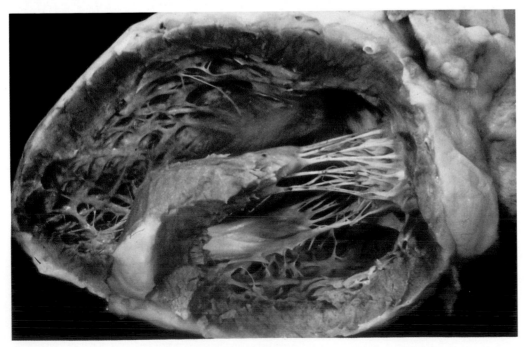

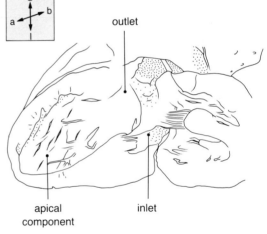

Fig. 2.34 *This specimen, viewed in anatomic orientation, shows the three components of the morphologically left ventricle.*

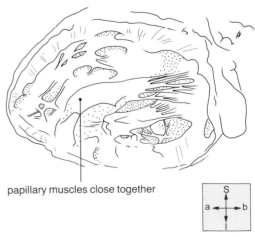

Fig. 2.35 *In this specimen, viewed from behind after the parietal wall of the left ventricle has been removed, the anterolateral and postero-medial papillary muscles are seen to be adjacent.*

fan-like left bundle branch cascades down this surface. The landmark of its descent is the membranous septum, specifically immediately beneath the commissure between right coronary and non-coronary leaflets of the aortic valve (Fig. 2.22). Initially, the bundle descends as a relatively narrow solitary fascicle, but soon divides into three interconnected fascicles that radiate into anterior, septal, and posterior divisions. The interconnecting radiations do not fan out to any degree until the bundle itself has descended to between one-third and one-half of the septal length.

Aortic Valve

As with the pulmonary valve, the leaflets of the aortic valve do not have an annulus, in the sense of a circular arrangement of collagenous tissue. Instead, the leaflets are attached in semilunar fashion across the anatomic ventriculo–aortic junction. This valve forms the keystone of the heart and is related to each of the other cardiac chambers and valves. Its morphology is described in detail in Chapter 3.

The Aorta

Ascending Aorta

The ascending aorta begins at the distal extremity of the three aortic sinuses, the so-called aortic bar, which lies at the opening line of the free edge of the valvar leaflets (Fig. 2.37). It runs its short course passing superiorly, obliquely to the right, and slightly forward toward the sternum. It is contained within the fibrous peri-cardial sack, so its surface is covered with serous pericardium. Its anterior surface abuts directly on the pulmonary trunk, which is also covered with serous pericardium. Together the two vessels make up the so-called vascular pedicle (Fig. 2.21). The ascending aorta is related antero-medially to the right atrial appendage, and posterolaterally to the right ventricular outflow tract and the pulmonary trunk. Extrapericardially, the thymus gland lies between it and the sternum. The medial wall of the right atrium, the superior caval vein, and the right pleura relate to its right side. On the left, its principal relationship is with the pulmonary trunk. Posterior to the ascending aorta lies the transverse sinus of the pericardium (Fig. 2.2), which separates it from the 'roof' of the left atrium and the right pulmonary artery.

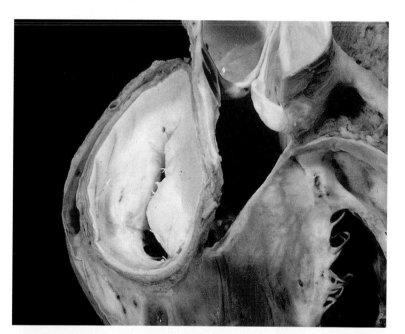

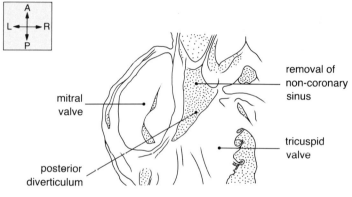

Fig. 2.36 *This dissection of a heart, seen in anatomical orientation, was made by removing the atrial musculature and the non-coronary sinus of the aorta to illustrate the location of the atrioventricular septum.*

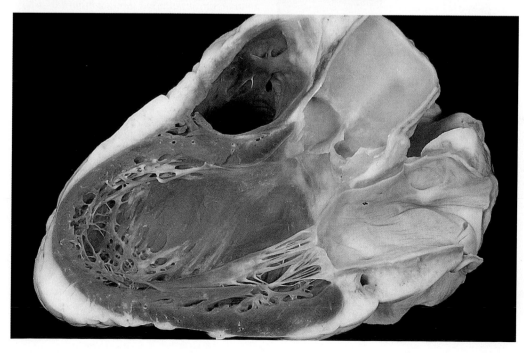

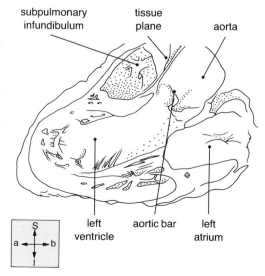

Fig. 2.37 *This long axis section of the left ventricle shows the aortic bar and the origin of the aorta.*

Aortic Arch

The arch of the aorta begins at the superior attachment of the pericardial reflection just proximal to the origin of the brachio-cephalic (innominate) artery (Fig. 2.38). It continues superiorly before coursing posteriorly and to the left, crossing the lateral aspect of the distal trachea and finally terminating on the lateral aspect of the vertebral column. Here it is tethered by the parietal pleura and the arterial ligament. During its course, it gives rise to the brachiocephalic, the left common carotid, and the left subclavian arteries. Bronchial arteries may arise from the arch and can be the source of troublesome bleeding if not carefully identified in the presence of aortic coarctation. The left phrenic and vagus nerves run over the anterolateral aspect of the arch just beneath the mediastinal pleura. The left recurrent laryngeal nerve originates from the vagus and curls superiorly around the arterial ligament before passing on to the posteromedial side of the arch (Fig. 1.12). Here the arch relates to the tracheal bifurcation and oesophagus on its medial border, but also to the left main-stem bronchus and the left pulmonary artery inferiorly.

Descending Aorta

The descending aorta continues from the arch, running an initial course lateral to the vertebral bodies and reaching an anterior position at its termination. Throughout its course it gives off many branches to the organs of the thorax, as well as the prominent lower nine pairs of intercostal arteries. These latter vessels are of critical concern for the cardiac surgeon. In aortic coarctation, they serve as primary collateral vessels which bypass the obstructed aorta, accounting for the rib notching seen in older children with this lesion. These vessels and their branches to the chest wall can be a source of troublesome bleeding if not properly secured when such patients undergo surgery. The surgeon must also remember that the dorsal branches of the intercostal vessels contribute a branch that is important in supplying blood to the spinal cord. Because it is difficult to predict

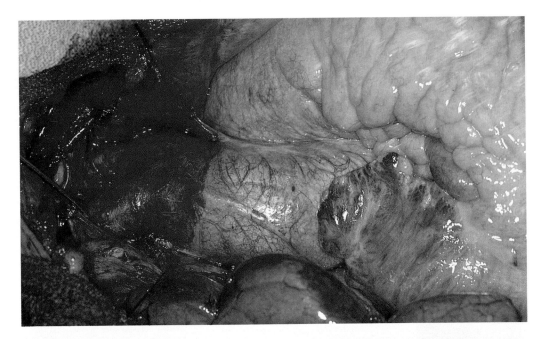

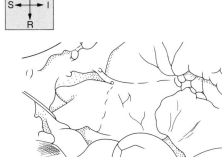

Fig. 2.38 *Operative view through a median sternotomy showing the beginning of the aortic arch. The aortic arch gives rise to the brachio-cephalic and left common carotid arteries just distal to the detached pericardial reflection. The origin of the left subclavian artery is not seen.*

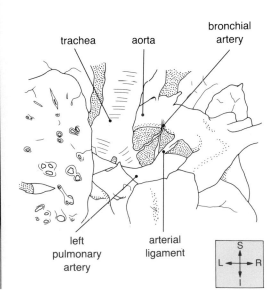

Fig. 2.39 *This dissection viewed from behind in anatomic orientation shows a bronchial artery arising from the aorta in the midline and dividing to supply both bronchuses.*

trachea   aorta   bronchial artery

left pulmonary artery   arterial ligament

exactly from where these vital branches will arise, the surgeon must make every attempt to protect their origin from permanent occlusion.

The important bronchial arteries (Fig. 2.39) also arise from the descending segment of the thoracic aorta. These vessels can become dilated in the presence of pulmonary atresia, when they serve as a source of pulmonary vascular supply. Acquired dilatation of bronchial arteries, however, must be distinguished from that of the major aorto–pulmonary collateral arteries that often supply blood to the lungs in tetralogy with pulmonary atresia (see Chapter 6).

The Pulmonary Arteries

Pulmonary Trunk

The pulmonary trunk is a short vessel, usually less than 5 cm long in the adult (Fig. 2.40). It is contained completely within the pericardium and, similar to its running mate, the ascending aorta, is covered with a layer of serous pericardium except where the two vessels abut each other in the vascular pedicle. It originates from the most anterior aspect of the heart, lying just behind the lateral edge of the sternum and the second left intercostal space. Initially, the pulmonary trunk

overlies the aorta and left coronary artery, but it soon moves to a side-by-side relationship with the ascending aorta. The left coronary artery turns abruptly and anteriorly to lie between the left atrial appendage and the pulmonary trunk. The arterial ligament extends from the aorta to the very end of the pulmonary trunk as the latter divides into left and right pulmonary arteries (Fig. 2.41).

Left Pulmonary Artery

The left pulmonary artery courses laterally in front of the descending aorta and the left main-stem bronchus before it sends

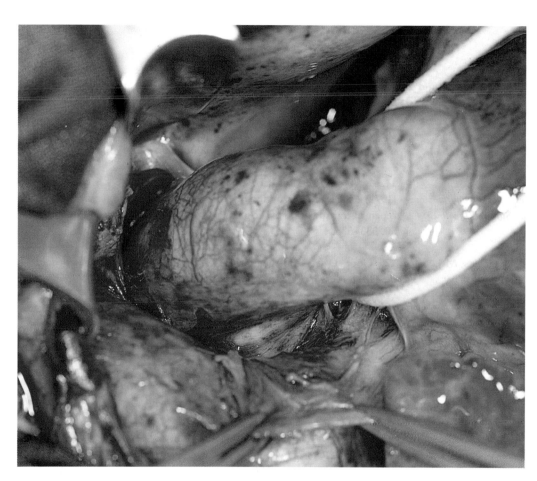

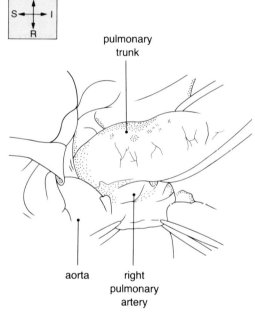

Fig. 2.40 *Operative view through a median sternotomy showing the short course of the pulmonary trunk to its bifurcation.*

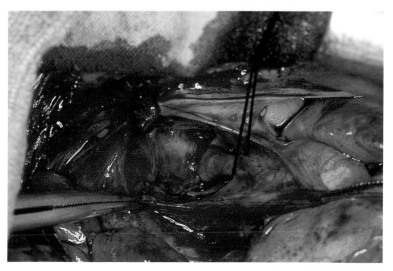

Fig. 2.41 *Operative view through a median sternotomy showing the arterial duct running from the pulmonary trunk to the aorta. Note its encirclement by the left recurrent laryngeal nerve.*

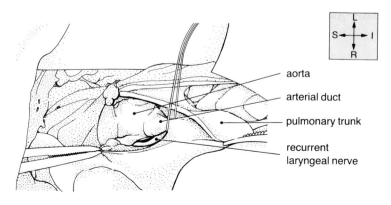

Introduction

It is axiomatic that a thorough knowledge of valvar anatomy is a prerequisite for successful surgery, be it valvar replacement or reconstruction. The surgeon will also require a firm understanding of other aspects of cardiac anatomy to ensure safe access to a diseased valve or valves. These anatomical features were described in Chapter 2. Knowledge of the surgical anatomy of the valves must be founded on an appreciation of their relationship to each other. This requires an understanding of the basic orientation of the cardiac valves, emphasizing the intrinsic features that make each valve distinct from the others. This information must then be supplemented by emphasizing the relationships of the valves to other structures that the surgeon must avoid, specifically, the conduction tissues and the major channels for the coronary circulation. Throughout the narrative, the presence of a normally structured heart will be presumed, lying in its usual position without any congenital cardiac malformations.

Position of the Valves within the Heart

The close proximity of the valves to each other is shown by studying the cylindrical short axis of the heart through the atrioventricular and ventriculo–arterial junctions (Fig. 3.1). All four valves are contained within this cylinder. When considering the position of each valve relative to the body, the pulmonary valve is the most anterior and superior; the tricuspid valve the most inferior; the mitral valve the most posterior of the four; while the central position of the aortic valve is readily evident.

This section also shows a crucial landmark, namely the crux of the heart. This is the point which bisects the posterior margins of the atrioventricular junctions. In the normally structured heart, it is the crossing point of the septal structures and the posterior atrioventricular groove.

Central Fibrous Body and Fibrous Skeleton

It is often presumed, and pictured, that all four valves are contained within the fibrous skeleton of the heart; but this is not so. Parts of the leaflets of the aortic valve are in fibrous continuity with those of the mitral and tricuspid valves. The confluence of these three valves is identified as the central fibrous body. The pulmonary valve has no fibrous continuity with the other valves, and its leaflets do not contribute either to the fibrous skeleton or the central fibrous body.

The fibrous skeleton, along with the atrioventricular junctions, serves two purposes. One is to anchor the junctional attachments of the atrioventricular valves. The other is to provide electrical insulation for the atrial myocardium from the ventricular myocardium, allowing conduction to occur only at the site of penetration of the atrioventricular bundle.

The fibrous trigones are two components of the attachments of the aortic valvar leaflets, and are the best formed and strongest components of the fibrous skeleton (Fig. 3.2). In contrast, those portions of the aortic valvar leaflets that face the pulmonary valve, together with all the leaflets of the pulmonary valve, have no attachments to the fibrous skeleton.

Arterial Valves

It is incorrect to speak of a ring for either the aortic or pulmonary valves. Rather than being attached in a circular fashion to a ring (or an *annulus*), the leaflets of these arterial (as opposed to atrioventricular) valves have semilunar attachments (Figs 3.3 and 3.20). The only circular feature of the valve is the anatomic junction of the arterial trunks to the supporting ventricular structures. The semilunar attachments of the leaflets cross this junction, the upper commissural extremity being attached to the arterial wall at a level that is up to 16–21 mm higher (in the adult) relative to the deepest part of the leaflets attached to the ventricles[1]. This is of considerable significance, since the triangular areas of outflow tract subjacent to the apices of the three commissures of the arterial valves all point to the outside of the heart. Although composed of arterial wall, they are part of the ventricles haemodynamically.

In the case of the aortic valves, the two posterior intercommissural triangles are in relation to the transverse sinus of the pericardium, while the anterior, or facing, triangle relates to a potential space between the aortic root and the right ventricular infundibulum (Fig. 3.4). Dissection in this area shows a discrete extracardiac plane often containing septal perforating branches of the anterior interventricular

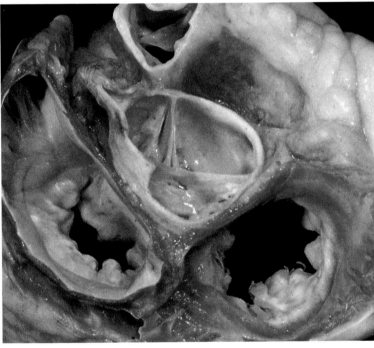

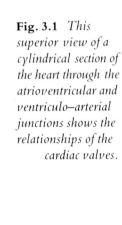

Fig. 3.1 *This superior view of a cylindrical section of the heart through the atrioventricular and ventriculo–arterial junctions shows the relationships of the cardiac valves.*

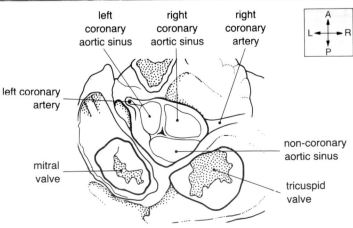

left coronary aortic sinus

right coronary aortic sinus

right coronary artery

left coronary artery

mitral valve

non-coronary aortic sinus

tricuspid valve

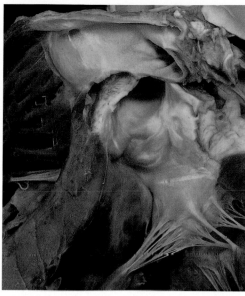

Fig. 3.2 *This view of the aortic valve in anatomic orientation shows the area of fibrous continuity with the mitral valve, which is thickened at both ends to form the fibrous trigones. Note that the leaflets of the aortic valve and pulmonary valve four which face each other are attached to the musculature of the ventricle.*

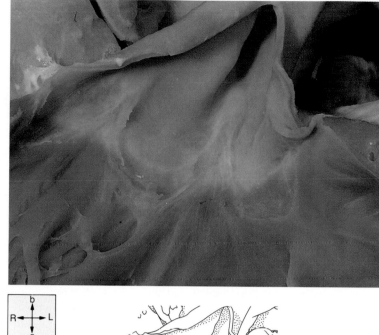

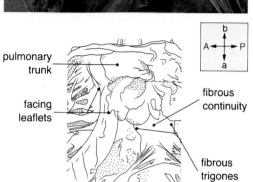

pulmonary trunk

facing leaflets

fibrous continuity

fibrous trigones

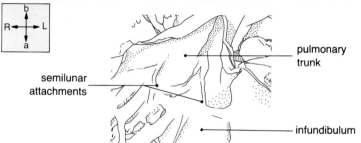

semilunar attachments

pulmonary trunk

infundibulum

Fig. 3.3 *In this anatomic specimen, the leaflets of the pulmonary valve have been removed to demonstrate their semilunar attachment.*

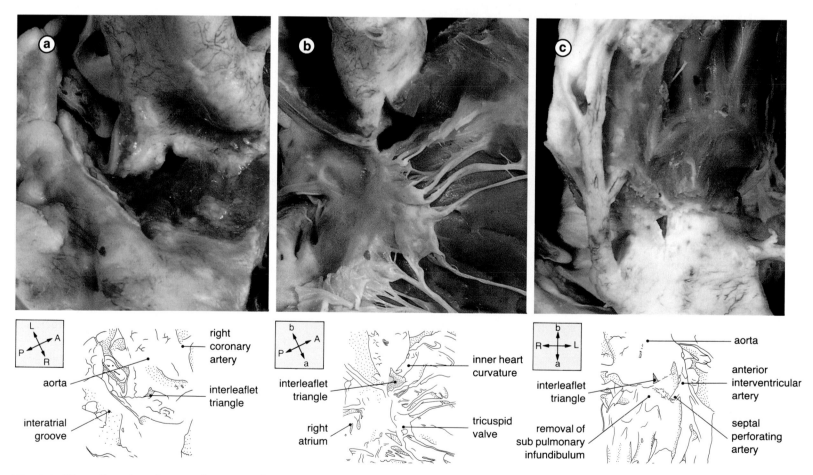

right coronary artery

aorta

interleaflet triangle

interatrial groove

inner heart curvature

interleaflet triangle

right atrium

tricuspid valve

aorta

anterior interventricular artery

interleaflet triangle

removal of sub pulmonary infundibulum

septal perforating artery

Fig. 3.4 *These dissections show a sub-aortic outflow tract such as demonstrated in Fig. 3.2. The interleaflet triangles of the aortic valve **(a)** between the non-coronary and left coronary leaflets **(b)** between the non-coronary and right coronary leaflets and **(c)** between the right and left coronary leaflets have been removed to show their relationships to adjacent structures.*

coronary artery (Fig. 3.2). Thus, the leaflets of the aortic valve are attached in part to the muscular component of the left ventricular outflow tract and to the area of fibrous continuity (Fig. 3.20). In the case of the pulmonary valve, the attachments are exclusively to the musculature of the right ventricular outflow tract (Fig. 3.3).

Atrioventricular Valves

The two atrioventricular valves are attached to the atrioventricular junction in the fashion of an annulus, but, even in this respect, there is a marked difference between the mitral and tricuspid valves in the extent to which this annulus is part of the fibrous skeleton. As described above, the strongest parts of the skeleton are the two areas of fibrous continuity, the right and left fibrous trigones (Fig. 3.2). Between these two trigones is a region of fibrous continuity between the leaflets of the aortic valve and those of the mitral valve. This region is called the aortic–mitral curtain.

The fibrous skeleton forming the ring of the mitral valve extends septally and parietally from the two trigones, usually as a complete collagenous structure. It is not always cord-like, often having a linear structure. Its structure varies markedly at different points around the junction, and it usually tends to fade out or become attenuated in the segment opposite the aortic–mitral curtain.

The right fibrous trigone brings both the mitral and aortic valves into fibrous continuity with the tricuspid valve. This part of the fibrous skeleton includes the membranous septum, which separates the left ventricular outflow tract from the chambers of the right heart (Fig. 3.5). Usually, the attachment of the septal leaf of the tricuspid valve extends obliquely across the membranous septum, dividing it into atrioventricular and interventricular components. It is the right fibrous trigone, together with the membranous septum, that make up the central fibrous body (Fig. 3.6). The remainder of the attachment of the tricuspid valve, around the right atrioventricular junction, is the most weakly constructed part of the cardiac skeleton, particularly in its parietal part. Thus, it is rarely possible to dissect a complete collagenous ring supporting the leaflets of the tricuspid valve.

Basic Morphology of the Atrioventricular Valves

Common Anatomical Features

There are several anatomic features common to both the mitral and tricuspid valves. The first feature has already been described, namely the attachments of the valvar leaflets to the fibrous skeleton. Another common feature is the histological arrangement of the leaflets. These structures have a spongy atrial and a fibrous ventricular layer. The atrial myocardium inserts for varying distances between the endocardium and the spongy layer. On rare occasions, rudimentary fibres of ventricular musculature may extend into the fibrous layer, most often in association with the basal cords (see below). In normal valves, blood vessels are found only within the segment of leaflet containing muscular fibres. The leaflets are supported by the tendinous cords, which insert into the papillary muscles or directly into the ventricular myocardium. These cordal attachments are the third feature common to both tricuspid and mitral valves, although there are fundamental differences in the way each of the cordal units is arranged. This is also the case with the fourth feature, namely the papillary muscles. The differences in these various features readily permit the morphological differentiation of the valves. Before describing these differences, it is important to emphasize those features of the leaflets and their tension apparatus that are common to both valves.

Valvar Leaflets

Considered as a whole, the leaflets form a continuous skirt that hangs from the atrioventricular junction. The skirt is divided into discrete components, and it is these individual components that are described as the leaflets. There is no consensus as to how many leaflets there are in each valve, or as to what constitutes the point of separation of one leaflet from the other. Traditionally, the tricuspid valve, as implied by its name, has been considered to have three leaflets. The alternative name for the mitral valve is the bicuspid valve, although it has been suggested that the mitral valve is better considered as having four leaflets[2].

Leaflets in atrioventricular valves are distinguished by identifying the commissures between them. This necessitates defining a commissure. Some[3] have suggested that a commissure is a breach in the skirt of valve tissue, supported by a

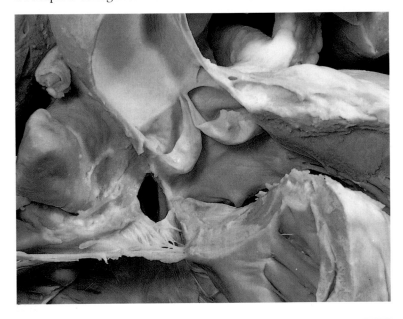

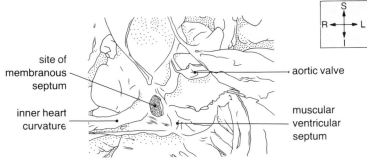

Fig. 3.5 *In this heart, the front of the right ventricle and the top of the ventricular septum have been removed to show the site of the membranous septum.*

fan-shaped commissural cord, such a cord then inserting into a major papillary muscle or group of papillary muscles. Since it is probably better not to define one structure in terms of another, we prefer to consider the commissures simply as the space between separate and identifiable components of the skirt of leaflet tissue. The leaflets are then supported by cords, while commissures are usually supported by fan-shaped cords attached to the free edge of the valvar leaflets (Fig. 3.7). The free edge away from the commissure is also supported by cords attached directly to the free edge (Fig. 3.8).

As indicated in the discussion[4] of the exquisitely complex categorization of cords proposed by the Toronto group[5], if any of these cords supporting the free edge are cut, the valve may become regurgitant. As suggested by Frater[4], it is sufficient to distinguish such cords supporting the free edge from those supporting the rough zone, avoiding the detailed classification proposed by the Toronto group[5]. The cords from the rough zone are prominent structures that extend from the papillary muscles to the ventricular aspect of the

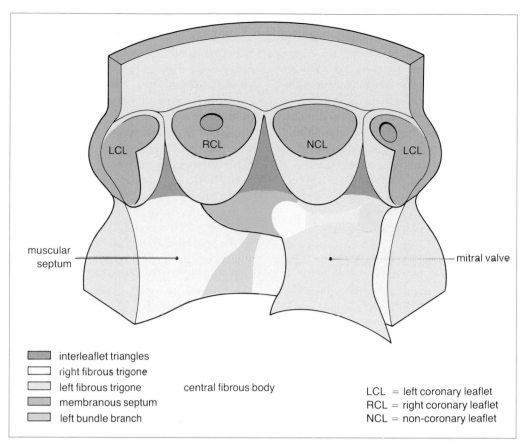

interleaflet triangles
right fibrous trigone
left fibrous trigone · · · · · · · · · · · · central fibrous body
membranous septum
left bundle branch

LCL = left coronary leaflet
RCL = right coronary leaflet
NCL = non-coronary leaflet

Fig. 3.6 *This diagram illustrates the fibrous structures which make up the central fibrous body.*

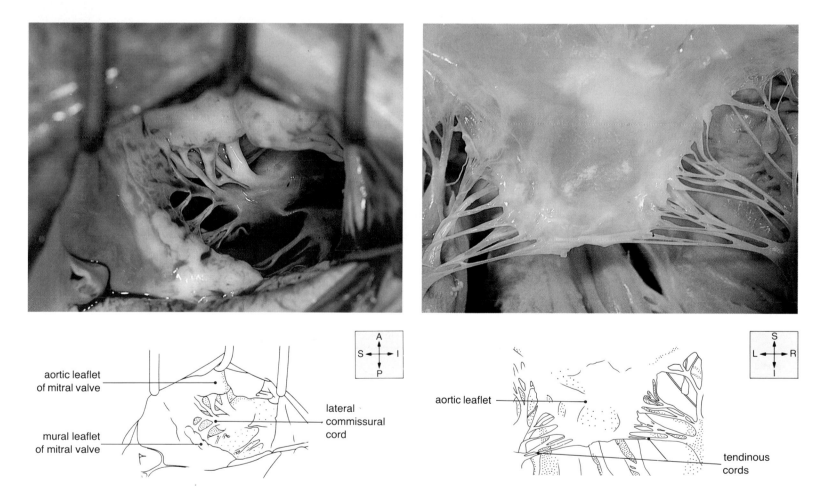

Fig. 3.7 *This operative view of a rheumatic mitral valve, taken through a left atriotomy, shows a fan-shaped commissural cord arising from the tip of its papillary muscle.*

Fig. 3.8 *This anatomic specimen, viewed from the inlet aspect, shows the aortic leaflet of the mitral valve with extensive tendinous cords attached to the free edge of the valve.*

leaflets. Some cords to the rough zone are particularly prominent and are called strut cords (Fig. 3.9). There is then a third type of cord that extends from the ventricular wall close to the atrioventricular junction and inserts into the ventricular aspect of the leaflet. These are the basal cords. There is little point in further characterizing the branching pattern and generations of these cords as long as it is appreciated that, normally, all parts of the leaflets receive good cordal support. The lack of cordal support focally may be a mechanism leading to the prolapse of a leaflet[6,7].

Functional Anatomy

As has been emphasized in describing the mitral valve[8], the different components of an atrioventricular valve (that is, the junction, leaflets, cords, papillary muscles and ventricular myocardium) function in concert to produce a competent valvar mechanism. The reason that the atrioventricular valves have such a complex tension apparatus is that, while in their closed position, they must withstand the full brunt of systolic ventricular pressure. A lesion of any of the valvar components can result in regurgitation. Thus, it is essential that the atrioventricular junction be of normal size and not overly dilated.

The leaflets must coapt snugly when they are partly everted into the atrium during ventricular systole. This demands an area of overlap. To this end, the closure point of the leaflets is about one-third of the distance from the free edge to the annular margin (Fig. 3.10). The point of closure at this position gives a considerable margin of safety for dilatation of the valvar orifice. Often, particularly in aged valves, this point of closure is marked by a series of nodules.

Equally significant to competent closure is the support of the leaflet by cords attached to the free edge. As discussed previously, this feature is very important in preventing the prolapse of the valve leaflets. It has been suggested[9] that prolapse of the leaflets of the mitral valve is one of the most common congenital lesions. There is, as yet, no consensus as to the etiology of such a prolapse. Morphologic observations[6,7] certainly suggest that the lack of cordal support to the free edge of the leaflets can contribute to prolapse: nonetheless, it is premature to label what is probably a variation of normal anatomy as a congenital cardiac malformation. Be that as it may, uniform support of the free edges of the leaflets is an integral part of a normal valve.

Also important in the maintenance of competence is the correct action of the papillary muscles and the ventricular

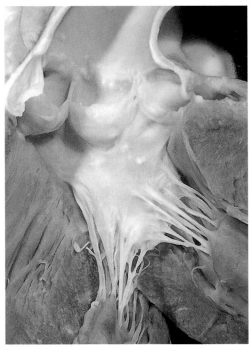

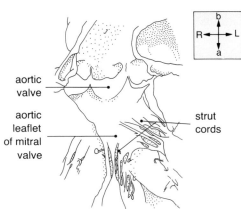

Fig. 3.9 *Some cords to the rough zone are particularly prominent, as shown in this illustration, and are defined as strut cords.*

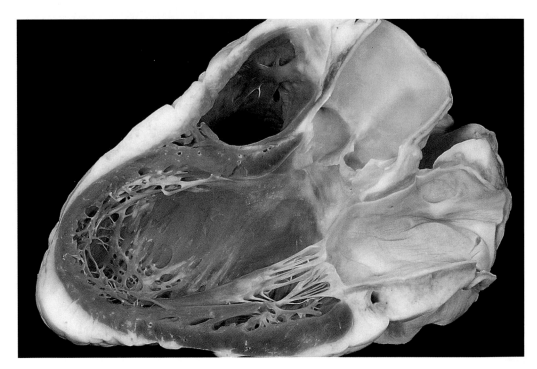

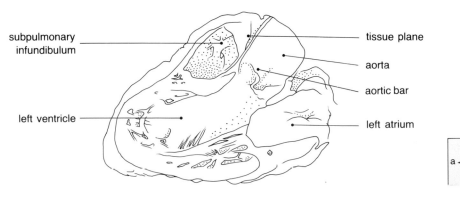

Fig. 3.10 *This long axis section through the left ventricle shows the closure line of the leaflets of the mitral valve at approximately one-third of the distance from the free edge to the annular margin.*

myocardium. Not only must the papillary muscles be viable, but they must also be in their appropriate position of mechanical advantage relative to the axis of the valve. Taken together, all parts of the valvar unit are significant in the normal function of the valve.

The Mitral Valve

Aortic and Mural Leaflets

The mitral valve has two major leaflets (Fig. 3.11) typically supported by paired papillary muscles. The two leaflets have widely dissimilar circumferential lengths. The ends of the commissure between them, together with the papillary muscles, are positioned in postero-medial and antero-lateral positions within the left ventricle, so that there is an angle between the axis of

opening of the valve and the plane of the inlet septum. The posterior extension of the subaortic outflow tract is wedged into this angle. This arrangement is important in terms of the disposition of the atrio-ventricular conduction tissue axis (see Chapter 5).

The leaflets to either side of the commissure are frequently described as being *anterior* and *posterior*. This description takes no account of the position of the leaflets in the heart when considered relative to the body. The axis of the valvar opening has considerable obliquity relative to the various anatomical axes. For this reason, it is much more useful to describe the leaflets as being *aortic* and *mural*, this accounting well for both their morphology and position.

The aortic leaflet is attached to only one-third of the annular circumference. It is

trapezoidal, or more semicircular, in shape than the mural leaflet. The mural leaflet, attached to two-thirds of the annulus, is a long, rectangular structure, although its middle component can also be somewhat semicircular.

It is the segments of the mural leaflet closest to the ends of the commissure that show the most variation in morphology. Often these segments are almost completely separate from the central component, producing the so-called scallops of the mural leaflet. Others refer to these scallops as commissural leaflets. Yacoub[2] has gone so far as to nominate them as separate leaflets of a quadrifoliate valve. This latter suggestion overlooks the marked variability that normally occurs in the valve, since sometimes the mural leaflet is comprised of four, five or even more scallops[10]. Suffice it to say that usually there are three scallops within the mural leaflet, and that each of these may function as a separate unit, notably in the setting of a prolapse.

Cordal Attachments

The cords supporting the leaflets attach them either to the papillary muscles (cords to the free edge and rough zone) or else directly to the wall of the ventricle (basal cords). The cords at either end of the commissure attach adjacent sides of the leaflets to the apex of the prominent papillary muscles (Fig. 3.12). Supplementary heads of both papillary muscles then support other cords to the free edge, which usually attach uniformly along the leading edge of the leaflets, although the degree of support can be quite variable.

The cords supporting the divisions between the scallops of the mural leaflet often have a fan-shaped appearance. When attached to a prominent supplementary head of a papillary muscle, they can be markedly similar to the cords supporting the two ends of the commissure.

Papillary Muscles

Almost always, the papillary muscles of the mitral valve are prominent paired structures located on postero-medial and antero-lateral aspects of the parietal ventricular wall. Although detailed study reveals considerable variation in the precise morphology of each muscle[6], neither arises from the septum, in contradistinction to the attachments of the tricuspid valve within the right ventricle. When the valve is dissected in its natural position within the left ventricle, the muscles can be seen to be adjacent to each other at the junction of the apical and middle third of the parietal ventricular wall.

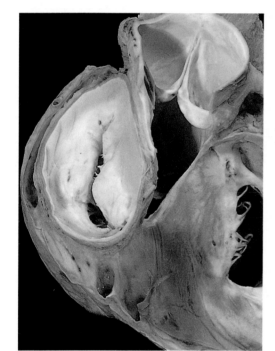

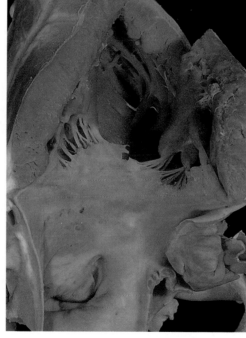

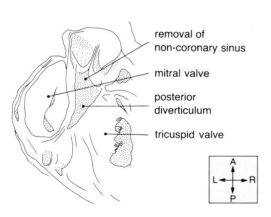

removal of non-coronary sinus

mitral valve

posterior diverticulum

tricuspid valve

A
L — R
P

Fig. 3.11 *This operative view of the mitral valve through a left atriotomy shows the arrangement of the aortic and mural leaflets.*

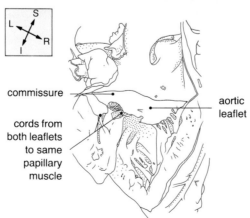

S
L — R
I

commissure

cords from both leaflets to same papillary muscle

aortic leaflet

Fig. 3.12 *This anatomic specimen, seen from behind, shows the mitral valve with the cords supporting the free edge of both leaflets attached to the same papillary muscles.*

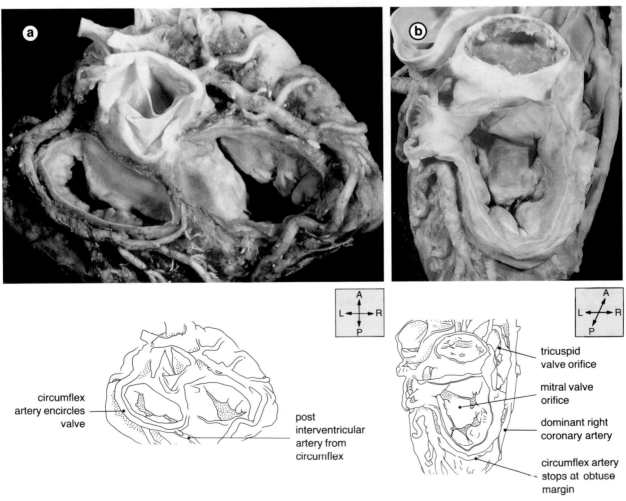

central fibrous body

aortic root

sinus node

antero-lateral commissure

circumflex coronary artery

atrioventricular node

postero-medial commissure

coronary sinus

atrioventricular nodal artery

circumflex artery encircles valve

post interventricular artery from circumflex

tricuspid valve orifice

mitral valve orifice

dominant right coronary artery

circumflex artery stops at obtuse margin

Fig. 3.14 *These dissections show the variable relationships of the circumflex artery to the mitral valve when (a) the left coronary artery and (b) when the right coronary artery supply the crux of the heart.*

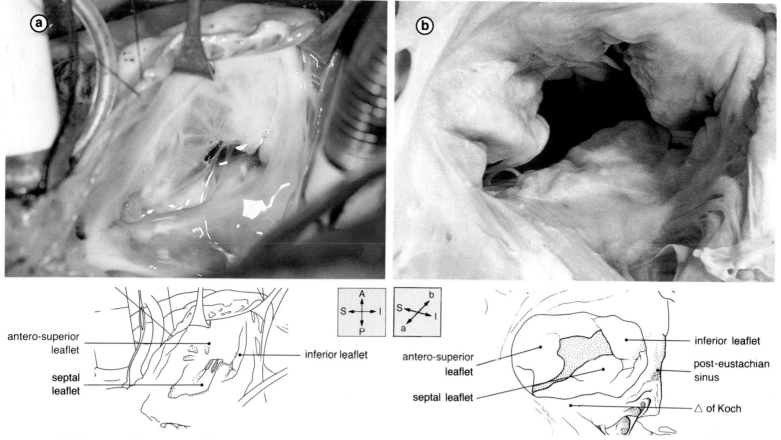

Fig. 3.15 *(a) A surgical dissection and (b) an anatomic specimen viewed in surgical orientation to show the three leaflets of the tricuspid valve.*

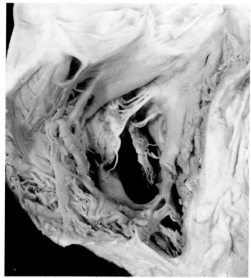

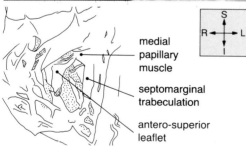

Fig. 3.16 *This outlet view of the right ventricle in surgical orientation shows the medial papillary muscle supporting the antero-septal commissure of the tricuspid valve (see also Fig. 2.30). Note the antero-superior leaflet hanging between the inlet and outlet parts of the ventricle.*

Morphological Relationships

The area of the valvar orifice related to the right fibrous trigone and central fibrous body is most critical because within this area lies the atrioventricular node and penetrating bundle (Fig. 3.13). Additionally, between the two trigones, the area of the orifice that is more or less in the mid-portion of the aortic leaflet of the mitral valve is directly related to the commissure between the non-coronary and left coronary leaflets of the aortic valve. At this point the aortic root is tented up, and an incision from within the left atrium that is apparently through the atrial wall will extend into the subaortic outflow tract. If the incision is continued superiorly, the atrial wall will be penetrated into the transverse sinus of the pericardial cavity which lies superiorly to the aortic–mitral curtain. The deep inner curvature of the heart overlies and runs superiorly and to either side of this curtain and is lined by the pericardium of the transverse sinus.

Encircling the mural leaflet of the valve are the circumflex coronary artery from below and to the left, and the coronary sinus from below and to the right (Fig. 3.13). Also, in some cases, the atrioventricular nodal artery will run in close proximity to the right side of the mitral

orifice, arising from either the circumflex or right coronary artery. The margin directly related to the circumflex artery is somewhat variable but, when the left coronary artery reaches the crux, the entire attachment of the mural leaflet can be intimately related to the coronary artery (compare Figs 3.14a and b).

The Tricuspid Valve

Septal, Antero-superior and Inferior Leaflets

The tricuspid valve has three major leaflets (Fig. 3.15) which are supported by papillary muscles of grossly disproportionate size. The septal and antero-superior leaflets are the most apparent.

The septal leaflet extends from the somewhat indistinct and inconstant inferior papillary muscle to the much more constant medial papillary muscle (the muscle of Lancisi or the papillary muscle of the conus). Almost invariably, this latter attachment is found to originate from the posterior limb of the septomarginal trabeculation (Fig. 3.16). The attachment of the septal leaflet crosses the membranous septum, dividing it into the atrioventricular and interventricular components. The distal extent of the septal leaflet is attached by several cords running from the free edge directly to the septum (Fig. 3.17). As previously emphasized, this feature serves to distinguish it from the leaflets of the mitral valve, which lack any attachment to the septum. In the area where the septal leaflet extends across the membranous septum, the leaflet may be divided, resulting in a discrete cleft extending towards the central fibrous body.

The antero-superior leaflet descends from the underside of the ventriculo-infundibular fold and hangs like an extensive curtain between the inlet and outlet parts of the ventricle, its medial end being attached to the medial papillary muscle (Fig. 3.16). There is more variability in the arrangement of its lateral component. Usually the lateral commissure between the antero-superior and the

inferior leaflet is supported by the prominent anterior papillary muscle, which originates from the apical portion of the septomarginal trabeculation. The leaflet is then supported by cords to the free edge and rough zone (including strut cords) in a fashion comparable with that seen in the aortic leaflet of the mitral valve. Infrequently, the anterior papillary muscle attaches directly to the midpoint of the antero-superior leaflet, and the muscle supporting the lateral commissure is relatively indistinct. Frequently, there are extensions of muscle from either the papillary muscles or the ventriculo–infundibular fold into this leaflet.

The third leaflet of the tricuspid valve is the inferior or mural leaflet. It is much less constant than the other two, since the inferior papillary muscle is often indistinct

and variable. The leaflet is attached to the parietal part of the atrioventricular junction, while being supported distally by several cords to the free edge, attached either to small heads of muscle or directly to the ventricular wall. Often it is possible to distinguish two scallops in its extent.

Morphological Relationships
The entire parietal attachment of the tricuspid valve is usually encircled by the right coronary artery running within the atrioventricular groove (Fig. 3.18). As discussed previously, it is rare to find a well-formed collagenous tricuspid 'annulus'. Instead, the atrioventricular groove more or less folds itself directly into the leaflets of the tricuspid valve. The atrial and ventricular myocardial masses are then separated almost exclusively by the adipose tissue within the groove.

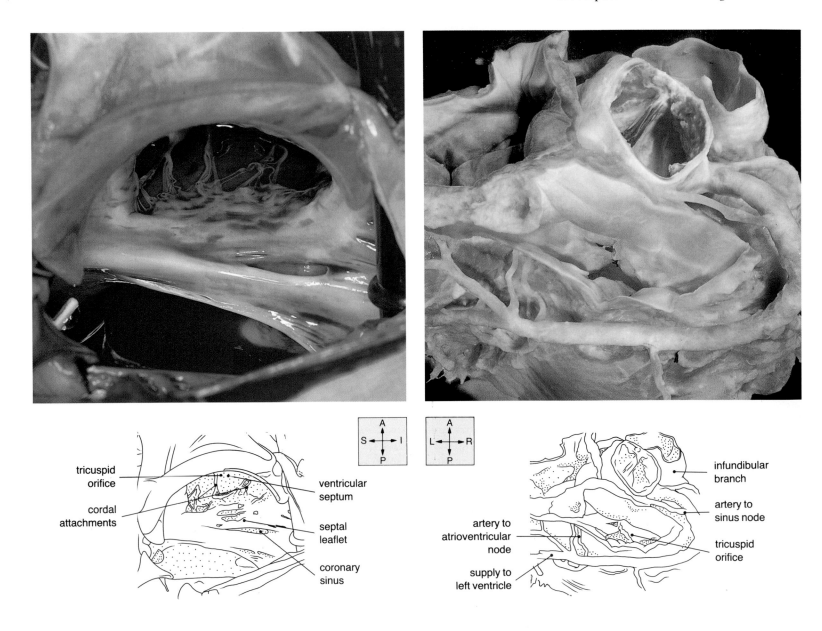

Fig. 3.17 *This operative view through a right atriotomy shows the cordal attachments to the septum of the septal leaflet of the tricuspid valve.*

Fig. 3.18 *This dissection of an anatomic specimen shows the relationship of the right coronary artery to the orifice of the tricuspid valve.*

Basic Morphology of the Arterial Valves

Valvar Leaflets

The arterial valves are much simpler structures than the atrioventricular valves, since they do not require an intricate tension apparatus to ensure their competence. Instead, their design is simplicity itself: three semilunar leaflets (Fig. 3.19) that open into the arterial sinuses during ventricular systole and collapse together during diastole. The semilunar leaflets are held in their closed position by the hydrostatic pressure of the column of blood they then support.

In terms of histological structure, the leaflets have a fibrous core with an endothelial lining. The fibrous core is thickened at the free edge, particularly at the central portion just short of the free edge where,

with age, a distinct fibrous nodule is seen (nodule of Arantius).

The leaflets of the valve do not close just at their free edge, rather the closure line extends some distance from the free edge towards the semilunar attachment. Not infrequently, the leaflets may be perforated beyond the line of closure in this outer component. Such perforations are a normal finding and do not affect valvar function.

The attached margin of the valve is a half-moon shape (Figs 3.3 and 3.20) so that, when the valve is removed from the heart, its seat can be seen to be arranged in the form of a coronet. The attachments of the leaflets at the apices of the commissures are significantly higher than the attachments at their mid portion. As already discussed, the site and nature of these attachments vary from aortic to pulmonary valve, being partly fibrous in the aorta and

exclusively muscular in the pulmonary trunk. In either case, it is incorrect to describe the arterial valves as having an annulus or ring. The only true ring is the area in which the fibrous walls of the arterial trunks are attached to the supporting ventricular structures. This is the anatomic ventriculo–arterial junction.

There is a marked discrepancy between this anatomic junction and the haemodynamic junction, the latter being marked by the semilunar attachment of the leaflets (Fig. 3.20). By virtue of this arrangement, part of the arterial wall is, haemodynamically, a ventricular structure. In contrast, part of the ventricle at the base of each sinus is within the arterial trunk. The commissures in the arterial valves, however, are comparable to those in the atrioventricular valves — they are simply the points of abutment of the semilunar leaflets (Fig. 3.20).

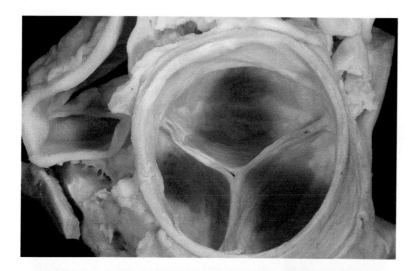

Fig. 3.19 *This view of the aortic valve from above shows the semilunar leaflets coapting snugly.*

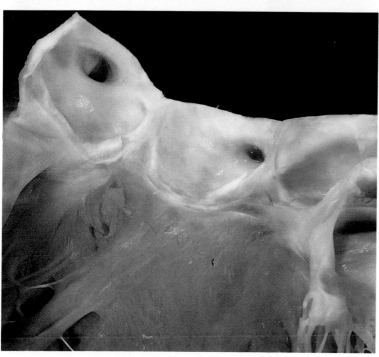

Fig. 3.20 *This dissection of the aortic valve shows how the semilunar attachments of the leaflets cross the circular anatomic ventriculo–arterial junction.*

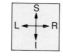

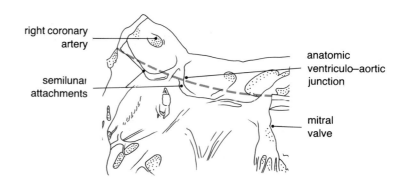

right coronary artery

semilunar attachments

anatomic ventriculo–aortic junction

mitral valve

Sinuses

Also of significance in the normal functioning of the arterial valves are the sinuses which are located at the origin of the arterial trunks. These dilatations are arranged in a clover-like fashion (Fig. 3.14a). They permit the valvar leaflets to retract during ventricular systole so that there is unrestricted blood flow from the ventricle to the arterial trunk. Two of the aortic sinuses are particularly important, since they give rise to the major coronary arteries. The coronary arterial origin is usually within the sinus, beneath the junction of sinus and ascending aorta (the aortic bar). There is, nonetheless, some variability in origin of the coronary arteries (see Chapter 4).

So far the account has presumed the presence of three leaflets of the arterial valve. In some instances, valves are found with four leaflets in either the aortic or pulmonary position[11, 12]. A more significant variation is a valve with two leaflets, either in the aortic (Fig. 7.63a) or pulmonary position. Indeed, this is probably the most common congenital cardiac malformation[9].

The Aortic Valve

Anatomical Features

As indicated above, the semilunar leaflets of the aortic valve are attached in part to the fibrous skeleton and in part to the muscular outlet portion of the left ventricle (Fig. 3.3). When naming the aortic leaflets, advantage can be taken of the fact that, almost without exception, the major coronary arteries originate from two of the aortic sinuses but not the third. Thus, the aortic leaflets can be described as being right coronary, left coronary, and non-coronary in position (Fig. 3.14a).

It is the right and left coronary leaflets that have a partly muscular origin from the left ventricular wall, the base of the myocardium being incorporated within the sinus. These leaflets face the pulmonary trunk. Their more distal adjacent parts originate from the free aortic wall and face the potential space between it and the pulmonary infundibulum and trunk (Fig. 3.2).

The attachment of the right coronary leaflet drops from this point towards the crest of the muscular part of the septum, near the membranous septum, and then rises again towards the apex of the commissure between the right and non-coronary leaflets. This posterior part of the right coronary leaflet is attached to the fibrous skeleton.

All of the non-coronary leaflet has a fibrous origin, and half of it, extending from the commissure with the right coronary leaflet, is attached in the region of the membranous septum (Fig. 3.21). The triangle between these leaflets is in close association with the right atrium and right ventricle (Fig. 3.4b).

The extensive posterior extension, or diverticulum, of the left ventricular outflow tract lies beneath the non-coronary leaflet, limited antero-laterally by the atrioventricular component of the membranous septum. Reaching its nadir at the attachment to the right fibrous trigone, the non-coronary leaflet then rises towards the apex of its commissure with the left coronary leaflet. The apex of this triangle between these leaflets is in close association with the transverse sinus (Fig. 3.4a).

The adjacent parts of both leaflets in this area are attached to the free aortic wall distally, and to the aortic leaflet of the mitral valve, thus forming the aortic–mitral curtain. As indicated, the commissural area of this curtain separates the left ventricular outflow tract, not from the left atrium, but from the transverse sinus of the pericardium. In other words, cutting through the sub-commissural curtain takes the surgeon outside the heart into the pericardial cavity (Fig. 3.22).

Beyond this area, the left coronary leaflet then adjoins a short segment of parietal myocardium before extending anteriorly to the facing commissure. The apex of this interleaflet triangle 'points' to the space between the aorta and the pulmonary trunk (Fig. 3.4c). The trough of the attachment of the left coronary leaflet is in close association with the area of the left fibrous trigone and the parietal wall of the left ventricle, while the anterior ascending component runs onto the free aortic wall posterior and superior to the ventricular septum.

The precise attachments of the aortic leaflets vary from heart to heart, particularly that portion of the commissure between the non-coronary and left coronary leaflets which is in close association with the aortic–mitral curtain[13]. The length of the sub-aortic fibrous curtain is also found to vary from heart to heart[14]. Additionally, in a small percentage of normal hearts, the aortic valve in this area has a complete muscular infundibulum[15]. These individual

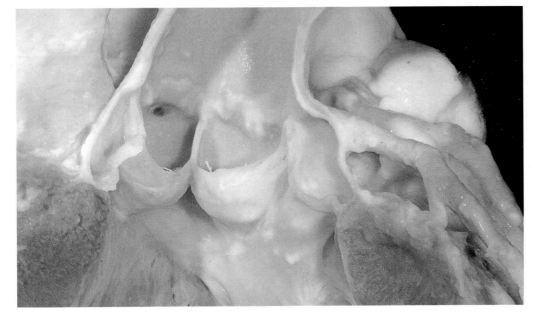

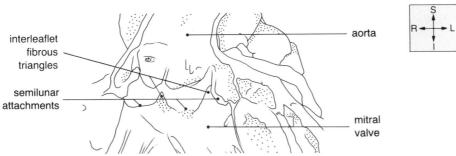

Fig. 3.21 *This view of the sub-aortic outflow tract in anatomical orientation shows the attachment of the three semilunar leaflets.*

variations do not distort the basic anatomical relationships as described above.

The non-coronary leaflet is attached above the extensive posterior diverticulum of the outflow tract. That is the part of the valve directly related to the right atrial wall (Figs 3.23 and 3.24). From the inferior attachment of the non-coronary leaflet in close relation to the right atrium, the valve tents up again to the commissure between the non-coronary and right coronary leaflets. Consequently, the ascending part of the non-coronary leaflet is positioned directly above that part of the atrial septum which contains the atrioventricular node, while the commissure itself is above the penetrating atrioventricular bundle and the membranous septum (Fig. 3.4b).

The commissure between the right and left coronary leaflets is usually positioned opposite a facing commissure of the pulmonary valve. The adjacent parts of these two leaflets, therefore, are attached to the outlet part of the ventricular septum and so are directly related to the infundibulum of the right ventricle, although a tissue plane interposes (Fig. 3.2). Incisions through the right ventricular outflow tract at this site, nonetheless, lead directly into the sub-aortic region (Fig. 3.24). This is

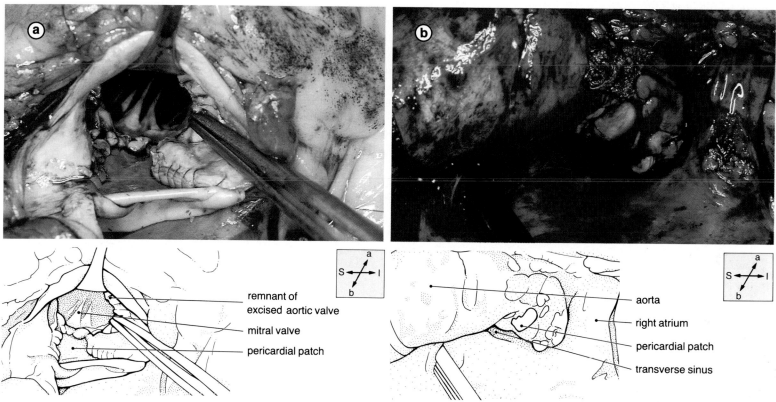

Fig. 3.22 *These operative views show the significance of the interleaflet triangle shown in Fig. 3.7a. An incision through the aortic–mitral curtain has been enlarged with a pericardial patch and is seen (a) through the aorta and (b) externally after closing the aorta.*

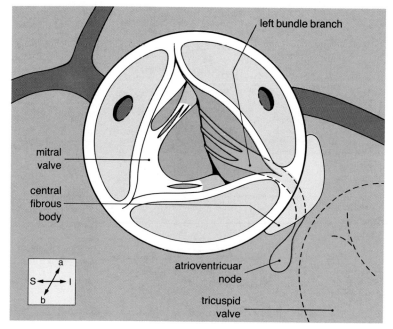

Fig. 3.23 *This diagram of the heart, in surgical orientation, shows the relationship of the aortic valve to the adjacent cardiac structures.*

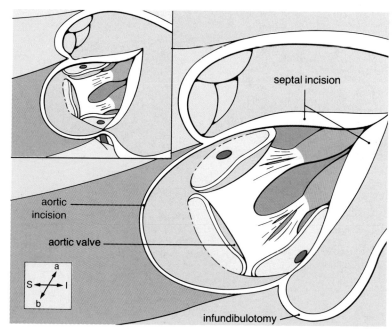

Fig. 3.24 *This diagram shows how incisions through the anterior part of the sub-aortic outflow tract lead directly to the infundibulum of the right ventricle.*

the basis of the right ventricular approach for relief of sub-aortic obstruction.

Beyond this point, the lateral part of the left coronary leaflet is the only part of the aortic valve not intimately related to another cardiac chamber. This is the part of the valve that originates from the lateral margin of the inner heart curvature and is, consequently, in relationship externally with the free pericardial space.

The Pulmonary Valve

The pulmonary valve in the normal heart has exclusively muscular attachments to the infundibulum of the right ventricle (Fig. 3.25a). Because of its oblique position, there is difficulty in naming the pulmonary leaflets according to their right/left and antero-posterior orientation. It is better to describe them according to their relationship to the aortic valve. As discussed above, the two leaflets of the aortic valve attached to the septum always face two leaflets of the pulmonary valve. Consequently, these two pulmonary valvar leaflets can be called the right and left facing leaflets. The third leaflet is then described simply as the non-facing leaflet.

The commissure between the two facing leaflets is usually thought to be attached to the outlet septum immediately above the anterior limb of the septomarginal trabeculation. In reality, it is attached to a sleeve of infundibular myocardium (Fig. 3.25b). As the right facing leaflet drops down from the apex of its facing commissure, it is supported by the inner curve of muscle that separates it from the tricuspid valve. This muscular mass is the supraventricular crest of the right ventricle. That particular part between the atrioventricular and arterial valves is called the ventriculo-infundibular fold. The commissure between the right and non-facing leaflets is then towards the parietal extent of this fold, and the non-facing leaflet is supported by the anterior parietal wall of the infundibulum.

The commissure between the non-facing and left facing leaflets extends from the parietal attachment back to the septum, so that the left facing leaflet runs from the parietal wall to the area of the septum.

When considered as a whole, the valve can be liberated from the right ventricle together with its infundibular sleeve without damaging any vital structures (Fig. 3.25b).

Relationships of the Valves to other Vital Cardiac Structures

As we have already discussed, positioned as they are mostly within the atrioventricular junction, the tricuspid, mitral, and aortic valves are intimately related to two vital cardiac subsystems, namely the atrioventricular conduction system and the coronary circulation. It is mandatory to avoid damage to these structures during surgery, so it is important to know their precise locations. This must be learned relative to landmarks within the valves themselves, since the conduction tissues are largely invisible and the course of the coronary vessels is likely to be hidden as the surgeon approaches the valves. Although we have mentioned these landmarks when discussing the individual valves, their importance is such that they justify a collective review.

The Atrioventricular Conduction Tissue Axis

In the normal heart, the penetrating atrioventricular bundle is the only muscular communication between the atrial and

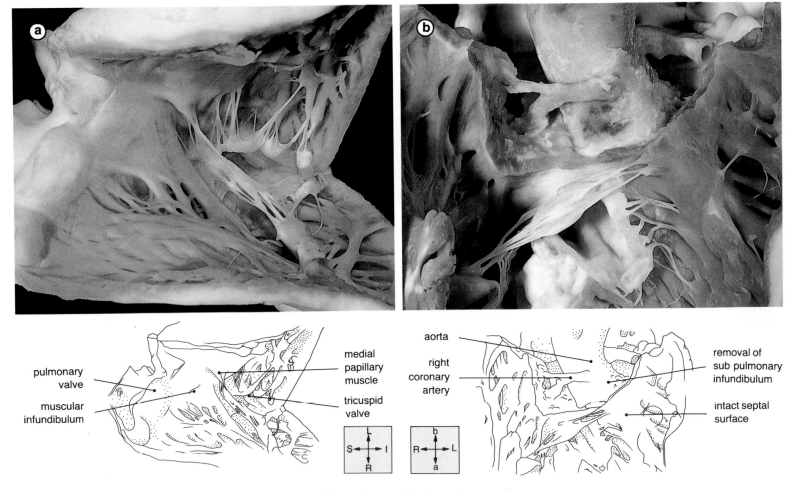

Fig. 3.25 *(a) This surgical orientation of the outflow tract of the right ventricle shows the muscular infundibulum supporting the leaflets of the pulmonary valve. (b) In this specimen the entire subpulmonary infundibulum has been removed without disturbing the structure of the left ventricle.*

ventricular muscle masses. Since the bundle penetrates through the membranous septal component of the central fibrous body, it is, of necessity, intimately related to the leaflets of the mitral, tricuspid, and aortic valves.

The conduction axis originates within the atrioventricular node and its atrial zones of transitional cells. Within the atrium, the components of the conduction axis are contained exclusively within the triangle of Koch (see Chapter 5). The inferior extent of the triangle is the junctional attachment of the septal leaflet of the tricuspid valve. As the axis penetrates the septum it immediately enters the sub-aortic region of the left ventricle (Fig. 3.26). The point of penetration is related to the postero-medial commissure of the mitral valve. In this area, the atrioventricular node lies within 5–10mm of the atrial attachment of the medial scallop of the mural leaflet. Having reached the left ventricular outflow tract, the conduction axis begins to branch either on the septal crest, where it is sandwiched between the crest and the interventricular membranous septum, or on the left ventricular aspect of the septum. This area is immediately beneath the commissure between the non-coronary and right coronary leaflets of the aortic valve, but the height of the commissure and the fibrous skeleton separates the valvar attachments from the conduction axis.

The Left and Right Bundle Branches

When seen from the left ventricle, the left bundle branch fans out as a continuous sheet on the smooth left septal surface beneath the commissure, splitting into its three divisions as it approaches the ventricular apex. The right bundle branch is the continuation of the axis beyond the branching bundle. This dips back across the septum as a thin, insulated cord that emerges on the right ventricular aspect in the area of the medial papillary muscle. Usually it then runs intramyocardially, within the structure of the septomarginal trabeculation to ramify at the ventricular apex.

When considered from the right side, the branching segment of the conduction axis can be imagined as a line joining the apex of the triangle of Koch to the medial papillary muscle. This is a relatively safe area for the surgeon, since the axis is carried on the left side of the septum. Nonetheless, the axis is within 5mm of the right ventricular septal surface.

The Vulnerable Coronary Circulation

The Coronary Sinus

On the venous side of the circulation, the coronary sinus is the only noteworthy structure related to the valves. The great cardiac vein joins with oblique and marginal venous branches in the postero-lateral left atrioventricular groove just beneath the left atrial appendage. This confluence becomes the coronary sinus (Fig. 3.27). It then proceeds in the fatty tissue of the posterior atrioventricular groove to empty into the right atrium. In an adult, its course may approach within 5–15mm of the medial attachment of the mural leaflet of the mitral valve (Fig. 3.28). Sutures placed deeply in this area during replacement of the mitral valve may lead to damage of the coronary sinus and extremely troublesome bleeding. When removing a prosthesis previously placed in the mitral position, care must also be taken not to enter the sinus with a scalpel or suture. The normal anatomy may well have been distorted by the earlier operation.

The Coronary Arteries

The coronary arteries are intimately related to both the mitral and tricuspid valves, since much of their course is within the atrioventricular groove.

The main stem of the left coronary artery branches in the angle of the left-sided ventriculo–infundibular fold immediately above the left fibrous trigone. The anterior interventricular artery descends away from the valves, although its septal perforating branches extend into the septum immediately beneath the left facing leaflet of the pulmonary valve. Consequently, they could be damaged by extensive dissection in this area. It is the circumflex branch of the left coronary artery that is most intimately related to the mitral valve, particularly when the left coronary artery is dominant. When the right coronary artery is dominant (that is, supplies the crux or part of the diaphragmatic surface of the left ventricle, and gives rise to the posterior interventricular artery, as occurs in about 85% of cases), the left circumflex is related only to the area around the lateral scallop of the mural leaflet of the mitral valve (Fig. 3.14b). When it is the circumflex branch which supplies the diaphragmatic surface of the left ventricle and the crux, its

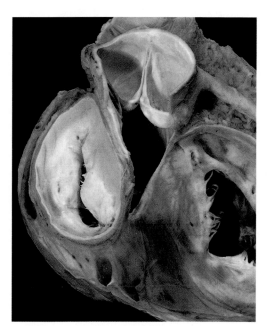

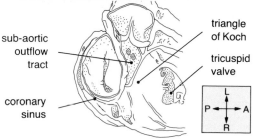

sub-aortic outflow tract

coronary sinus

triangle of Koch

tricuspid valve

Fig. 3.26 *This dissection of the heart, seen in anatomical orientation, demonstrates the relationship of the triangle of Koch and sub-aortic outflow tract of the left ventricle. Note also the course of the coronary sinus.*

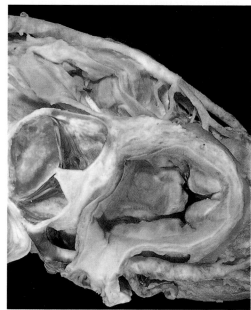

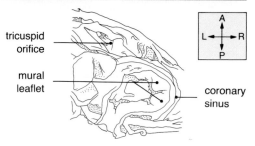

tricuspid orifice

mural leaflet

coronary sinus

Fig. 3.27 *This dissection, seen in anatomical orientation, shows the relationship of the coronary sinus to the mural leaflet of the mitral valve.*

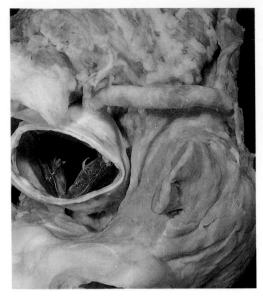

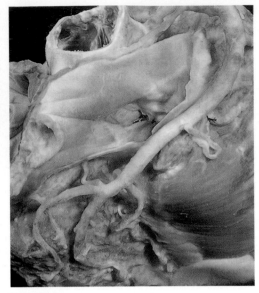

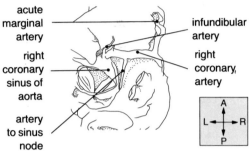

acute
marginal
artery

infundibular
artery

right
coronary
sinus of
aorta

right
coronary
artery

artery
to sinus
node

A
L — R
P

Fig. 3.28 *This dissection, seen in surgical orientation, shows the initial course of the right coronary artery.*

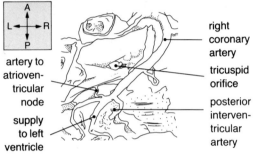

A
L — R
P

artery to
atrioven-
tricular
node

supply
to left
ventricle

right
coronary
artery

tricuspid
orifice

posterior
interven-
tricular
artery

Fig. 3.29 *This dissection, in anatomical orientation, shows the origin of the artery to the atrioventricular node from the right coronary artery.*

entire course is intimately related to all of the mural leaflet (Fig. 3.14a).

The right coronary artery always runs a circumferential course around the mural attachments of the tricuspid valve. The initial course of the artery is through the right atrioventricular groove (Fig. 3.29), where it lies on the epicardial aspect of the ventriculo–infundibular fold. It can be damaged by deeply placed sutures in this area[16]. The artery then encircles the attachment of the mural (inferior) leaflet of the tricuspid valve before, in the majority of cases, turning down to become the posterior interventricular artery. Just prior to its descent, the right coronary artery, when dominant, takes a prominent U-loop beneath the floor of the coronary sinus. From the apex of this loop it gives rise to the artery to the atrioventricular node (Fig. 3.30). In cases where the left circumflex gives rise to the posterior interventricular artery, then the atrioventricular nodal artery originates from that vessel (Fig. 3.14a). Whether arising from the left or right coronary artery, this small but important vessel is related to the posterior aspect of the annular attachment of the septal leaflet of the tricuspid valve and the annular attachment of the medial aspect of the mural leaflet of the mitral valve.

References

1. McAlpine, W.A. (1975) Heart and Coronary Arteries. In *An Anatomical Atlas for Clinical Diagnosis, Radiological Investigation, and Surgical Treatment.* Berlin: Springer–Verlag, pp. 22–23.

2. Yacoub, M. (1976) Anatomy of the mitral valve chordae and cusps. In *The Mitral Valve.* Edited by D. Kalmanson. London: Edward Arnold, pp. 15–20.

3. Lam, J.H.C., Ranganathan, N., Wigle, E.D. & Silver, M.D. (1970) Morphology of the human mitral valve. I. Chordae tendineae: a new classification. *Circulation,* **41,** 449–458.

4. Frater, R. (1976) Anatomy and physiology of the normal mitral valve. (Discussion) In *The Mitral Valve.* Edited by D. Kalmanson. London: Edward Arnold, p. 41.

5. Ranganathan, N., Lam, J.H.C., Wigle, E.D. & Silver, M.D. (1970) Morphology of the human mitral valve. II. The valve leaflets. *Circulation,* **41,** 459–467.

6. Becker, A.E. & de Wit, A.P.M. (1979) Mitral valve apparatus. A spectrum of normality relevant to mitral valve prolapse. *British Heart Journal,* **42,** 680–689.

7. Van der Bel-Kahn, J., Duren, D.R. & Becker, A.E. (1985) Isolated mitral valve prolapse: chordal architecture as an anatomic basis in older patients. *Journal of the American College of Cardiology,* **5,** 1335–1340.

8. Perloff, J.K. & Roberts, W.C. (1972) The mitral apparatus. Functional anatomy of mitral regurgitation. *Circulation,* **46,** 227–239.

9. Roberts, W.C. (1984) The two most common congenital heart diseases. (Editorial) *American Journal of Cardiology,* **53,** 1198.

10. Anderson, R.H. & Becker, A.E. (1980) In *Cardiac Anatomy – An Integrated Text and Colour Atlas.* London and Edinburgh: Gower–Churchill Livingstone, p. 4.6.

11. Feldman, B.J., Khandheria, B.K., Warnes, C.A., Seward, J.B., Taylor, C.L. & Tajik, A.J. (1990) Incidence, description and functional assessment of isolated quadricuspid aortic valves. *American Journal of Cardiology,* **65,** 937–938.

12. Becker, A.E. (1972) Quadricuspid pulmonary valve. Anatomical observations in 20 hearts. *Acta Morphology Neerlande Scandinavia,* **10,** 299–309.

13. Goor, D.A. & Lillehei, C.W. (1975) In *Congenital Malformations of the Heart.* New York: Grune and Stratton, p. 25.

14. Rosenquist, G.C., Clark, E.B., McAllister, H.A., Bharati, S. & Edwards, J.E. (1979) Increases in mitral–aortic separation in discrete subaortic stenosis. *Circulation,* **60,** 70–74.

15. Rosenquist, G.C., Clark, E.B., Sweeney, L.J. & McAllister, H.A. (1976) The normal spectrum of mitral and aortic valve discontinuity. *Circulation,* **54,** 298–301.

16. McFadden, P.M., Culpepper, W.S. III & Ochsner, J.L. (1982) Iatrogenic right ventricular failure in tetralogy of Fallot repairs: reappraisal of a distressing problem. *Annals of Thoracic Surgery,* **33,** 400–402.

SURGICAL ANATOMY OF THE CORONARY CIRCULATION 4

Introduction

The coronary circulation consists of the coronary arteries and veins, together with the lymphatics of the heart. Since the lymphatics are of very limited significance to operative anatomy, they will not be discussed further. Relatively speaking the veins are also of less interest, so, while the veins are discussed briefly, this chapter is concentrated upon those anatomic aspects of arterial distribution that are pertinent to the surgeon.

Aortic Sinuses

The coronary arteries are the first branches of the ascending aorta, arising from the aortic root immediately above its attachment to the heart. Normally, there are three sinuses at the aortic root, but only two coronary arteries. The sinuses can be named, therefore, according to whether or not they give rise to an artery, the normal arrangement being a right coronary, left coronary, and non-coronary sinus (Fig. 3.14). In this respect, the terms 'right' and 'left' refer to the coronary sinuses giving rise to the right and left coronary arteries, rather than to the position of the sinuses relative to the right–left coordinates of the body. This is important since, in the normal heart, the aortic root is obliquely situated, yet frequently in malformed hearts, the root is abnormally situated. Whatever the position of the aortic root, however, the two coronary arteries (when two are present) almost always originate from those aortic sinuses that face the sinuses of the pulmonary trunk. Because of this, it is more convenient, and more accurate, to term these sinuses the right-hand and left-hand facing sinuses (often called sinuses number 1 and 2 respectively). The point of reference is the observer standing within the non-facing sinus and looking towards the pulmonary trunk (Fig. 4.1). This convention, introduced by the group from Leiden[1], holds true irrespective of the relationships of the arterial trunks. Its value will become evident when we discuss coronary arterial origins in malformed hearts (see Chapter 8).

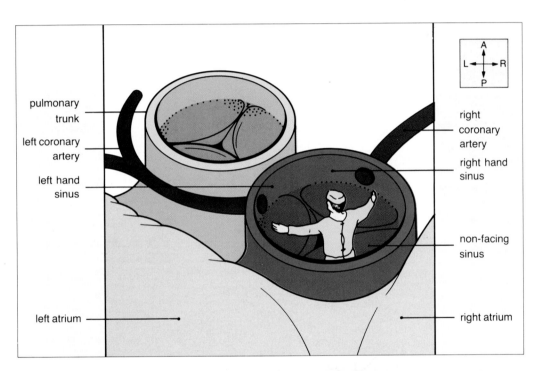

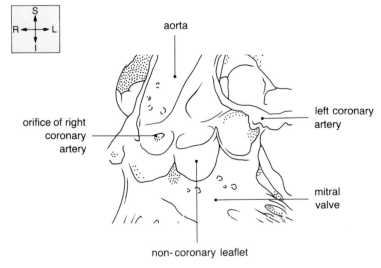

Fig. 4.1 *This diagram shows how the sinuses can be figuratively described as left- and right-handed, by conceptualizing the surgeon standing in the non-coronary sinus facing towards the pulmonary trunk.*

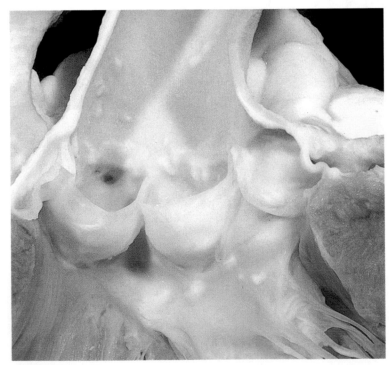

Fig. 4.2 *This specimen, seen in anatomical orientation, shows the normal origins of the coronary arteries. They originate from the two sinuses of the aorta, below the aortic bar. Note that there are two arterial orifices in the right coronary sinus.*

Origin of the Coronary Arteries in Normal Hearts

The coronary arteries usually arise from the aortic sinuses beneath the so-called aortic bar, the transitional zone between the aortic root and the tubular component of the ascending aorta (Fig. 4.2). The free edge of the leaflets of the aortic valve usually opens against this bar during ventricular systole. Deviations of origin of the coronary arteries relative to the aortic bar are not uncommon[2] and, indeed, are considered abnormal only when they are more than 1 cm from the bar. According to Barder[3] this occurs in 3.5% of hearts. The arterial opening can deviate either towards the ventricle, so that the artery arises deep within the aortic sinus, or towards the aortic arch, so that the origin is outside the sinus. Such displacement may lead to the artery taking an oblique course through the aortic wall, a so-called intramural course, which introduces the potential for luminal narrowing and disturbances in myocardial perfusion, particularly when the deviated origin is intimately related to a valvar commissure[4].

The left coronary artery almost always originates from a single orifice within the left-hand facing sinus. In contrast, in approximately 50% of hearts, there are two orifices within the right-hand facing sinus. In such instances, the orifices are unequal in size, the larger giving rise to the main trunk of the right coronary artery while the considerably smaller second orifice usually gives rise to an infundibular artery, or more rarely, to the artery supplying the sinus node. In the series reported by Becker[5], two orifices were found in the right-hand facing sinus in 46% of cases, three orifices in 7% and four orifices in 2%. These multiple orifices are of little surgical significance. In contrast, multiple orifices in the left-hand facing sinus, although extremely rare (Engel and his colleagues reported only 8 cases out of 4250 patients[6]), do have clinical significance, because they may create problems in the interpretation of coronary angiograms if unrecognized.

Rarely, the coronary arteries can also arise from a solitary orifice, usually within the right-hand facing sinus. The artery supplied from such a solitary orifice can follow two possible patterns. It can divide immediately into right and left coronary arteries (Fig. 4.3a), then the left artery passes either in front of or behind the pulmonary trunk before dividing into anterior interventricular (descending) and circumflex branches (Fig. 4.3b). Alternatively and less frequently, the single artery follows the path of the normal right coronary artery but continues beyond the crux, encircling the mitral orifice, to terminate as the anterior interventricular coronary artery.

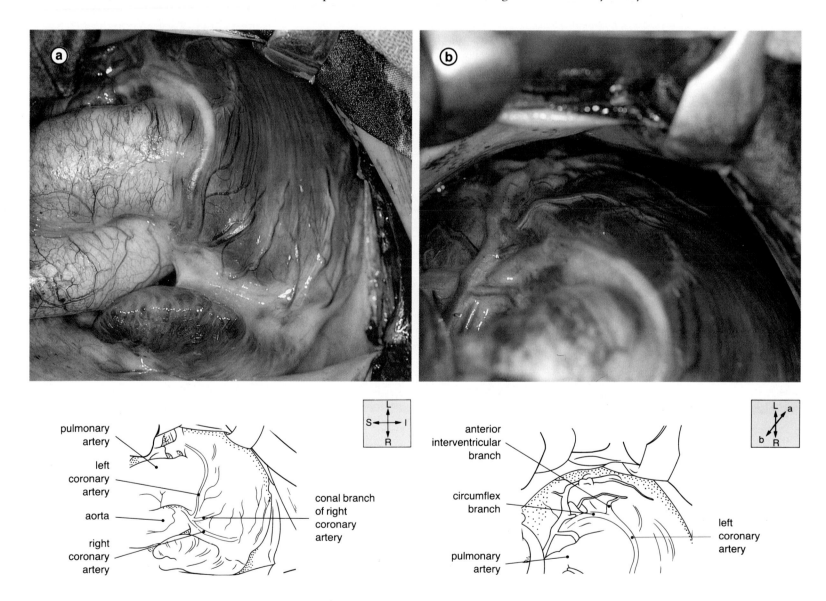

Fig. 4.3 *(a) This operative view, seen through a median sternotomy, shows a solitary coronary artery dividing immediately into right and left branches. (b) The left branch passes in front of the pulmonary trunk and divides into anterior descending and circumflex branches.*

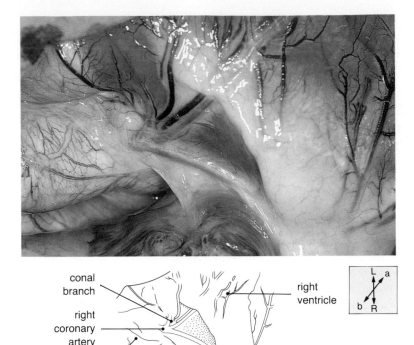

conal
branch

right
coronary
artery

aorta

right
ventricle

right atrial
appendage

Fig. 4.4 *In this operative view, seen through a median sternotomy, the right coronary artery emerges from its sinus into the right atrio-ventricular groove and immediately gives rise to an infundibular branch.*

Course of the Coronary Arteries

The epicardial course of the major coronary arteries follows the atrioventricular and interventricular grooves.

Right Coronary Artery and its Branches

The right coronary artery emerges from the right-hand facing aortic sinus and immediately enters the right atrioventricular groove, lying within the ventriculo–infundibular fold (Fig. 4.4). It then encircles the tricuspid orifice within the fat pad of the groove (Fig. 3.18). In approximately nine-tenths of cases, the right coronary artery gives rise to a posterior interventricular artery at the crux (that is when the right coronary artery is dominant). In a good proportion of these cases, the artery continues beyond the crux and supplies descending branches to the diaphragmatic surface of the left ventricle (Fig. 4.5). As the artery encircles the tricuspid orifice, it is most closely associated to the attachments of the valvar leaflets near the origin of its acute marginal branch.

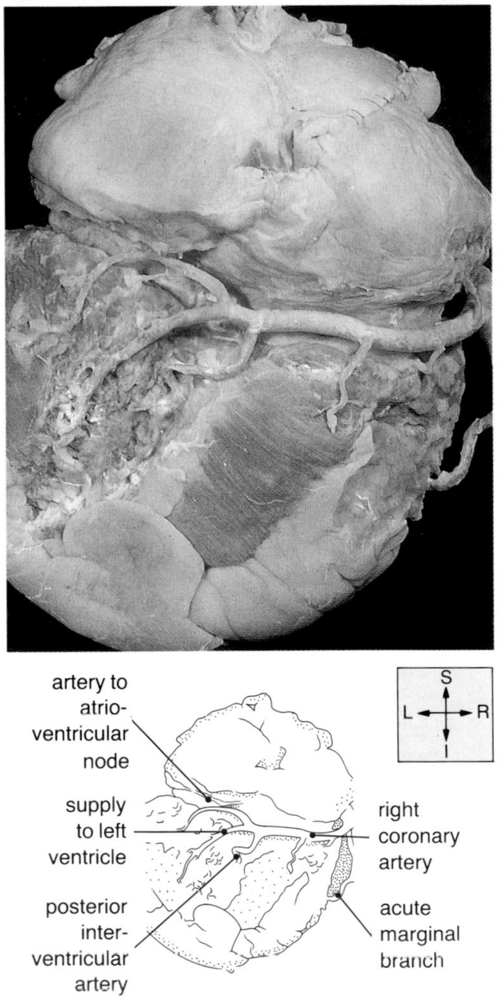

artery to
atrio-
ventricular
node

supply
to left
ventricle

posterior
inter-
ventricular
artery

right
coronary
artery

acute
marginal
branch

Fig. 4.5 *This view of the diaphragmatic surface of the heart, in anatomical orientation, shows the distribution of the dominant right coronary artery.*

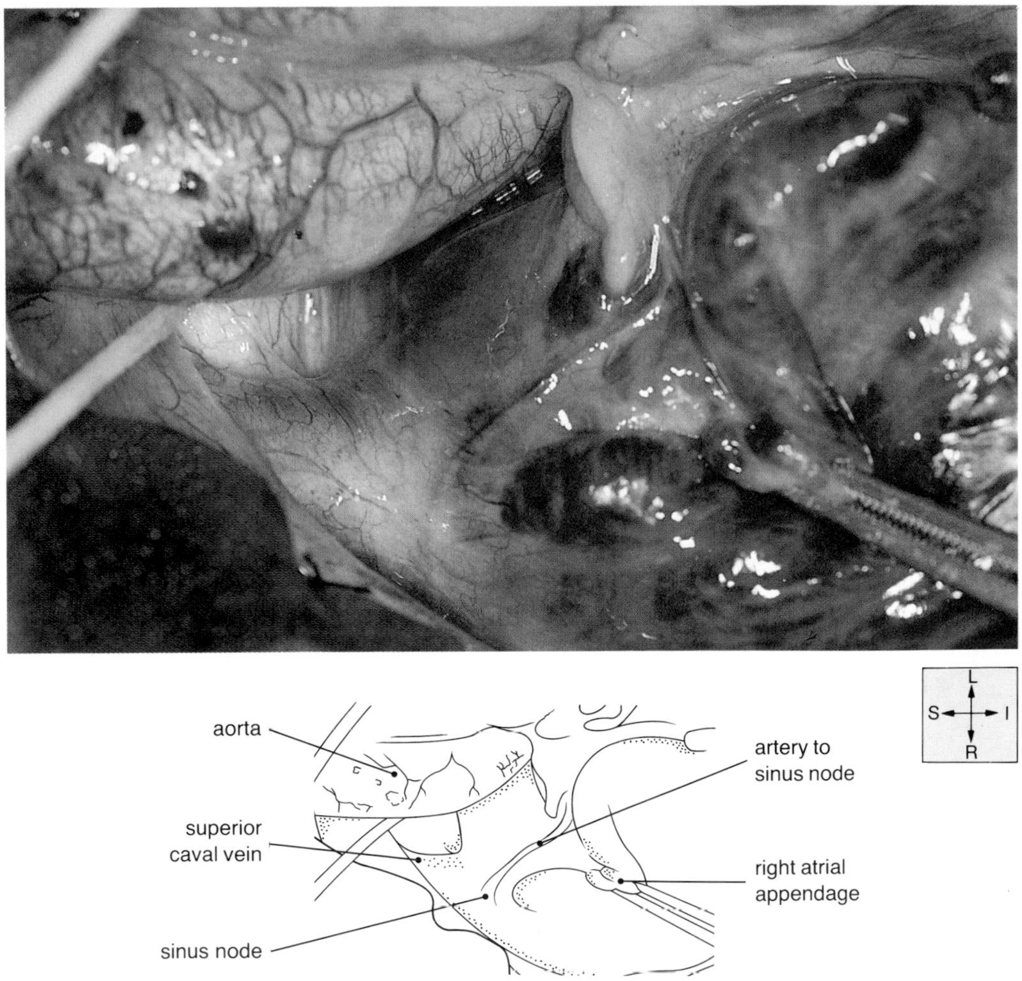

aorta

superior
caval vein

sinus node

artery to
sinus node

right atrial
appendage

Fig. 4.6 *This operative view shows there is also an artery to the sinus node arising proximally from the right coronary artery.*

Other important branches also originate from this encircling segment of the artery. Immediately after its origin, the artery lies in the right atrioventricular groove within the ventriculo–infundibular fold, where it gives rise to descending infundibular branches (which may also arise by separate orifices; see above) and in just over half of the cases, to the sinus node artery. Very rarely, the nodal artery can arise laterally from the right coronary artery, coursing over the lateral margin of the appendage to reach the terminal groove (Fig. 2.14). This case is of major significance for the operating surgeon. Even rarer are those instances when the node is supplied by both a proximal and a distal branch of the right coronary artery (Fig. 4.6).

Left Coronary Artery and its Branches

The main stem of the left coronary artery emerges from the left-hand facing sinus into the left margin of the ventriculo–infundibular fold, being positioned behind the pulmonary trunk and beneath the left atrial appendage. It is a very short structure, rarely extending beyond 1cm before branching into its anterior interventricular and circumflex branches (Fig. 4.7). In some hearts the main stem trifurcates and an intermediate branch is present between the two main branches (Fig. 4.8). The intermediate branch supplies the pulmonary surface (obtuse margin) of the left ventricle.

The anterior interventricular artery runs down within the anterior interventricular groove, giving off diagonal branches to the obtuse margin and the important perforating branches which pass posteriorly into the septum (Fig. 4.9). The first septal perforating branch is particularly important, since it is at major risk when the pulmonary valve is removed for use as a homograft. Then, the interventricular artery continues towards the apex, and frequently curves under the apex onto the diaphragmatic surface of the ventricles.

The circumflex branch of the left coronary artery passes backward to run in close relationship with the mitral orifice. Its relationship to the orifice is most extensive when it gives rise to the posterior interventricular artery at the crux (that is

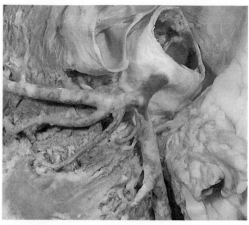

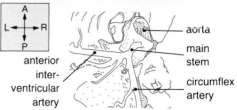

Fig. 4.7 *This dissection, in anatomical orientation, shows the left coronary artery branching into its anterior interventricular and circumflex branches. The appendage has been reflected to show the bifurcation.*

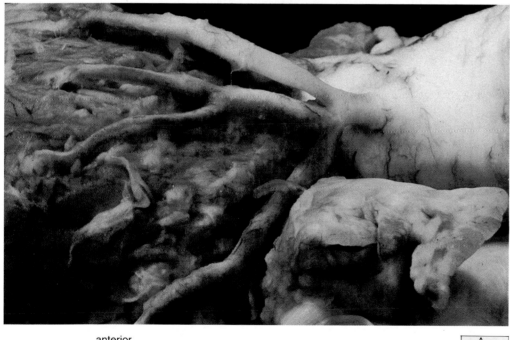

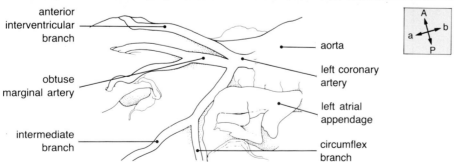

Fig. 4.8 *The left coronary artery in this anatomical specimen gives rise to three, rather than two, branches. The intermediate branch supplies the obtuse margin of the left ventricle. Courtesy of Prof. A.E. Becker.*

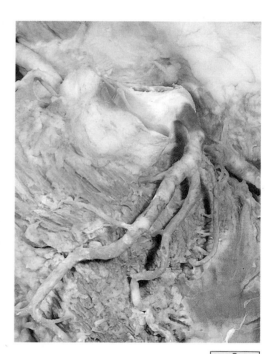

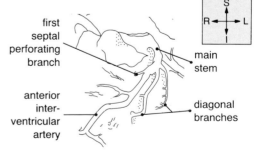

Fig. 4.9 *This dissection, in anatomical orientation, shows the course and branches of the anterior interventricular artery.*

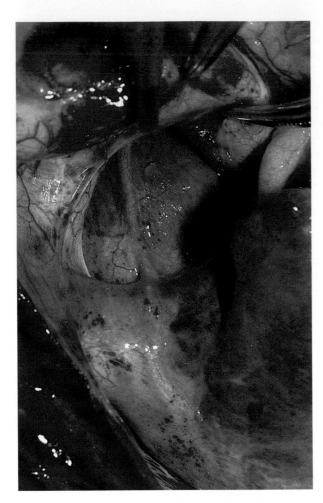

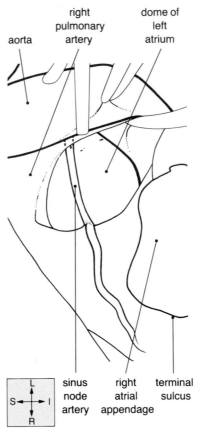

aorta | right pulmonary artery | dome of left atrium

sinus node artery | right atrial appendage | terminal sulcus

when there is a dominant left coronary artery; Fig. 3.14a). A dominant left coronary artery, however, is found in only about one-tenth of cases. When the left coronary is not dominant, the circumflex artery usually terminates by supplying descending branches to the pulmonary surface of the left ventricle. In approximately 45% of normal individuals, the circumflex artery also gives rise to the artery that supplies the sinus node (Fig. 4.10).

Myocardial Bridging

Throughout much of their epicardial course the arteries and their accompanying veins are encased in epicardial adipose tissue. In some hearts the myocardium itself may form a 'bridge' over segments of the artery. The role of these 'bridges' (Fig. 9.33) in the development of coronary arterial disease is not clear. They certainly can be an impediment to the surgeon in his effort to isolate the artery.

Fig. 4.10 *This operative view, through a median sternotomy, shows the course of the circumflex artery to the sinus node when arising from the proximal part of the artery.*

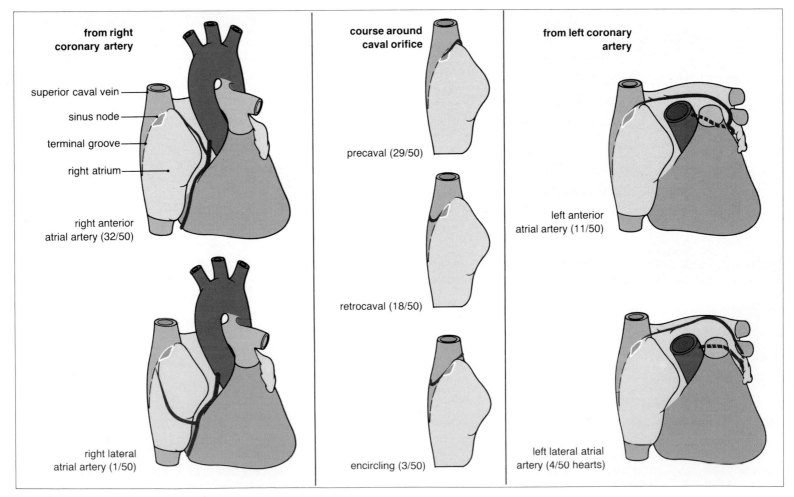

from right coronary artery

superior caval vein
sinus node
terminal groove
right atrium

right anterior atrial artery (32/50)

right lateral atrial artery (1/50)

course around caval orifice

precaval (29/50)

retrocaval (18/50)

encircling (3/50)

from left coronary artery

left anterior atrial artery (11/50)

left lateral atrial artery (4/50 hearts)

Fig. 4.11 *This diagram shows the variations in the origins of the artery to the sinus node and their incidence in a series of 50 normal hearts.*

Artery to the Sinus Node

The origin of the important sinus nodal artery has already been discussed. This, the largest of the atrial arteries, originates from the right coronary artery in 55% of individuals, and from the circumflex artery in virtually all the remainder (Fig. 4.10). There are, however, rare variants that must be recognized when present. The right lateral origin has already been discussed (Fig. 2.17). Equally rarely, the artery to the sinus node may take a lateral or terminal origin from the circumflex artery (Fig. 3.5). Although rare in normal individuals, our experience suggests that these variants are more frequent in congenitally malformed hearts[7].

It is also important to be aware of the course the artery to the sinus node takes relative to the cavoatrial junction. There are three possibilities (Fig. 4.11). Usually, the artery courses anterocavally across the crest of the appendage to reach the node (Fig. 4.10). Alternatively, it runs deep within Waterston's groove and passes retrocavally (Fig. 2.6a), being intimately related to the superior rim of the oval fossa. The third possibility is for the artery to branch and form a circle around the cavoatrial junction (Fig. 2.6b).

The Arterial Supply to the Ventricular Conduction Tissues

The arterial supply to the ventricular conduction tissues is also of surgical significance. The atrioventricular nodal artery arises from the dominant coronary artery at the crux, usually from a U-turn of this artery beneath the floor of the coronary sinus. Then, the nodal artery passes towards the central fibrous body, running into the fibrofatty plane of the atrio-ventricular groove (Fig. 4.12) to enter the node. In some hearts it perforates the fibrous atrioventricular junction to supply a good part of the branching atrioventricular bundle. The septal perforating arteries from the anterior interventricular artery always supply the anterior parts of the ventricular bundle branches and, occasionally, also supply the greater part of the posterior ventricular conduction tissues[8].

The Coronary Veins

The coronary veins drain blood from the myocardium to the right atrium. The smaller veins (anterior and smallest cardiac veins) which drain directly into the atrial cavity are not of surgical significance. The

larger veins accompany the major arteries and run into the coronary sinus. The great cardiac vein runs alongside the anterior interventricular artery and becomes the

coronary sinus as it encircles the mitral orifice to enter the posterior and leftward margin of the atrioventricular groove (Fig. 4.13). The coronary sinus then runs within

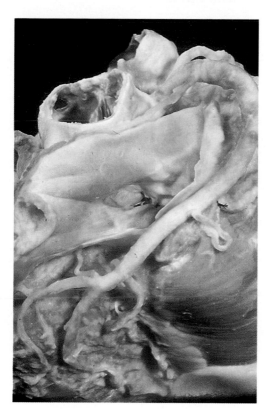

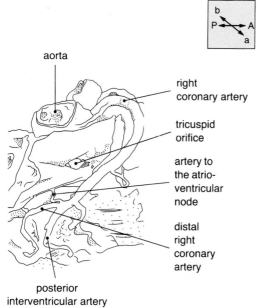

Fig. 4.12 *This dissection, in anatomical orientation, illustrates the artery to the atrioventricular node arising from the right coronary artery.*

- aorta
- right coronary artery
- tricuspid orifice
- artery to the atrio-ventricular node
- distal right coronary artery
- posterior interventricular artery

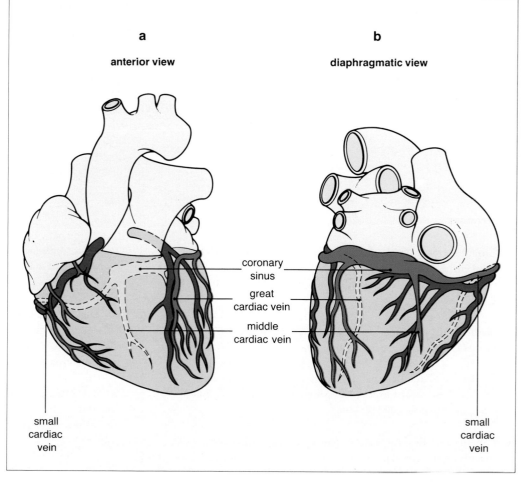

a
anterior view

b
diaphragmatic view

- coronary sinus
- great cardiac vein
- middle cardiac vein
- small cardiac vein
- small cardiac vein

Fig. 4.13 *This diagram, in anatomical orientation, shows the arrangement of the cardiac veins as seen from the (a) front and (b) back.*

the groove (Fig. 4.14), lying between the left atrial wall and the ventricular myocardium, before draining into the right atrium between the atrial septum and the post-Eustachian sinus. At the crux, the sinus receives the middle cardiac vein, which has ascended with the posterior interventricular artery, and the small cardiac vein, which has encircled the tricuspid orifice in company with the right coronary artery. Occasionally, these latter two veins drain directly to the right atrium.

Venous Valves

As with veins elsewhere in the body, the cardiac veins contain valves within their lumens. The orifice of the coronary sinus is guarded by the Thebesian valve (Fig. 4.15), which, on very rare occasions, may be imperforate. A prominent valve is also found in the great cardiac vein where it turns round the obtuse margin to become the coronary sinus. This is called the valve of Vieussens.

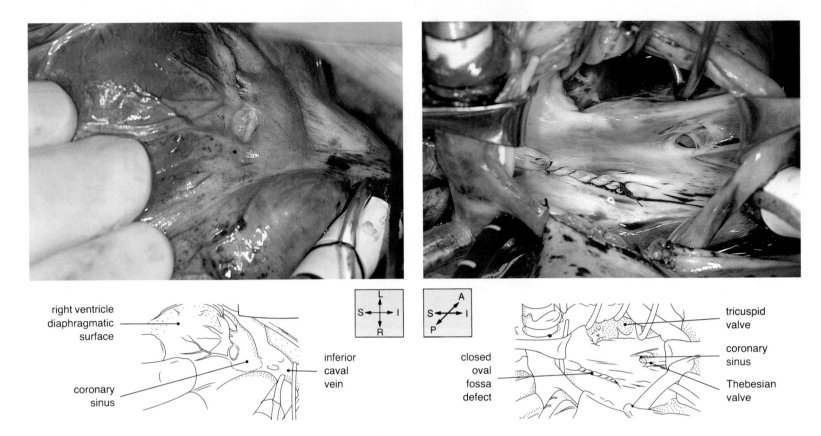

Fig. 4.14 *This operative view through a median sternotomy (with the apex of the heart lifted), shows the coronary sinus running through the left atrioventricular groove.*

Fig. 4.15 *This operative view, through a right atriotomy, shows the Thebesian valve guarding the orifice of the coronary sinus.*

References

1. Gittenberger-de Groot, A.C., Sauer, U., Oppenheim-Dekker, A. & Quaegebeur, J. (1983) Coronary arterial anatomy in transposition of the great arteries: a morphologic study. *Pediatric Cardiology*, Suppl.I, **4**, 15–24.

2. Neufeld, H.N. & Schneeweiss, A. (1983) *Coronary Artery Disease in Infants and Children*. Philadelphia: Lea & Febiger, pp.73–75.

3. Barder, G. (1963) Beitrag zur Systematic und Haufigkeit der Anomalien der Coronararterien des Menschen. *Virchow Archives of Pathology and Anatomy*, **337**, 88–96.

4. Gittenberger-de Groot, A.C., Sauer, U. & Quaegebeur, J. (1986) Aortic intramural coronary artery in three hearts with transposition of the great arteries. *Journal of Thoracic and Cardiovascular Surgery*, **91**, 566–571.

5. Becker, A.E. (1981) Variations in the main coronary arteries. In *Paediatric Cardiology*, Volume 3. Edited by A.E. Becker, G. Losekoot, C. Marcelletti & R.H. Anderson. Edinburgh: Churchill Livingstone, pp.263–277.

6. Engel, H.J., Torres, C. & Page, H.I.Jr. (1975) Major variations in anatomical origin of the coronary arteries: angiographic observations in 4250 patients without associated congenital heart disease. *Catheterization and Cardiovascular Diagnosis*, **1**, 157–169.

7. Barra Rossi, M., Ho, S.Y., Anderson, R.H., Rossi Filho, R.I. & Lincoln, C. (1986) Coronary arteries in complete transposition: the significance of the sinus node artery. *Annals of Thoracic Surgery*, **42**, 573–577.

8. Anderson, R.H. & Becker, A.E. (1980) *Cardiac Anatomy. An Integrated Text and Colour Atlas*. London and Edinburgh: Gower Medical Publishing – Churchill Livingstone, pp.6.28–6.29.

SURGICAL ANATOMY OF THE CONDUCTION SYSTEM

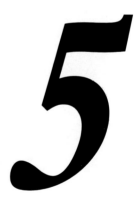

Introduction

The disposition of the conduction system in the normal heart has already been discussed (see Chapter 2). Additionally, the importance of avoiding the cardiac nodes and ventricular bundle branches as well as scrupulously protecting the blood supply to these structures has been described. In this chapter, the anatomy of these tissues relative to the surgical treatment of intractable rhythm problems will be considered. Abnormal dispositions of conduction tissue which are secondary to congenital cardiac lesions will be discussed in the appropriate sections devoted to those lesions.

Intractable Tachycardia

It may be necessary, in patients with intractable tachycardia, to ablate the atrioventricular bundle. Although this sometimes occurs inadvertently, it can be surprisingly difficult to divide the bundle intentionally. The landmark for this structure is the apex of the triangle of Koch (Fig. 5.1), that is, the point at which the tendon of Todaro inserts into the central fibrous body (Fig. 2.20b). At the apex of this triangle, the axis of atrioventricular conduction tissue gathers itself together and enters the fibrous body. It then penetrates to the left through the fibrous body.

As the axis passes through the fibrous tissue and divides into branches, it is crossed by the septal leaflet of the tricuspid valve which divides the membranous septum into atrioventricular and interventricular components. Often the interventricular component is occupied by the conduction tissue axis (Fig. 5.2). The axis may be found on the crest of the muscular septum immediately beneath the fibrous membranous septum. When viewed from the left ventricle, the bundle is intimately related to the subaortic outflow tract. It is the fibrous triangle separating the non-coronary and right coronary leaflets of the aortic valve that marks its location (Fig. 5.3).

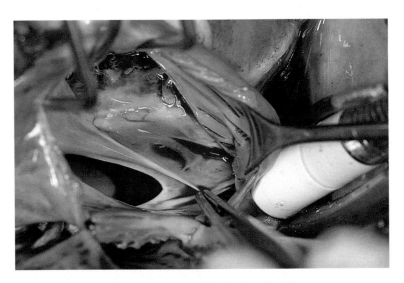

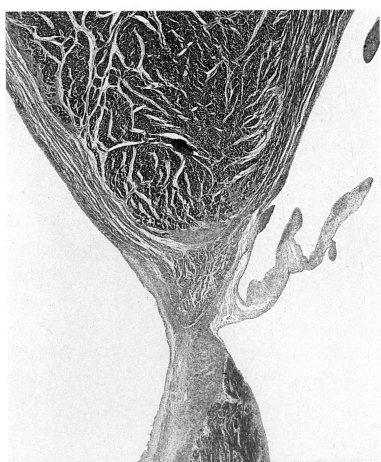

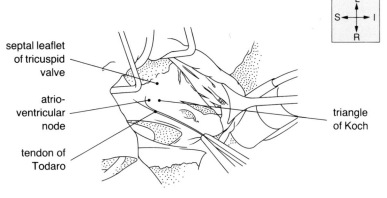

Fig. 5.1 *This operative view, through a right atriotomy, in a patient with an atrial septal defect in the oval fossa, demonstrates the land-marks of the triangle of Koch. Tension has been placed on the Eustachian valve to bring the tendon of Todaro into prominence.*

septal leaflet of tricuspid valve

atrio-ventricular node

tendon of Todaro

triangle of Koch

Fig. 5.2 *This histological section, in surgical orientation, shows the branching components of the conduction axis occupying the membranous septum immediately adjacent to the septal leaflet of the tricuspid valve. Courtesy of Prof. A.E. Becker.*

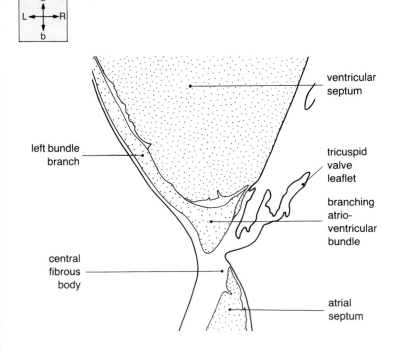

ventricular septum

left bundle branch

tricuspid valve leaflet

branching atrio-ventricular bundle

central fibrous body

atrial septum

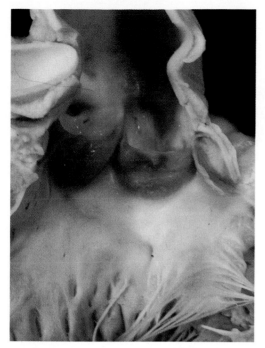

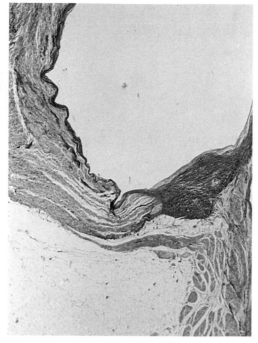

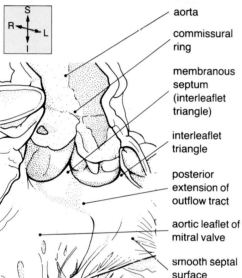

aorta

commissural ring

membranous septum (interleaflet triangle)

interleaflet triangle

posterior extension of outflow tract

aortic leaflet of mitral valve

smooth septal surface

Fig. 5.3 *This dissection of the left ventricular outflow tract, in anatomical orientation, shows the triangle between the non-coronary and right coronary leaflet of the aortic valve that is the landmark to the point of descent of the left bundle branch.*

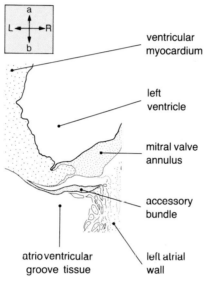

ventricular myocardium

left ventricle

mitral valve annulus

accessory bundle

atrioventricular groove tissue

left atrial wall

Fig. 5.4 *This histological section, in surgical orientation, shows the typical left-sided accessory muscular atrioventricular connexion. (Elastic stain. Courtesy of Prof. A.E. Becker.)*

Sometimes, the branching bundle lies below the septal crest, being carried on the left ventricular aspect of the septum[1]. From the left side, the right bundle branch then burrows intramyocardially to reach the right side of the septum. Taken together, these features indicate that the apex of the triangle of Koch is the most appropriate marker for locating the bundle. The node, which is within the triangle, is positioned some distance above the attachment of the septal leaflet of the tricuspid valve and its location is well anterior to the orifice of the coronary sinus.

Ventricular Preexcitation

Ventricular preexcitation is the other frequent rhythm problem that necessitates knowledge of the pertinent anatomy if optimae surgical treatment is to be achieved. Preexcitation is an abnormal cardiac rhythm where all or part of the ventricular myocardium is excited earlier than would be expected if the impulse had reached the ventricles by way of the normal atrioventricular conduction system[2]. There are various anatomical pathways, proven and hypothetical, that

could produce this phenomenon. Essentially, they are pathways that short-circuit part or all of the normal delay induced by the atrioventricular conduction tissues. Most of this delay is effected within the atrioventricular node, but an increment is also imparted as the impulse traverses the ventricular conduction branches, since these structures are insulated from the septal myocardium. Accessory pathways between the atrium and the atrioventricular bundle, and those between the conduction axis and the ventricular septum, are not yet amenable to surgical division.

Wolff–Parkinson–White Syndrome

The accessory atrioventricular pathways that produce the Wolff–Parkinson-White syndrome, probably the most common form of preexcitation, are very amenable to surgical division[3,4]. These pathways, often inappropriately called bundles of Kent[5], connect the atrial and ventricular myocardial muscle masses outside the area of the specialized conduction tissues. They can be found anywhere around the atrioventricular junction and can be categorized conveniently as left-sided, right-sided, and septal pathways. The anatomy of each group shows significant differences.

Left-sided Pathways

Left-sided pathways are found at any point around the mitral orifice, although they are exceedingly rare in the area of aortic–mitral valvar continuity. The pathways almost always run from atrial to ventricular muscle masses outside a well-formed fibrous annulus (Fig. 5.4). The atrial origin of the bundle is very close to the fibrous junction, and usually the bundle itself skirts very close to the fibrous tissue, often branching into several roots which then insert into the ventricular myocardium[6]. The bundles are rarely thicker than 1–2mm in diameter and are composed of ordinary myocardium. Frequently there may be more than one bundle in the same patient. The surgical significance of this anatomy is that, if approached from within the atrium[7], incisions that divide the atrial myocardium above the origin of the leaflets of the mitral valve are unlikely to divide the accessory muscle bundle itself. In order to ablate the accessory connexion, it is usually necessary to dissect within the fat pad on the epicardial aspect of the annulus (Fig. 5.5). Alternatively, the pathway can be approached from the epicardium. It is then necessary to reflect the coronary vessels to expose the accessory muscle bundles.

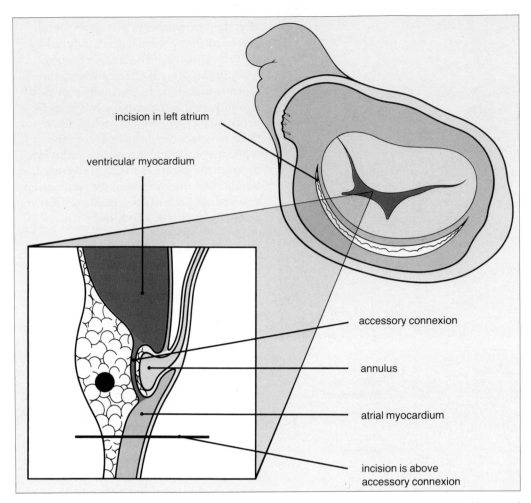

incision in left atrium

ventricular myocardium

accessory connexion

annulus

atrial myocardium

incision is above
accessory connexion

Fig. 5.5 *This surgically orientated diagram shows the endocardial incision advocated for ablation of muscular atrioventricular connexions. The incision itself does not divide the connexion (inset). Compare with Fig. 5.4.*

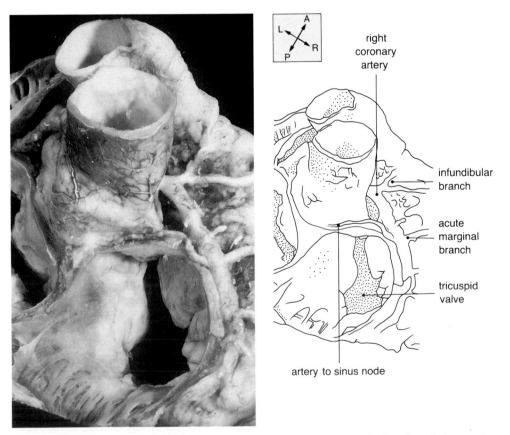

right coronary artery

infundibular branch

acute marginal branch

tricuspid valve

artery to sinus node

Fig. 5.6 *This dissection, in anatomic orientation, shows the sites at which right-sided muscular atrioventricular connexions can cross the tricuspid orifice.*

Right-sided Pathways

Right-sided accessory pathways may also pass through the fat pad to connect the atrial and ventricular myocardial masses, but these are more frequently found some distance away from the attachment of the leaflets of the tricuspid valve. This attachment is rarely to a firm and well-formed fibrous junction as is seen on the mitral side. Right-sided connexions can be multiple and coexist with left-sided pathways. They are frequently associated with Ebstein's malformation. They can be found at any point in the anterolateral aspect of the tricuspid orifice from the site of the membranous septum to the coronary sinus (Fig. 5.6). The same rules for their ablation apply as discussed for left-sided connexions.

Septal Pathways

Connexions within the atrioventricular septum constitute the greatest surgical challenge[7]. When viewed from the right atrium, they can cross from the atrial to the ventricular myocardium at any point in the septum between the coronary sinus mouth and the membranous septum. They present problems to the surgeon, firstly, because they may run deep within the septum as viewed from the right atrium, and secondly, because the atrioventricular node and bundle are also found within this area. The anatomy of the area is exposed by dissecting the coronary sinus floor. This reveals a continuation of the atrioventricular groove extending beneath the sinus to reach the central fibrous body (Fig. 5.7). The artery to the atrioventricular node courses forwards within this tissue plane (Fig. 5.8) to the node in the anterior region. Accessory connexions may cross this plane at any point from the attachment of the mitral valve to the tricuspid valvar attachment to the septum. Indeed, the only connexion that has been identified within the septum[8] was located at the insertion of the tricuspid valve (Fig. 5.9). The tissue plane can be entered via the right atrial cavity or can be reached from the epicardial aspect. Incisions within this area of the atrioventricular septum, which interrupt the muscular approaches to the atrioventricular node, have also been shown to be capable of interrupting reciprocating atrioventricular nodal tachycardias[9]. It must be remembered, however, that the triangle of Koch contains both the atrioventricular node and its nutrient artery, so that surgical incisions may produce complete atrioventricular dissociation unless performed with care.

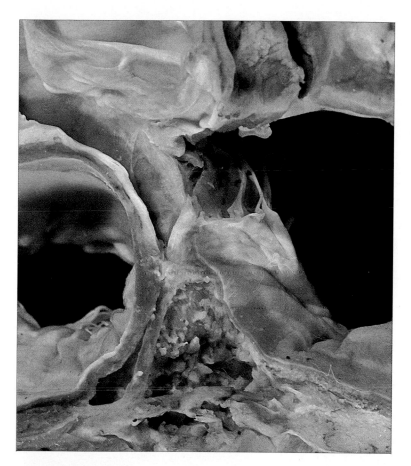

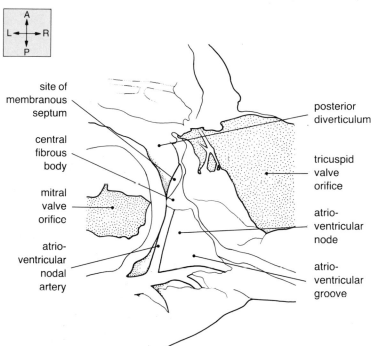

Fig. 5.7 *This dissection shows the plane occupied by adipose tissue running forward beneath the mouth of the coronary sinus. It carries the artery to the atrioventricular node, in this case from a dominant left coronary artery.*

site of membranous septum

central fibrous body

mitral valve orifice

atrio-ventricular nodal artery

posterior diverticulum

tricuspid valve orifice

atrio-ventricular node

atrio-ventricular groove

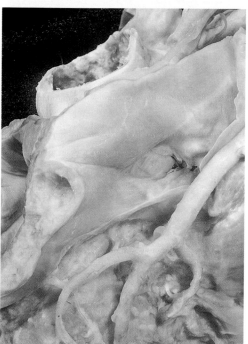

Fig. 5.8 *This dissection, in anatomical orientation, shows the plane of adipose tissue between the floor of the coronary sinus and the ventricular myocardium. In this heart it carries the artery to the atrioventricular node from a dominant right coronary artery.*

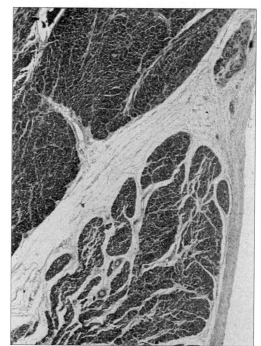

Fig. 5.9 *This histological section, in surgical orientation, shows a muscular accessory atrioventricular connexion extending from the distal insertion of the atrial myocardium into the septal leaflet of the tricuspid valve. (Trichrome stain. Courtesy of Prof. A.E. Becker.)*

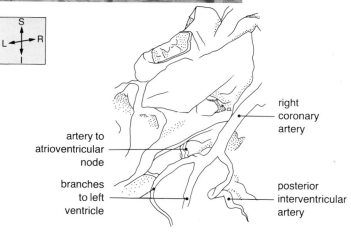

artery to atrioventricular node

branches to left ventricle

right coronary artery

posterior interventricular artery

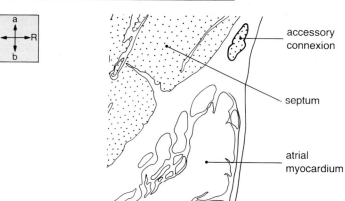

accessory connexion

septum

atrial myocardium

The So-called 'Anterior Septum'

It should also be noted in this context that surgeons operating for relief of arrhythmias have often referred to the 'anterior septum'[10,11]. By this, they mean the area of the right atrioventricular junction lying anterior to the site of the membranous component of the septum. It is a mistake to describe this part of the right junction as 'septal'. In reality, it is the medial margin of the ventriculo–infundibular fold.

Muscular connexions in this area join the atrial wall to the supraventricular crest of the right ventricle (Fig. 5.10). Recent experience has also shown that muscular connexions running to the lateral margin of the supraventricular crest can produce the electrocardiographic pattern associated with nodoventricular (or so-called, Mahaim) fibres[12]. These connexions, when removed surgically, have then been shown to resemble histologically the atrioventricular node tissues[12]. The atrial

component of these connexions is remarkably reminiscent of the illustrations provided by Kent when he argued that such tissues were the pathway for normal atrioventricular conduction. We know now that Kent was mistaken in this opinion[5], but it does seem that, under abnormal circumstances[12], his 'nodes' can indeed function as muscular accessory connexions and produce ventricular preexcitation.

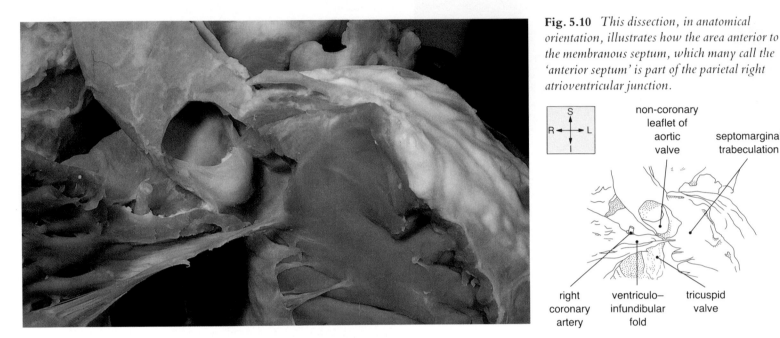

Fig. 5.10 *This dissection, in anatomical orientation, illustrates how the area anterior to the membranous septum, which many call the 'anterior septum' is part of the parietal right atrioventricular junction.*

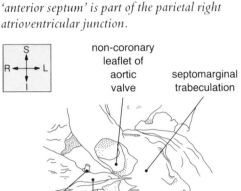

References

1. Massing, G.K. & James, T.N. (1976) Anatomical configuration of the His bundle and bundle branches in the human heart. *Circulation*, **53**, 609–621.

2. Durrer, D., Schuilenburg, R.M. & Wellens, H.J.J. (1970) Preexcitation revisited. *American Journal of Cardiology*, **25**, 690–698.

3. Sealy, W.C., Gallagher, J.J. & Pritchett, E.L.C. (1978) The surgical anatomy of Kent bundles based on electrophysiological mapping and surgical exploration. *Journal of Thoracic and Cardiovascular Surgery*, **76**, 804–815.

4. Sealy, W.C. (1983) Surgical treatment of the two types of tachycardia caused by Kent bundles with only retrograde function. *Journal of Thoracic and Cardiovascular Surgery*, **85**, 746–751.

5. Anderson, R.H. & Becker, A.E. (1981) Stanley Kent and accessory atrioventricular connexions. *Journal of Thoracic and Cardiovascular Surgery*, **81**, 649–658.

6. Becker, A.E. & Anderson, R.H. (1980) Anatomic substrates of ventricular preexcitation. In *Medical and Surgical Management of Tachyarrhythmias*. Edited by W. Bircks, E. Loogen, H.D. Schulte & L. Seipel. Berlin: Springer-Verlag, pp. 81–93.

7. Sealy, W.C. & Gallagher, J.J. (1980) The surgical approach to the septal area of the heart based on experience with 45 patients with Kent

bundles. *Journal of Thoracic and Cardiovascular Surgery*, **79**, 542–551.

8. Becker, A.E., Anderson, R.H., Durrer, D. & Wellens, H.J.J. (1978) The anatomical substrates of Wolff–Parkinson–White Syndrome: a clinico-pathologic correlation in seven patients. *Circulation*, **57**, 870–879.

9. Johnson, D.C., Ross, D.L. & Uther, J.B. (1990) The surgical cure of atrioventricular junctional reentrant tachycardia. In *Cardiac Electrophysiology from Cell to Bedside*. Edited by D.P. Zipes & J. Jalife. London: W.B. Saunders Company, pp. 921–923.

10. Guiraudon, G.M., Klein, G.J., Sharma, A.D., Yee, R., Pineda, E.A. & McLellan, D.G. (1988) Surgical approach to anterior septal accessory pathways in 20 patients with the Wolff–Parkinson–White syndrome. *European Journal of Cardio-thoracic Surgery*, **2**, 201–206.

11. Guiraudon, G.M., Klein, G.J., van Hemel, N., Guiraudon, C.M., Yee, R. & Vermeulen, F.E.E. (1990) Anatomically guided surgery to the AV node. AV nodal skeletonization: experience in 46 patients with AV nodal reentrant tachycardia. *European Journal of Cardio-thoracic Surgery*, **4**, 461–465.

12. Guiraudon, C.M., Guiraudon, G.M., & Klein, G.J. (1988) "Nodal ventricular" Mahaim pathway: histologic evidence for an accessory atrioventricular pathway with an AV node-like morphology. *Circulation*, **78**, II:40 *abstract*.

ANALYTIC DESCRIPTION OF CONGENITALLY MALFORMED HEARTS

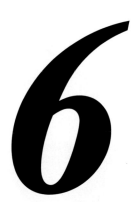

Introduction

Previous systems for describing congenital cardiac malformations have frequently been based upon embryological concepts and theories. As useful as these systems have been, often they have confused the clinician rather than clarifying the basic anatomy of a given lesion. An effective system for describing this anatomy must be based upon the observed morphology. At the same time, it must be capable of accounting for all known congenital cardiac conditions, even those that, as yet, have not been encountered. To be clinically useful, the system must be broad and accurate as well as clear and consistent. The terminology used should be unambiguous and as simple as possible. The sequential segmental approach[1] is such a system which is more useful because it emphasizes surgical applications.

The basic philosophy of the system is to describe separately the architectural make-up of the atrial mass, the ventricular mass, and the arterial segment, along with the nature of the junctional arrangement and the interrelationships of cardiac structures (Fig. 6.1). This provides the basic framework within which all other associated malformations can then be catalogued. As indicated, such an approach is particularly useful to the surgeon, for it focuses on demonstrable anatomical derangements rather than diverting one's attention to speculative embryological theory.

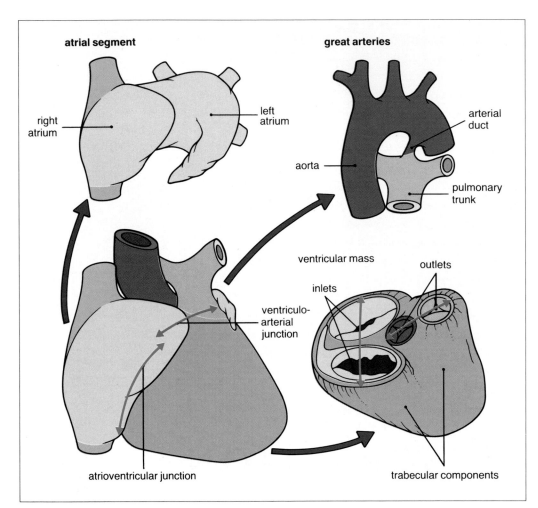

Fig. 6.1 *This diagram shows the component parts of the heart and their junctions.*

The Sequential Segmental Approach

Atrial Arrangement

The first step in analyzing any malformed heart is to determine the arrangement of the chambers within the atrial mass. Such analysis is based on the anatomy of their appendages, which are their most constant components. The atrial chambers can then be classified as morphologically right or left in type. As described in Chapter 2, the morphologically right appendage has a broad triangular shape, whereas the morphologically left appendage is finger-like and much narrower (Fig. 6.2) with several constrictions along its length.

The appendages can be arranged in only four topological ways within the atrial mass (Fig. 6.3). Almost always, the atrium possessing the morphologically right appendage is right-sided and the one with the morphologically left appendage is left-sided. This usual arrangement is also called *situs solitus*. Rarely, the appendages can be disposed in a mirror-image fashion, that is the so-called *situs inversus* arrangement. More common than the mirror-image variant, but still infrequent, is where the appendages of both chambers in the atrial mass have the same morphology. This can

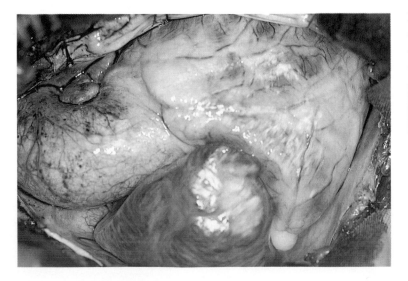

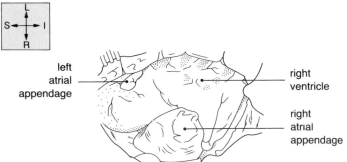

Fig. 6.2 *This operative view through a median sternotomy shows the differences between the broad triangular morphologically right atrial appendage and the narrow finger-like morphologically left atrial appendage.*

occur in two forms, with morphologically right (Fig. 6.4) or morphologically left (Fig. 6.5) appendages on both sides.

Traditionally, these bilaterally symmetrical topologic arrangements (or isomeric types) have been named according to the arrangement of the abdominal organs, particularly the spleen, since they usually exist with a jumbled up arrangement of the abdominal organs ('visceral heterotaxy')[2,3]. It is far more convenient to designate them in terms of their own intrinsic morphology[4,5], particularly since this can readily be determined by the surgeon in the operating room. It is useful to know that isomerism of the right appendages is almost always found with absence of the spleen (asplenia) and right bronchial isomerism, while isomerism of the left appendages is found with multiple spleens (polysplenia) and left bronchial isomerism.

The topologic arrangement of the atrial appendages can be predicted with a high degree of accuracy by studying the relationships of the abdominal great vessels with cross-sectional ultrasonography[6]. Identification of isomerism of the atrial appendages is of value in two additional ways. First, it gives an indication of unusual dispositions of the sinus node. In right isomerism, for example, the sinus node is duplicated as it is a morphologically right atrial structure. Consequently, a node is found laterally in each of the terminal grooves[7]. In left isomerism, in contrast, there are no terminal grooves (Fig. 6.5) and the sinus node is a poorly formed structure without a constant site. Usually it is found in the anterior inter-atrial groove close to the atrioventricular junction[8].

The second advantage of recognizing isomeric appendages is that they are known to be harbingers of complex intra-cardiac lesions. Hearts with isomerism of either type tend to have bilateral superior caval veins, common atrial chambers, and common atrioventricular valves. Right isomerism is almost invariably associated with a totally anomalous pulmonary venous connexion. Frequently, it is also seen with pulmonary stenosis or atresia and in association with a univentricular atrioventricular connexion. In a majority of cases, left isomerism is associated with the interruption of the inferior caval vein with continuation through the azygos system of veins.

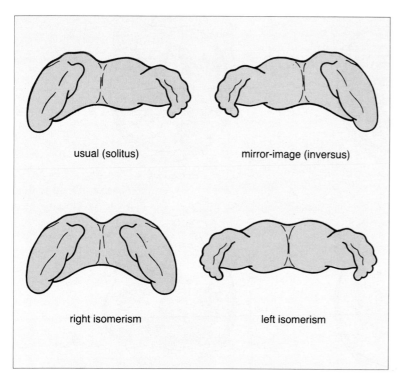

usual (solitus) mirror-image (inversus)

right isomerism left isomerism

Fig. 6.3 *This diagram shows the four possible topological arrangements of the morphologically right and left atrial appendages. Note that the veno-atrial connections are variable.*

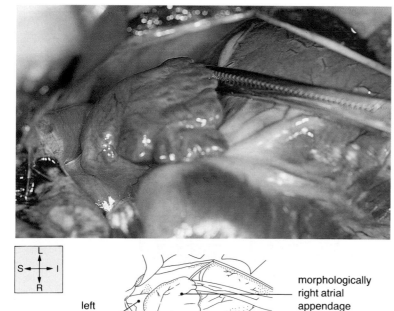

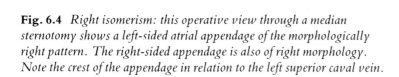

left superior caval vein

morphologically right atrial appendage

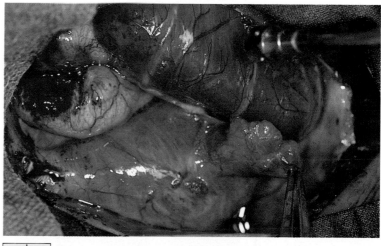

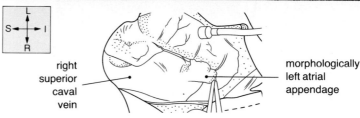

right superior caval vein

morphologically left atrial appendage

Fig. 6.4 *Right isomerism: this operative view through a median sternotomy shows a left-sided atrial appendage of the morphologically right pattern. The right-sided appendage is also of right morphology. Note the crest of the appendage in relation to the left superior caval vein.*

Fig. 6.5 *Left isomerism: this operative view through a median sternotomy in a patient with a left-sided morphologically left atrial appendage shows that the right-sided appendage is also of left morphology. Note the absence of any terminal groove.*

The Atrioventricular Junction

Once the arrangement of the atrial appendages has been established, it is then necessary to analyze the atrioventricular junction. For this, one needs to know how the atrial chambers are (or are not) connected to the ventricular mass, and the morphology of the valves that guard the atrioventricular junction.

Morphology of the Connexion

There are five distinct and discrete ways in which the atrial chambers may be connected to the ventricular mass, the final one having two subtypes (Fig. 6.6). Most often, the chambers are connected to the morphologically appropriate ventricles. This pattern is called concordant connexions. When each atrium is connected

in this way, there is rarely any difficulty in distinguishing the morphology of the ventricles, even when the ventricles themselves are unusually related (see below). In the second arrangement, which is called discordant connexions, each atrium is connected with a morphologically inappropriate ventricle.

Concordant and discordant connexions can exist with either the usual or mirror-

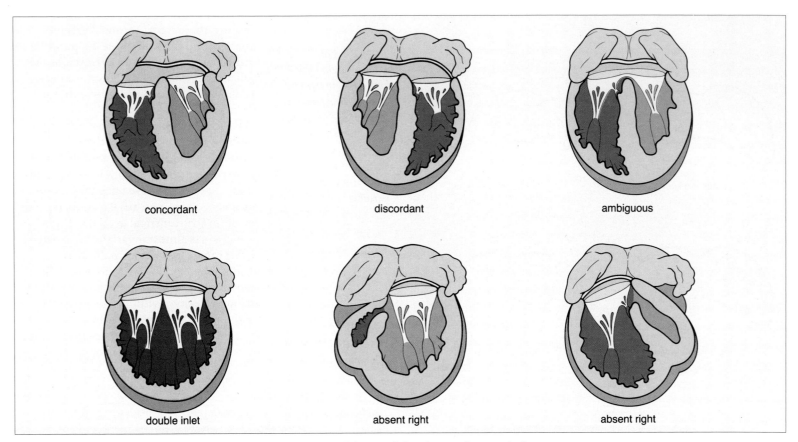

Fig. 6.6 *This diagram shows the possible anatomic connexions of the atrial chambers to the ventricular mass.*

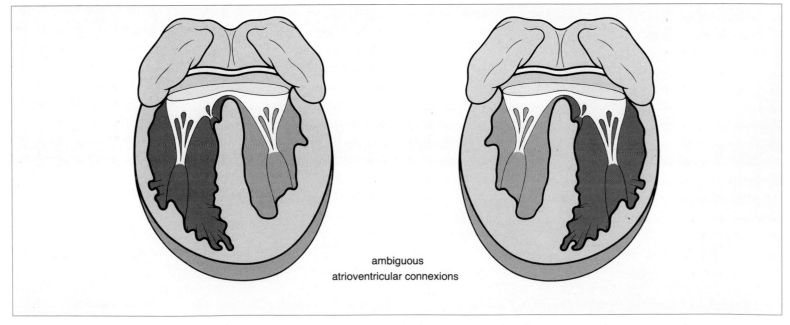

Fig. 6.7 *This diagram shows that, when the atrial appendages are isomeric (in this example with right isomerism), the atrioventricular connexion when each atrium is connected to a separate ventricle, must be ambiguous irrespective of the ventricular topology.*

image arrangement of atrial appendages, but not with isomeric appendages. This is because, when the appendages are isomeric and each atrium is connected to its own ventricle, it is inevitable that half the junction will be concordantly connected while the other half will be discordantly connected (Fig. 6.7). This will occur irrespective of the topologic pattern of the ventricular mass (see below). This is a third type of connexion, therefore, and is called a biventricular and ambiguous atrioventricular connexion.

In the three connexions described so far, each atrium is connected to its own ventricle. The essential feature in the remaining two types of atrioventricular connexion is that the atrial chambers connect to only one ventricle. In one of these patterns, both atrial chambers connect to the same ventricle, making a double inlet atrioventricular connexion. In the other, one of the atrial chambers is connected to a ventricle but the other has no connexion with the ventricular mass at all. This arrangement can be divided into two subtypes, as the lack of connexion can be found in either the right-sided (Fig. 6.8) or the left-sided (Fig. 6.9) atrioventricular junction.

Considerable controversy has been associated with hearts where the atrial chambers connect to only one ventricle, whether it be due to a double inlet or to absence of one connexion. Previously, such hearts have been classified as single ventricle or common ventricle, but more recently they have been categorized as univentricular hearts. This is despite the fact that, usually, the ventricular mass contains more than one chamber. By focusing on the fact that the atrioventricular connexion is to one ventricle only, a satisfactory solution is achieved for this dilemma in nomenclature. These hearts are best described, therefore, in terms of whether there is a univentricular or a biventricular atrioventricular connexion.

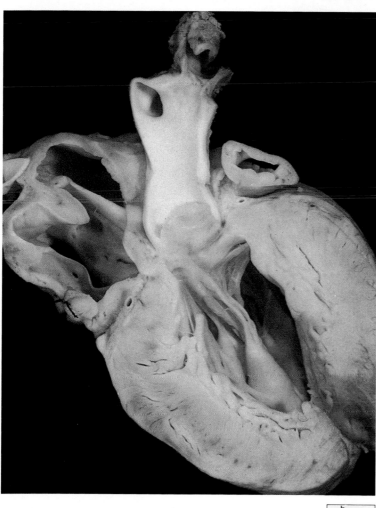

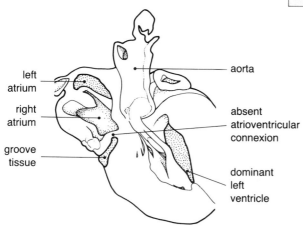

Fig. 6.8 *This section through a specimen in 'four-chamber' orientation shows an absence of the right atrioventricular connexion (tricuspid atresia). Note that the left atrium is connected to a dominant right ventricle.*

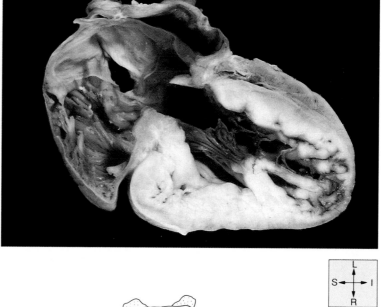

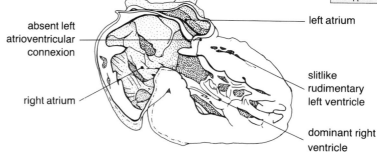

Fig. 6.9 *This section through a specimen in 'four-chamber' orientation shows an absence of the left atrioventricular connexion (mitral atresia). Note that the right atrium is connected to a dominant right ventricle.*

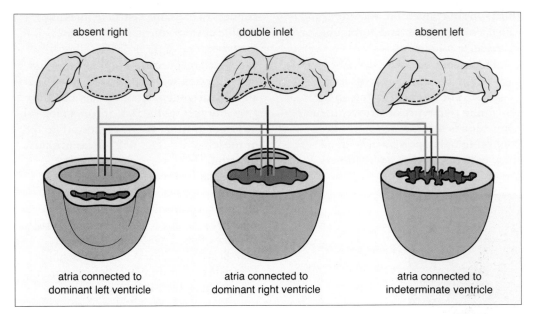

Fig. 6.10 *This diagram shows how hearts with a univentricular atrioventricular connexion (double inlet or absent right-sided or left-sided atrioventricular connexion) can be found when the atrial chambers are connected to a dominant left, a dominant right, or a solitary and indeterminate ventricle.*

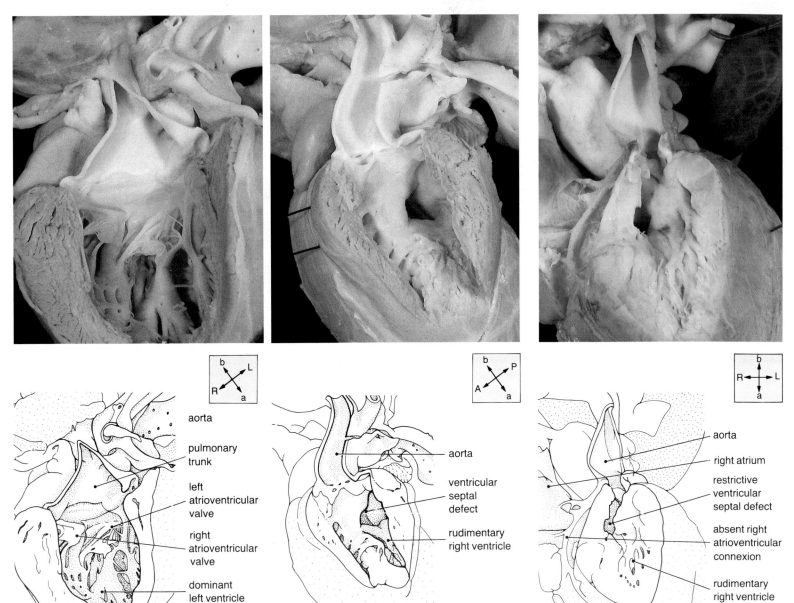

Fig. 6.11 *This rudimentary and incomplete morphologically right ventricle, possessing only apical trabecular and outlet components, exists in a heart with a double inlet to a dominant left ventricle.*

Fig. 6.12 *This rudimentary and incomplete morphologically right ventricle with only apical trabecular and outlet components is from a heart with an absent right atrioventricular connexion, with the left atrium connected to a dominant left ventricle (tricuspid atresia).*

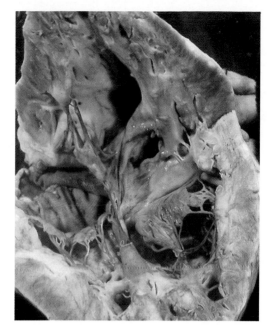

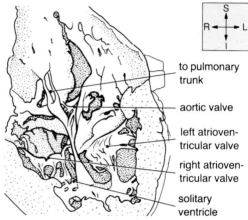

to pulmonary trunk

aortic valve

left atrioventricular valve

right atrioventricular valve

solitary ventricle

Fig. 6.13 *This heart has double inlet to, and double outlet from, a solitary and indeterminate ventricle.*

Ventricular Morphology in Hearts with Univentricular Connexion

The ventricle(s) to which the atrial chamber(s) is (are) connected may have one of three morphologies: right, left, or indeterminate (Fig. 6.10). Most frequently, the atrial chambers are connected to a morphologically left ventricle, as determined from the pattern of its apical trabecular component. Almost always, there will then be a complementary right ventricle, but without an atrioventricular connexion (or in other words, without an inlet portion). Such incomplete right ventricles are always found antero-superiorly relative to the dominant left ventricle, irrespective of whether there is double inlet (Fig. 6.11), absent right (Fig. 6.12), or absent left atrioventricular connexion.

More rarely, the atrial chambers may be connected to a dominant right ventricle. This happens most frequently in the absence of the left atrioventricular connexion (Fig. 6.9), but can be found with double inlet or, rarely, with absent right atrioventricular connexion. When only the right ventricle is connected to the atrial chambers, it is the left ventricle that exists in an incomplete and rudimentary form, lacking an atrioventricular connexion

and, hence, an inlet portion. Invariably it will be found in a posteroinferior position, though it may be left-sided (usual) or right-sided (rare).

The third morphological configuration found with double inlet or, rarely, with absence of either atrioventricular connexion, is where the atrial chambers connect to a solitary ventricle that has indeterminate apical trabecular morphology (Fig. 6.13). Incomplete and rudimentary second ventricles are never found in this variant of univentricular atrioventricular connexion.

Valvar Morphology

Atrioventricular valvar morphology is largely independent of the way in which the atrial chambers connect with the ventricles and, so, is a separate feature of the atrioventricular junction (Fig. 6.14). With concordant, discordant, ambiguous, or double inlet connexions, both atrial chambers are connected to the ventricular mass. These two atrioventricular junctions can be guarded by two separate atrioventricular valves or by a common valve. When there are two valves, either can be imperforate. An imperforate valve must be distinguished from absence of an atrioventricular connexion, since either can

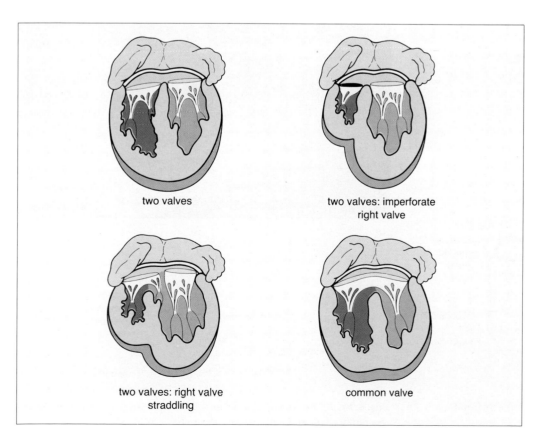

two valves

two valves: imperforate right valve

two valves: right valve straddling

common valve

Fig. 6.14 *This diagram shows the variations in atrioventricular valvar morphology, that can be found when both atrial chambers are connected to the ventricular mass.*

produce atrioventricular valvar 'atresia'. With an imperforate valve, the connexion has formed but is blocked by a valvar membrane (Fig. 6.15). When the connexion is absent, the floor of the atrium involved is completely separated from the ventricular mass by the fibrofatty tissue of the atrioventricular groove (see Fig. 6.9).

Either one of the two atrioventricular valves, or a common valve, can straddle a septum within the ventricular mass. In this respect, straddling of the valvar tension apparatus is distinguished from overriding of its annulus. Straddling is considered to be present when the tension apparatus is attached to each side of a septum (Fig. 6.16). Overriding is present when the junction is connected to both ventricles. The degree of override, which usually coexists with straddling, determines the precise nature of the atrioventricular connexion. So as to adjudicate the connexion in the presence of overriding, the overriding junction is assigned to the ventricle connected to its greater part (the '50% law'; Fig. 6.17). The possible arrangements are much more limited when one atrioventricular connexion is absent. In this case, the solitary valve present can either be committed in its entirety to one ventricle, or else it can straddle and override.

Ventricular Morphology and Topology

From the discussion above, it will be appreciated that the nature of an atrioventricular connexion is inextricably linked with the architectural arrangement of the ventricular mass. Concordant or discordant atrioventricular connexions cannot be defined until the morphology of the ventricles is known. Although ambiguous, double inlet, and absent connexions can all be identified without mention of ventricular morphology, it is always necessary to give more information concerning the arrangement of the ventricular mass. For instance, in the case of an ambiguous connexion, it is important to specify the pattern (topology) in which the morphologically right ventricle is structured relative to the morphologically left ventricle. This is because there is an ambiguous connexion when the right-sided atrium (with either a right or left appendage) is connected to either a morphologically right or a morphologically left ventricle (see Fig. 6.7).

When there is right atrial isomerism, and the right-sided atrium is connected to a morphologically right ventricle, the ventricular mass is almost invariably as in hearts with concordant atrioventricular connexions and usual atrial arrangement. In contrast, when there is right atrial isomerism and the right-sided atrium is connected to a morphologically left ventricle, the ventricular mass is as usually found in the presence of discordant atrioventricular connexions and usual atrial arrangement.

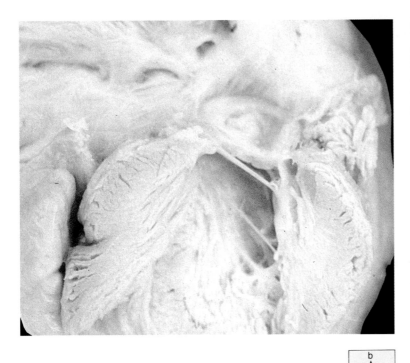

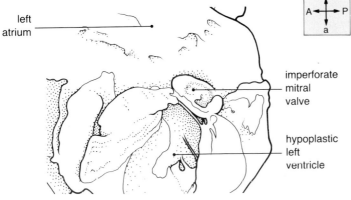

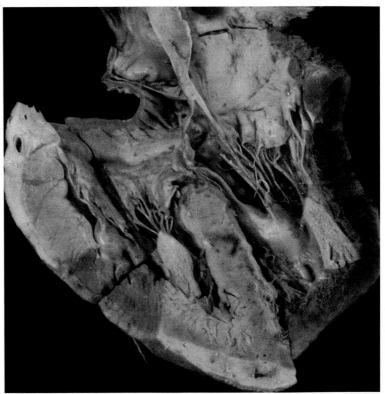

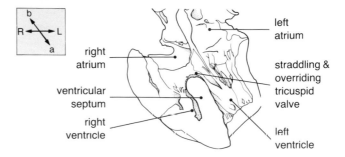

Fig. 6.15 *In this heart, the left side of concordant atrioventricular connexions is blocked by an imperforate mitral valve.*

Fig. 6.16 *In this heart sectioned in its 'four-chamber' orientation, there is straddling of the right atrioventricular valve.*

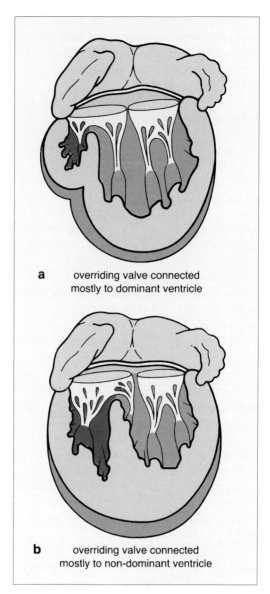

a overriding valve connected mostly to dominant ventricle

b overriding valve connected mostly to non-dominant ventricle

These two basic patterns of topology can be described figuratively in terms of the way in which a hand can be placed palm downwards upon the septal surface of the morphologically right ventricle. The other hand will then fit in the morphologically left ventricle in similar fashion, but it is the arrangement of the right ventricle that is chosen for descriptive purposes. When the ventricles are found with the usual atrial arrangement and concordant atrioventricular connexions, only the right hand can be placed so that the thumb is in the ventricular inlet and the fingers are in the outlet. When the usual atrial arrangement exists with discordant atrioventricular connexions, only the left hand can be placed in this manner. These two patterns[9] are respectively called 'right-hand' and 'left-hand' patterns of ventricular topology (Fig. 6.18). The significance of this feature in hearts with ambiguous connexion is that the ventricular topology determines the disposition of the atrioventricular conduction tissues[8]. This topic is discussed further in Chapter 8.

When the atrial chambers connect to only one ventricle, the morphology of that ventricle must always be described because, as already stated, the dominant ventricle may be of left ventricular, right ventricular, or solitary (indeterminate) pattern. It is also necessary to determine whether a rudimentary and incomplete ventricle is present and, if present, to describe its relationship to the dominant ventricle.

Ventricular Relationships

Generally, ventricular relationships, as opposed to ventricular topology, should be described as a separate feature of the heart. Where each atrium is connected to its own ventricle, the relationships are almost always in harmony with both the connexion and topology present. When the atrial chambers are in their usual position with concordant atrioventricular connexions, the observed relationships are usually for the morphologically right ventricle to be right-sided, anterior, and inferior to the morphologically left ventricle. In the mirror-image atrial arrangement, with concordant atrioventricular connexions, the morphologically right ventricle is almost invariably left-sided, anterior, and inferior to the morphologically left ventricle.

With the atrial chambers in their usual arrangement and discordant atrioventricular connexions, there is almost always a left-hand pattern of ventricular

Fig. 6.17 *An overriding valve is assigned to the ventricle connected to its greater part, giving a spectrum between* **(a)** *double inlet and* **(b)** *biventricular atrioventricular connexions.*

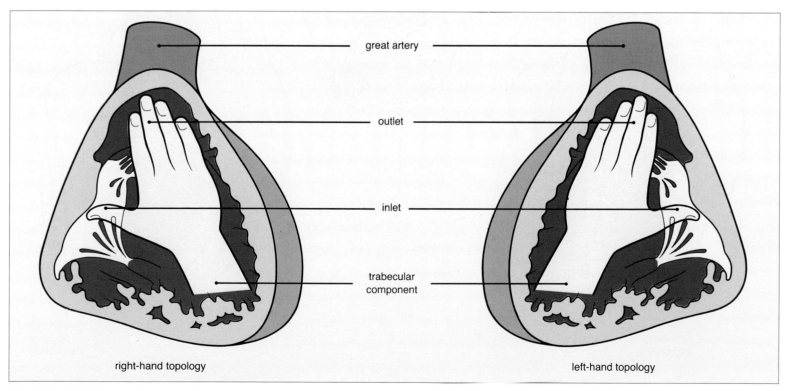

right-hand topology

left-hand topology

Fig. 6.18 *This diagram shows how the patterns of ventricular topology can be described figuratively in terms of the ways that the palmar surface of the hands can be placed upon the septal surface of the morphologically right ventricle.*

topology, and the usual relationship is for the morphologically right ventricle to be left-sided, anterior and inferior. When discordant atrioventricular connexions accompanies a mirror-image atrial arrangement, there is usually right-hand topology and the ventricular relationships are similar to those in the normal heart.

When the relationships are as anticipated, it is unnecessary to describe them. But, very occasionally, the relationships of the ventricles are not as anticipated for the connexion present. These disharmonious relationships underscore the anomaly known as the 'criss-cross heart'[9,10]. With these hearts, and also those with so-called 'superoinferior ventricles'[11], connexions and relationships must be described separately, using as much detail as necessary for unambiguous categorization. The essence of the 'criss-cross heart', therefore, is that the ventricular relationships are not as expected for the given atrioventricular connexion (Fig. 6.19). Even more rarely, the ventricular topology may be disharmonious with the atrioventricular connexions[12]. All features must then be described.

In hearts with a univentricular atrioventricular connexion, the relationship of the incomplete and rudimentary ventricle, if present, must be described. With a dominant left ventricle, the incomplete right ventricle is always anterosuperior but can be right- or left-sided. The sidedness of the ventricle does not affect the basic disposition of the atrioventricular conduction tissues in these hearts. With a dominant right ventricle, the incomplete and rudimentary left ventricle, if present, is always posteroinferior but again can be right- or left-sided. In this case, the sidedness of the rudimentary ventricle does affect the disposition of the atrioventricular conduction tissue (see below).

Thus, in summary, when considering the atrioventricular junction, there are four different features to take into account, namely the way the atrial myocardium is connected to the ventricular mass, the morphology of the atrioventricular valves guarding the junctions, the ventricular morphology and topology, and the ventricular relationships. All are of importance to the surgeon because they influence the disposition of the atrioventricular conduction axis.

Ventriculoarterial Junction

Analysis of the ventriculoarterial junction proceeds as described for the atrioventricular junction, with morphology of the connexion, the valvar morphology, and the relationships of the arterial trunks being different facets requiring separate description in mutually exclusive terms. It is also necessary to take account of infundibular morphology.

Ventriculoarterial Connexions

There are four discrete ways in which the arterial trunks can be connected to the ventricular mass, namely in concordant, discordant, double outlet, and single outlet fashion (Fig. 6.20). Concordant ventriculoarterial connexions exist when the arterial trunks are connected to morphologically appropriate ventricles. Discordant connexions account for the trunks being connected with morphologically inappropriate ventricles. A double outlet connexion exists when both great arteries are connected to the same ventricle, which may be of right, left, or indeterminate morphology. A single outlet arrangement is where only one arterial trunk is connected to the heart (Fig. 6.21). This may be a common trunk, supplying directly the systemic, pulmonary, and coronary arteries, or it may be an aortic or pulmonary trunk when the complementary arterial trunk is atretic and its connexion to a known ventricle cannot be established. Rarely, in the absence of intrapericardial

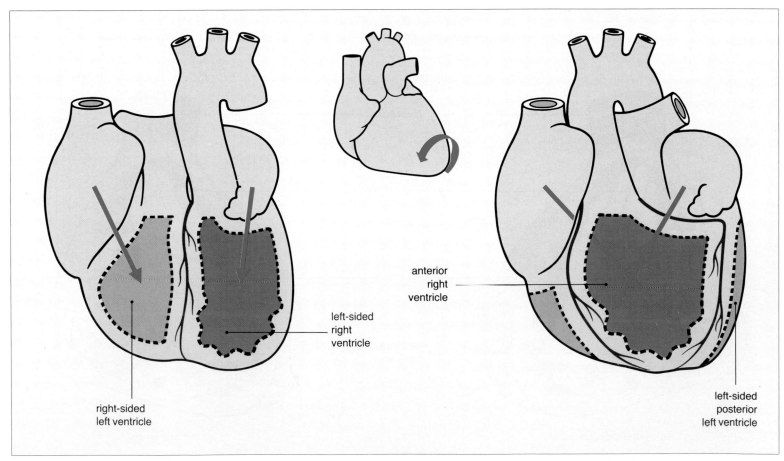

anterior right ventricle

left-sided right ventricle

right-sided left ventricle

left-sided posterior left ventricle

Fig. 6.19 *This diagram shows how a criss-cross heart is produced by rotation of the ventricular mass around its long axis. This example shows a criss-cross pattern in a heart with usually arranged atrial chambers and a discordant atrioventricular connexion.*

pulmonary arteries, it may be more accurate to describe an arterial trunk as solitary rather than common (Fig. 6.21).

Arterial Valvar Morphology

The morphological arrangement of the arterial valves is limited because they have no tension apparatus. Furthermore, a common valve can exist only with a common trunk and as an integral part of the connexion. The different patterns involve one or two arterial valves. Usually both valves are perforate, but either or both may override the ventricular septum. When a valvar orifice is overriding, the '50% law' can again be applied to assign the valve to the ventricle that is connected to its greatest part, thus avoiding the need for intermediate categories.

The other pattern of valvar morphology is when one of the arterial valves is imperforate. As in the case of the atrioventricular junction, an imperforate arterial valve must be distinguished from the absence of a ventriculoarterial connexion, since both can produce arterial valvar 'atresia'.

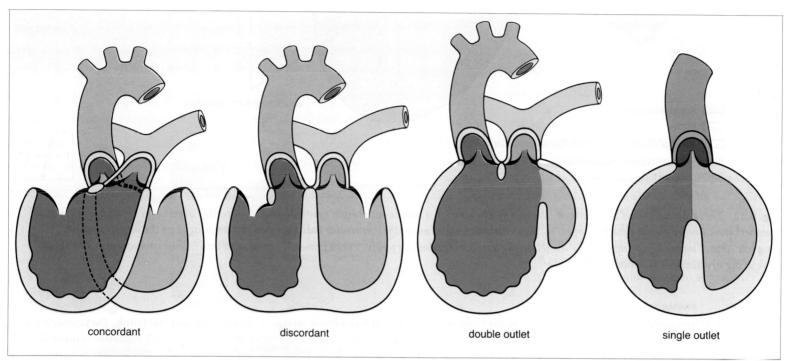

Fig. 6.20 *This diagram shows the four different types of ventriculoarterial connexion.*

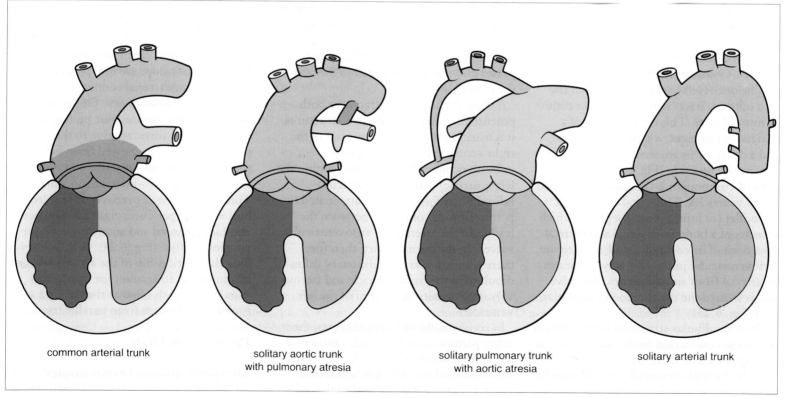

Fig. 6.21 *This diagram shows the four patterns that produce single outlet from the ventricular mass.*

4. Macartney, F.J., Zuberbuhler, J.R. & Anderson, R.H. (1980) Morphological considerations pertaining to recognition of atrial isomerism. Consequences for sequential chamber localisation. *British Heart Journal*, **44**, 657–667.

5. Sharma, S., Devine, W., Anderson, R.H. & Zuberbuhler, J.R. (1988) The determination of atrial arrangement by examination of appendage morphology in 1842 autopsied specimens. *British Heart Journal*, **60**, 227–231.

6. Huhta, J.C., Smallhorn, J.F. & Macartney, F.J. (1982) Two dimensional echocardiographic diagnosis of situs. *British Heart Journal*, **48**, 97–108.

7. Van Mierop, L.H.S. & Wigglesworth, F.W. (1962) Isomerism of the cardiac atria in the asplenia syndrome. *Laboratory Investigations*, **11**, 1303–1315.

8. Dickinson, D.F., Wilkinson, J.L., Anderson, K.R., Smith, A., Ho, S.Y. & Anderson, R.H. (1979) The cardiac conduction system in situs ambiguus. *Circulation*, **59**, 879–885.

9. Van Praagh, S., LaCorte, M., Fellows, K.E., Bossina, K., Busch, H.J., Keck, E.W., Weinberg, P.M. & Van Praagh, R. (1980) Superioinferior ventricles: anatomic and angiographic findings in ten postmortem cases. In *Etiology and Morphogenesis of Congenital Heart Disease*. Edited by R. Van Praagh & A. Takao. New York: Futura Publishing Company, pp. 317–378.

10. Anderson, R.H., Shinebourne, E.A. & Gerlis, I.M. (1974) Criss-cross atrioventricular relationships producing paradoxical atrioventricular concordance or discordance. Their significance to nomenclature of congenital heart disease. *Circulation*, **50**, 176–180.

11. Anderson, R.H. (1982) Criss-cross hearts revisited. *Pediatric Cardiology*, **3**, 305–313.

12. Anderson, R.H., Smith, A. & Wilkinson, J.L. (1987) Disharmony between atrioventricular connexions and segmental combinations – unusual variants of 'criss-cross' hearts. *Journal of the American College of Cardiology*, **10**, 1274–1277.

LESIONS IN NORMALLY CONNECTED HEARTS

7

Septal Defects

Introduction

Understanding the anatomy of septal defects is greatly facilitated if the heart is thought of as having three distinct septal structures: the atrial septum, the atrioventricular septum and the ventricular septum (Fig. 7.1).

Atrial Septum

The atrial septum is a relatively small structure comprising, for the most part, the floor of the oval fossa. It is limited superiorly, anteriorly and posteriorly by the rim of the fossa, which is formed by infolding of the adjacent right and left atrial walls (Fig. 2.17a). Inferiorly, the septum is continuous with the atrioventricular septum, the atrial component overlapping the muscular ventricular septum in this area (Fig. 3.27) (see below).

Atrioventricular Septum

The atrioventricular septum is a fibromuscular structure best viewed from the right atrium. It corresponds, roughly, to the triangle of Koch (Fig. 7.2). The medial portion of this septum is the atrial aspect of the membranous septum and the central fibrous body. The part that extends laterally and inferiorly to the mouth of the coronary sinus is muscular in nature. It is formed by the lower part of the atrial septum overlapping the upper component of the ventricular septum by virtue of the differential attachments of the leaflets of the tricuspid and mitral valves (Fig. 7.1).

Ventricular Septum

Usually the surgeon only views the ventricular septum from the right ventricular aspect. For this reason, and other reasons discussed below, ventricular septal defects are best considered in terms of right ventricular landmarks.

The ventricular septum is composed of a small fibrous element, the membranous septum, and a much larger muscular part. It is more complex geometrically than the other septal structures, which lie almost completely in a coronal plane. The muscular part of the septum can, at first sight, seem to be simply divided into inlet, apical trabecular and outlet components, each of these parts abutting on the membranous septum (Fig. 7.3). Closer inspection shows that such analysis is simplistic rather than simple. This is because, by virtue of the deeply wedged location of the sub-aortic outflow tract, much of the so-called inlet septum, delimited on the right ventricular aspect by the septal leaflet of the tricuspid valve, separates the right ventricular inlet from the left ventricular outlet (Fig. 7.4). The outlet component is much smaller than it appears because most of the subpulmonary infundibulum is a free-standing muscular sleeve (Fig. 7.5). The small outlet septal component, together with the much more

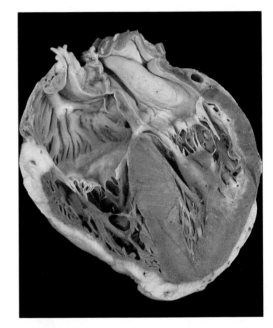

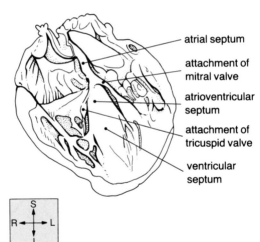

Fig. 7.1 *This 'four-chamber' cut through the heart, in anatomic orientation, shows the three distinct septal structures.*

atrial septum

attachment of mitral valve

atrioventricular septum

attachment of tricuspid valve

ventricular septum

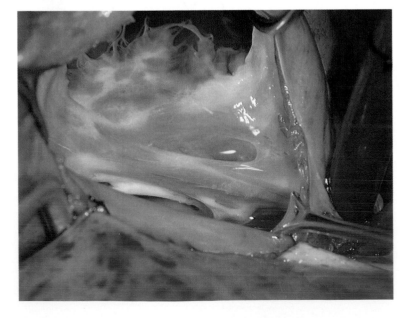

Fig. 7.2 *This surgical view through a right atriotomy shows the landmarks of the triangle of Koch that occupy the atrial aspect of the muscular atrioventricular septum.*

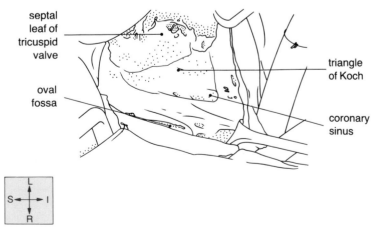

septal leaf of tricuspid valve

oval fossa

triangle of Koch

coronary sinus

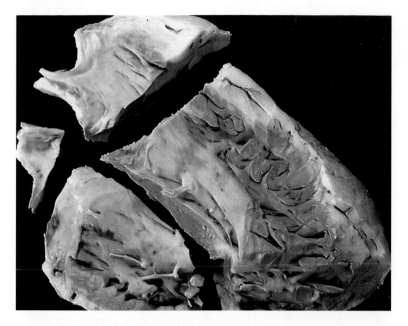

Fig. 7.3 *In this dissection, seen in anatomic orientation, the ventricular septum has been separated from the remainder of the heart and is divided into fibrous and muscular parts. The muscular part is then further divided into segments corresponding to the components of the right ventricle.*

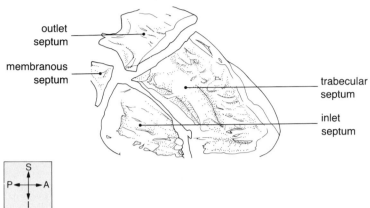

Fig. 7.4 *This section, simulating the oblique subcostal echocardiographic cut, shows how the muscular septum separates the right ventricular inlet from the left ventricular outlet.*

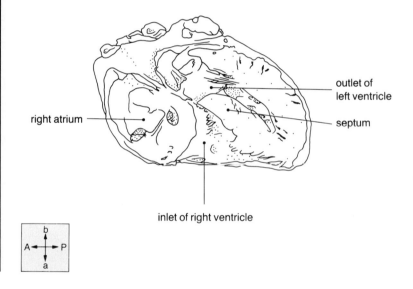

Fig. 7.5 *This dissection of the ventricular outflow tracts, in anatomic orientation, shows the free-standing sleeve of infundibulum that supports the pulmonary valvar leaflets.*

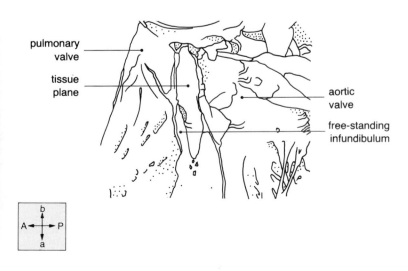

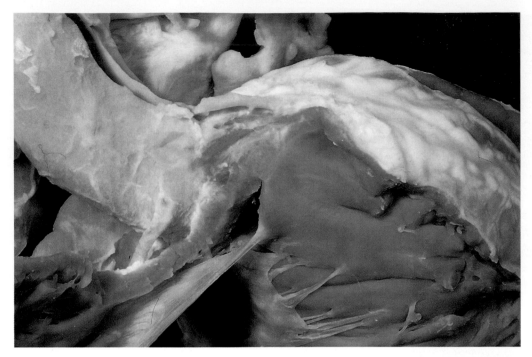

extensive ventriculo–infundibular fold, form the supraventricular crest (Fig. 7.6). The apical trabecular septum, therefore, accounts for the greater part of the muscular septum, extending in a curvilinear fashion, reflecting the fact that the right ventricle wraps itself around the conical left ventricle. An important landmark for the description of defects within the ventricular septum is the septomarginal trabeculation, the extensive muscular strap which overlies the apical trabecular septum with its limbs extending to the base of the heart.

Atrial Septal Defects

There are several lesions which permit interatrial shunting (Fig. 7.7). Although collectively termed 'atrial septal defects', they are not all within the confines of the normal atrial septum (see Fig. 2.10). The so-called secundum defect, or, as is preferred, the oval fossa defect, is a true deficiency of the atrial septum. The 'ostium primum' defect is due to a deficiency of the atrio-ventricular septum and will be considered in the next section. Sinus venosus defects, most frequently associated with partial anomalous pulmonary venous drainage, are found at the mouths of the caval veins. Finally, there is the rare defect of the orifice of the coronary sinus, occurring when the sinus itself is unroofed in the left atrium.

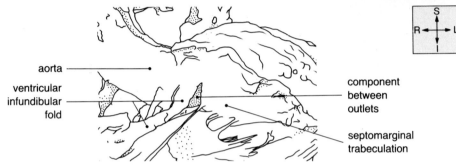

aorta
ventricular infundibular fold
component between outlets
septomarginal trabeculation

Fig. 7.6 *This dissection, seen in anatomic orientation, shows how most of the supraventricular crest is formed by the ventriculo– infundibular fold. Only a small part of the subpulmonary outlet, removed in this dissection, separates the ventricular outlets.*

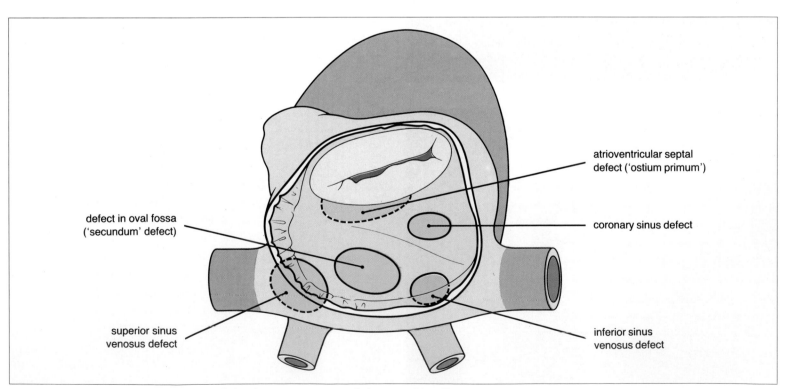

atrioventricular septal defect ('ostium primum')
coronary sinus defect
defect in oval fossa ('secundum' defect)
inferior sinus venosus defect
superior sinus venosus defect

Fig. 7.7 *This diagram shows the various holes that permit interatrial shunting. Not all are true deficiencies of the atrial septum.*

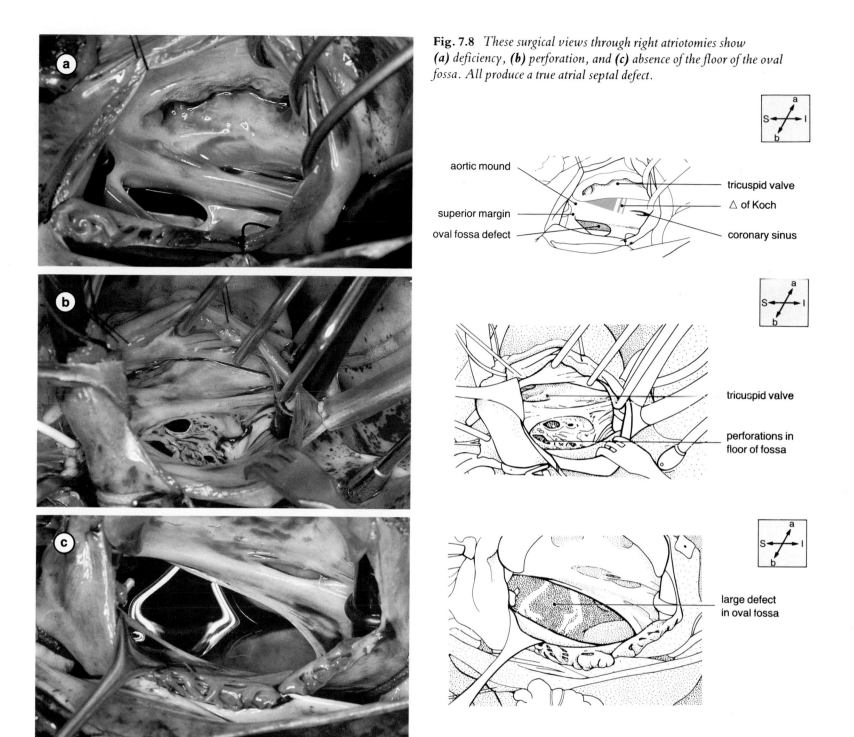

Fig. 7.8 *These surgical views through right atriotomies show* **(a)** *deficiency,* **(b)** *perforation, and* **(c)** *absence of the floor of the oval fossa. All produce a true atrial septal defect.*

aortic mound
tricuspid valve
△ of Koch
superior margin
oval fossa defect
coronary sinus

tricuspid valve
perforations in floor of fossa

large defect in oval fossa

Fig. 7.9 *This dissection shows the relationship of the artery to the sinus node to the superior rim of the oval fossa.*

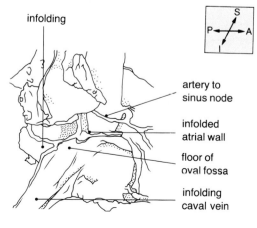

infolding
artery to sinus node
infolded atrial wall
floor of oval fossa
infolding caval vein

Oval Fossa Defects

Defects within the oval fossa, or 'secundum' defects, are by far the most common. They are due to deficiency (Fig. 7.8a), perforation (Fig. 7.8b), or absence (Fig. 7.8c) of the floor of the fossa (the flap-valve of the oval foramen). When the haemodynamics of the shunt across such a defect dictate surgical closure, the hole is unlikely to be small enough to permit direct suture. If attempted, the results may so distort atrial anatomy as to result in dehiscence. Since the edge of the fossa is almost always intact, a patch can be readily secured to its margins. It is important to note, nonetheless, that the superior margin is an infolding of the atrial wall. Consequently the potential danger (Fig. 7.9) is to the sinus nodal artery, which sometimes courses intramyocardially through this superior margin, and to the aorta, which underlies the cephalad margin (the aortic mound).

In some cases, the postero-inferior edge of the fossa is deficient, extending the defect into the mouth of the inferior caval vein (Fig. 7.10). It is possible in this circumstance to mistake a well formed Eustachian valve for the postero-inferior margin of the defect. Because a patch attached to this valve would connect the inferior caval vein to the left atrium, it is always prudent to ensure continuity of the inferior caval vein and right atrium following placement of the patch.

Sinus Venosus Defects

Sinus venosus defects are rarer than defects within the oval fossa and present greater problems in repair. The inferior defect is extremely rare. It opens into the mouth of the inferior caval vein posterior to the confines of the oval fossa, which is usually intact (Fig. 7.11). The right inferior pulmonary vein is usually in close proximity to the interatrial defect. A defect at the mouth of the superior caval vein occurs much more frequently (Fig. 7.12). It, too, is outside the confines of the oval fossa and may be intimately related to the orifice of the right superior pulmonary vein. Indeed, this vein frequently drains

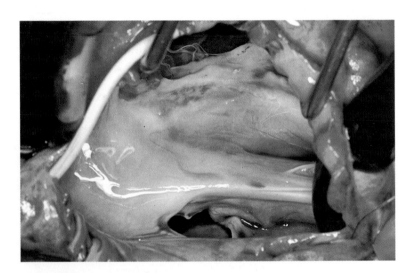

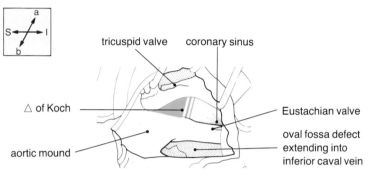

Fig. 7.10 *This surgical view through a right atriotomy shows a defect within the oval fossa extending into the mouth of the inferior caval vein.*

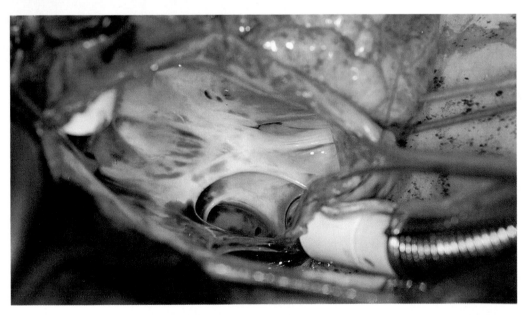

Fig. 7.11 *This surgical view through a right atriotomy shows an inferior sinus venosus defect. Note that the oval fossa is intact and the inferior edge of the atrial septum is malaligned with the inferior caval vein.*

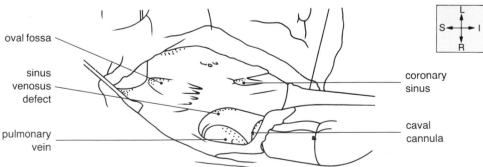

directly into the superior caval vein (Fig. 7.13) and often through more than one orifice.

The key to diagnosis of sinus venosus defects, however, is that the caval vein is connected to both atria, overriding the margin of the atrial septa[1]. The difficulty during surgical repair relates to the need to construct a repair that redirects the venous return and closes the interatrial communication without obstructing venous flow or, in the case of a superior defect, damaging the sinus node. As described in Chapter 2, the sinus node is related to the anterolateral quadrant of the cavoatrial junction and lies immediately subepicardially within the terminal groove (Fig. 2.10). The sinus node should not be at risk with a simple closure of the atrium (Fig. 7.14). The problem arises with the necessity either to suture in the area of the node when redirecting the pulmonary venous return or to enlarge the caval venous orifice. The former risk can be minimized with the judicious placement of the sutures; the latter problem is much greater. Because the artery to the sinus node may pass either in front of or behind the caval vein, the entire cavoatrial junction is a potentially dangerous area. Determining the course of the nodal artery beforehand would facilitate the design of an operation least likely to damage the node or its artery.

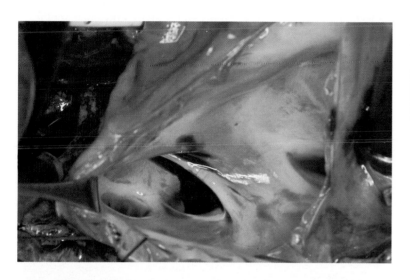

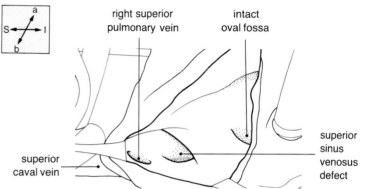

Fig. 7.12 *This surgical view through a right atriotomy shows a superior sinus venosus defect outside the confines of the oval fossa.*

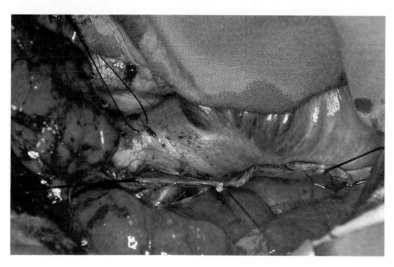

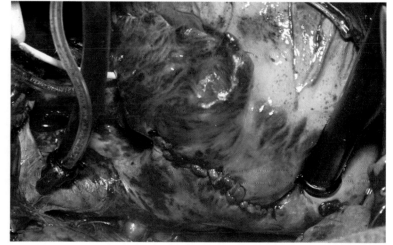

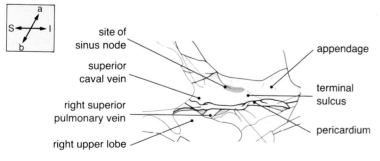

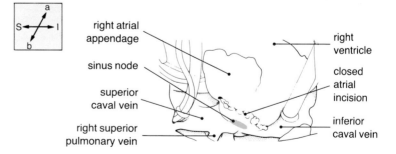

Fig. 7.13 *This surgical view, through a median sternotomy of the heart shown in Fig. 7.12, illustrates the anomalous connexion of the right superior pulmonary vein and the site of the sinus node.*

Fig. 7.14 *This view of a heart with a superior sinus venosus defect, seen through a median sternotomy, shows how the incision into the atrium to allow repair can be made without placing the sinus node, or its arterial supply, at risk.*

Unroofed Coronary Sinus

The final defect which permits interatrial shunting is part of a constellation of lesions, and is probably best termed 'unroofed coronary sinus'[2]. In this combination, a persistent left superior caval vein usually drains directly to the left atrial roof, between the appendage and the left pulmonary veins (Fig. 7.15a), and there is a large hole at the site of the coronary sinus (Fig. 7.15b). Often, there is evidence of the course the vein should have taken between the atrial roof and the left side of the coronary sinus orifice, but sometimes the hole can exist in isolation without a persistent left caval vein. Surgical treatment depends upon the presence and connexions of the left superior caval vein. If it is in free communication with the right superior caval vein, or if there is no left-sided vein, the orifice of the coronary sinus can simply be closed and the vein, if present, ligated. If the left-sided channel has no anastomoses with the right side, it may be better to construct a channel in the posterior wall of the left atrium that connects the mouth of the left-sided vein with the interatrial communication at the orifice of the coronary sinus.

Atrioventricular Septal Defects

Introduction

'Atrioventricular septal defects' is the most accurate collective term for the anomalies variously described as 'endocardial cushion defects', 'atrioventricular canal defects', and 'persistent atrioventricular canal'[3]. This is because, in anatomic terms, the malformations are primarily due to the absence of the usual atrioventricular septal structures.

As noted above, the normal heart contains both a membranous septum (Fig. 7.16a) and a muscular septum separating the cavity of the right atrium from the left ventricle (Fig. 7.16b). The latter exists because the attachment of the tricuspid valvar leaflet to the septum is further towards the apex than is the septal attachment of the mitral valvar leaflets. A defect at the site of these structures (Fig. 7.17) is the essence of the atrioventricular septal defect, irrespective of the arrangement of the leaflets of the valve or valves guarding the atrioventricular junction[3,4].

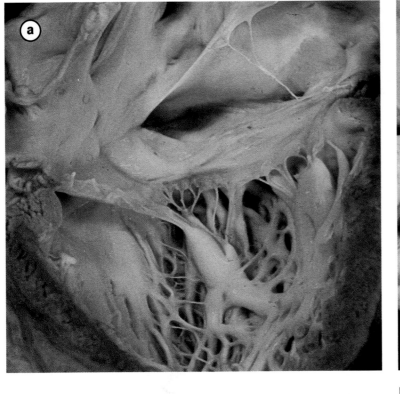

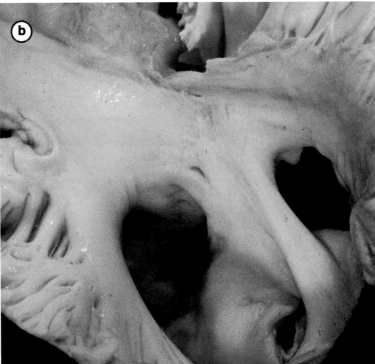

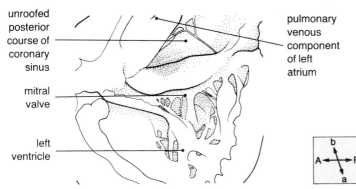

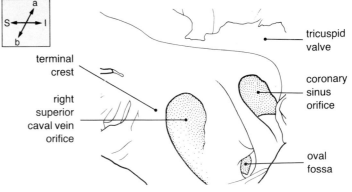

Fig. 7.15 **(a)** *This anatomic orientation of the left atrium shows the unroofed course of a persistent left superior caval vein along the posterior wall of the left atrium, where filigreed remnants show the initial wall that separated the sinus from the left atrium.*

(b) *This surgical orientation shows the enlarged mouth of the sinus opening to the right atrium and functioning as an interatrial communication outside the confines of the septum.*

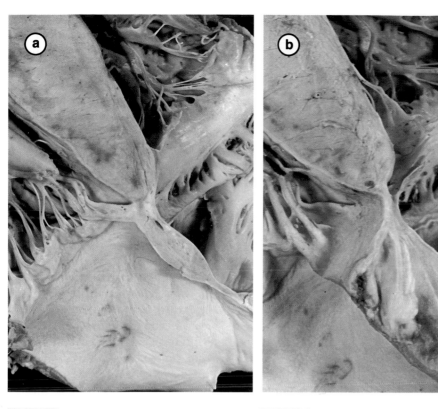

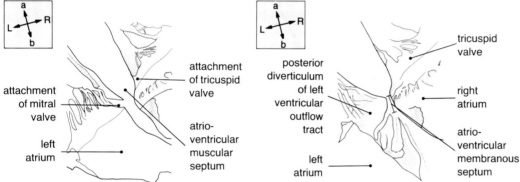

Fig. 7.16 *These 'four-chamber' sections, orientated in surgical fashion, show (a) the membranous septum crossed on the right side by the tricuspid valvar leaflet, which divides it into atrioventricular and interventricular components, and (b) the off-setting of the attachments of the mitral and tricuspid valvar leaflets which produce the normal muscular atrioventricular septum.*

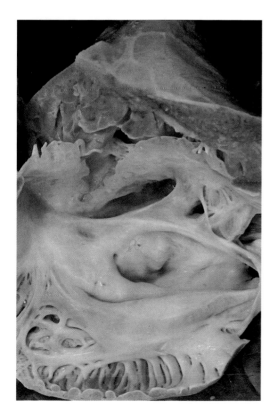

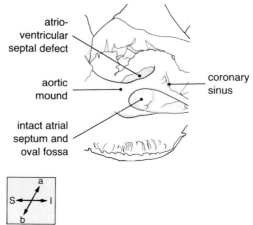

Fig. 7.17 *This surgical orientation of the right side of the heart with a deficient atrioventricular septation and separate right and left atrioventricular orifices ('ostium primum' defect) shows how the hole is at the site of the normal atrioventricular septal structures. Note that the structure of the atrial septum is virtually normal, although its leading edge is bowed away from the defect.*

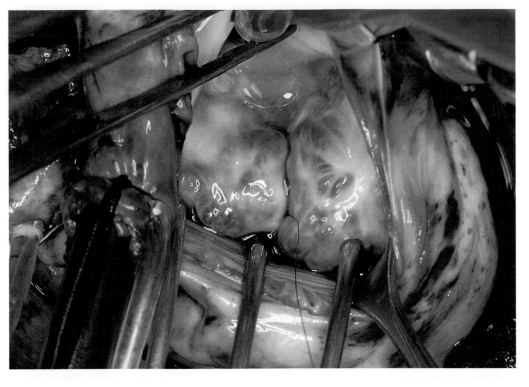

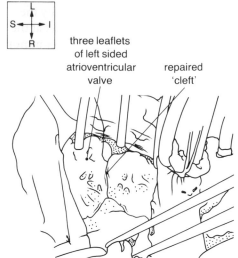

Fig. 7.22 *This operative view through a right atriotomy shows the typical three-leaflet formation of the left atrioventricular valve in an atrioventricular septal defect. It bears no resemblance to the formation of the leaflets seen in the normal mitral valve.*

three leaflets
of left sided
atrioventricular
valve

repaired
'cleft'

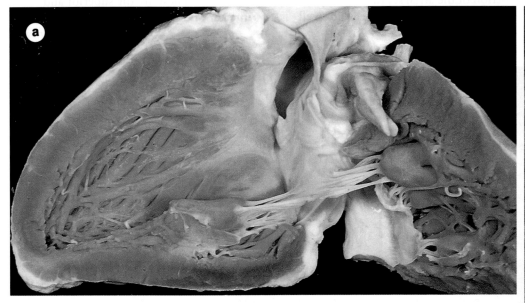

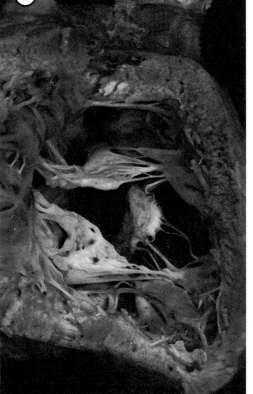

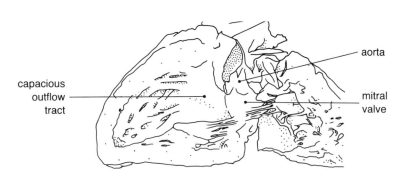

capacious
outflow
tract

aorta

mitral
valve

outflow tract

left ventricular
components of
superior and
inferior bridging
leaflets

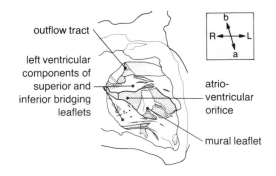

atrio-
ventricular
orifice

mural leaflet

Fig. 7.23 *(a) This view of the left ventricle, taken from the apex with the chamber opened in clam-like fashion, shows the interrelationship of the normal mitral valve and the outflow tract to the aorta. Note the position of the papillary muscles supporting the commissure of the mitral valve. (b) This view of the left atrioventricular valve and the outflow tract in a heart with atrioventricular septal defect is taken in comparable fashion to the normal heart seen in (a). Note that the left valve in the heart with deficient atrioventricular septation has three leaflets, with papillary muscles in markedly different orientation from the normal heart.*

entirely contained within the right ventricle: the antero-superior and mural (lateral) leaflets. The final leaflet is contained exclusively within the left ventricle, and is also a mural leaflet.

Although the two right ventricular leaflets are comparable to similar leaflets seen in the normal heart, the left ventricular side of a common atrioventricular valve bears no resemblance to a normal mitral valve (Fig. 7.22). The commissures and papillary muscles of the normal mitral valve are situated posteroseptally and anterolaterally beneath the orifice (Fig. 7.23a), producing an extensive mural leaflet guarding two-thirds of the circumference of the valve. In atrioventricular septal defects, the left ventricular papillary muscles are deviated laterally so that the mural leaflet is, in comparison to the normal, relatively insignificant, guarding less than one-third of the overall circum-

ference. The left orifice is, in effect, guarded by a valve with three leaflets, these being the small mural leaflet and the left ventricular components of the superior and inferior bridging leaflets. The papillary muscles are also abnormal, being situated laterally within the ventricle (Fig. 7.23b).

Until recently, conventional wisdom[7] held that the morphology of the valve in the presence of a common orifice reflected the presence of four leaflets with a cleft in the 'common anterior leaflet'. Close examination of this supposed 'cleft' (Fig. 7.24a) shows that, on its infundibular aspect, it is supported by the medial papillary muscle of the right ventricle (Fig. 7.24b). When seen from the outflow tract, this junction is virtually indistinguishable from the anteroseptal commissure of a normal tricuspid valve (Fig. 7.24c). This arrangement, therefore, represents minimal bridging of the superior leaflet of

a five-leaflet valve into the right ventricle, with the commissure between it and the antero-superior leaflet of the right ventricle supported by the medial papillary muscle. The variability noted by Rastelli and co-workers[8] in hearts with a common valvar orifice is then readily explained by increased commitment of the superior bridging leaflet to the right ventricle, with concomitant diminution in the size of the antero-superior leaflet and the movement of the papillary muscle which supports the commissure towards the right ventricular apex[9] (Fig. 7.25). A further difference between the hearts at either end of this spectrum is that, with minimal bridging, the superior bridging leaflet is usually tethered by cords to the crest of the ventricular septum whereas, with extreme bridging, the leaflet tends to be free-floating.

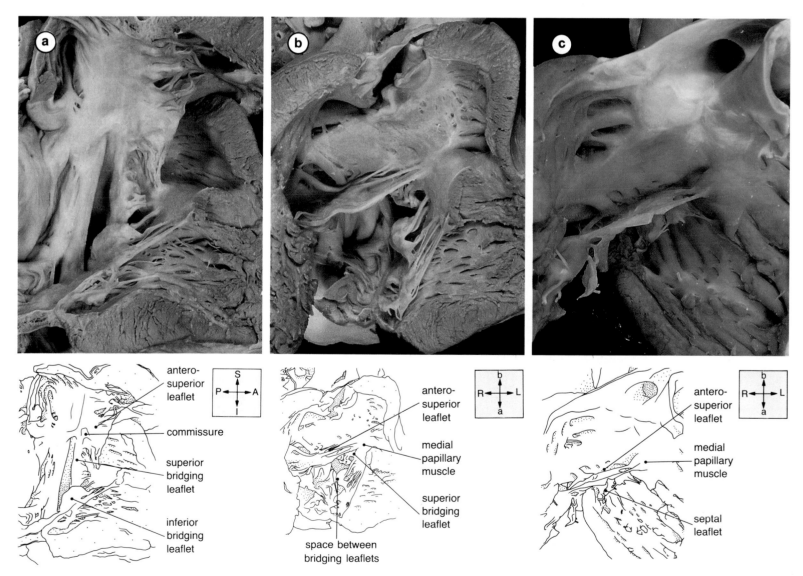

Fig. 7.24 *These illustrations show the commissure between the superior bridging and antero-superior leaflets of the common atrioventricular valve in an atrioventricular septal defect with common orifice. (a) The commissure from the inlet aspect, with minimal bridging of the superior leaflet, the so-called Rastelli type A. (b) The same commissure seen from the infundibular aspect, and as shown in (c) the normal heart seen in comparable orientation, the structures are directly comparable.*

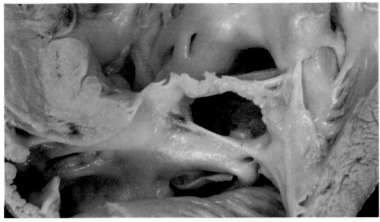

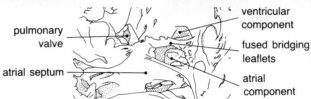

pulmonary valve

atrial septum

ventricular component

fused bridging leaflets

atrial component

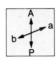

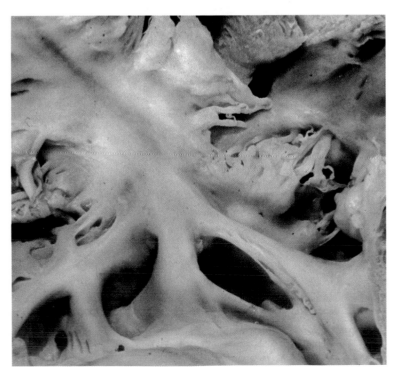

Fig. 7.30 *In this atrioventricular septal defect, again with separate valvar orifices, and seen in surgical orientation, the bridging leaflets and the connecting tongue float free of both atrial and ventricular septal structures so that there are both atrial and ventricular defects.*

Fig. 7.31 *This figure, based on the measurements taken by Ebels and his colleagues[12], shows how the extent of 'scooping' of the ventricular septum is greater when there is a common valvar orifice than when the junction is guarded by separate right and left atrioventricular orifices.*

percent of cases / percent of outlet

☐ common orifice (97)   ☐ separate orifice (40)

potential exists, nonetheless, for the leaflets to be free-floating with separate valvar orifices (Fig. 7.30). Rarely, the leaflets may be attached firmly to the septal structures in the presence of a common valvar orifice.

As discussed, if this variability in terms of shunting is described together with the presence of a common valvar orifice or separate right and left orifices, then there is no need to confuse the categorization of these hearts with the introduction of so-called intermediate or transitional variants.

Ventricular Conduction Pathways
It is evident from our discussion that the basic morphology of the ventricular septum is comparable in all atrioventricular septal defects. It is this disposition which determines the course of the ventricular conduction pathways. Although the hallmark of the malformation is absence of the atrioventricular muscular and membranous septal structures, there is also hypoplasia to a greater or lesser extent of the muscular ventricular septum. The degree of hypoplasia determines how much the septum appears to be 'scooped out', this being greater in hearts with a common valvar orifice than in those with separate right and left orifices[12] (Fig. 7.31). The non-branching bundle runs down the crest of this part of the scooped out septum and is covered by the inferior bridging leaflet. Often the inferior leaflet is divided by

Fig. 7.32 *In this surgical orientation of an atrioventricular septal defect with common valvar orifice, the course of the atrioventricular conduction axis has been shown.*

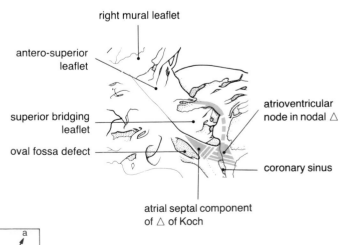

right mural leaflet

antero-superior leaflet

superior bridging leaflet

oval fossa defect

atrioventricular node in nodal △

coronary sinus

atrial septal component of △ of Koch

a midline raphe immediately above the vulnerable non-branching bundle.

The branching component of the conduction axis is found astride the mid-portion of the septal crest, usually covered by the connecting tongue and leaflet tissue in hearts with separate right and left valvar orifices, but sometimes exposed in the presence of a common orifice and free-floating leaflets. The right bundle branch then runs towards the medial papillary muscle. Anterior to this point, the septum is devoid of conduction tissue (Fig. 7.32).

Left Ventricular Outflow Tract
Although not readily evident to the surgeon during operation, the left ventricular outflow tract in atrioventricular septal defects is intrinsically narrow. It is much longer in hearts with separate orifices because of the attachment of the superior bridging leaflet (Fig. 7.33). This may become manifest as obstruction of the left ventricular outflow tract postoperatively and may require enlargement of this area. The obstruction may be due either to naturally occurring lesions[13] or to injudi-

cious placement of a prosthesis used to replace the left atrioventricular valve. If a prosthesis must be employed, the anatomy dictates the insertion of a model with low profile, or else resection of the shelf between the initial hinge-point of the superior leaflet and the attachment of the aortic valve[14]. It is also possible in hearts with separate valvar orifices to liberate the superior bridging leaflet from the septal crest and to insert a gusset so as to enlarge the outflow tract (Fig. 7.34).

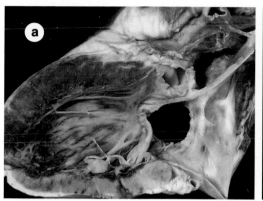

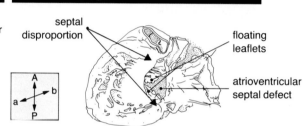

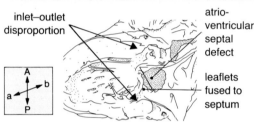

Fig. 7.33 *These hearts, shown in anatomical orientation, have been dissected to show the structures forming the narrowed outflow tract in hearts with atrioventricular septal defects. The tract is longer in hearts with (a) separate valvar orifices than when there is (b) a common orifice, because of the tethering of the superior bridging leaflet.*

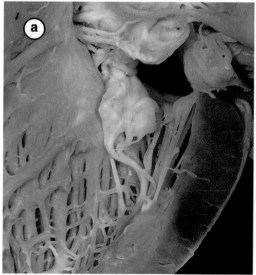

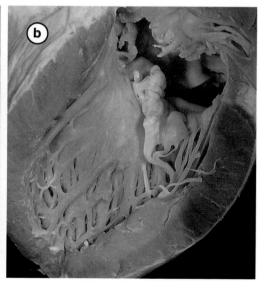

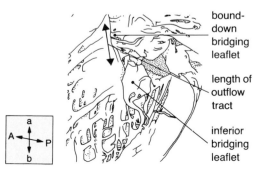

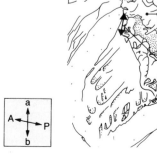

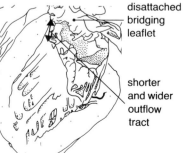

Fig. 7.34 *These dissections, viewed (a) in surgical and (b) in anatomical orientation, show how liberation of the superior bridging leaflet from the septal crest in hearts with separate valve orifices ('ostium primum' defects) gives the opportunity of enlarging the left ventricular outflow tract.*

Ventricular Dominance

There is also variability in the commitment of the common atrioventricular junction to the ventricular mass. Usually it is shared equally, giving a balanced arrangement, but, if the orifice favours one ventricle (right or left ventricular dominance), the other ventricle is often severely hypoplastic. This can have a major influence on the outcome of surgery and should always be assessed preoperatively.

Malalignment of Atrial and Ventricular Septal Structures

The morphology underscoring ventricular disproportion can also reflect malalignment between the atrial septum and the muscular ventricular septum (Fig. 7.35). This produces an arrangement analogous to straddling of the tricuspid valve (see below). The malalignment of the atrial and ventricular septal structures means that the connecting atrioventricular node can no longer be found at the crux. Instead, it is found where the ventricular septum meets the atrioventricular junction. This arrangement must be identified preoperatively, since it can be exceedingly difficult to recognize during the operation. If unrecognized, it is likely that the repair will damage the conduction axis. Septal malalignment, therefore, should be excluded in all cases of atrioventricular septal defect with left ventricular dominance[15]. This arrangement should also be distinguished from those hearts in which the sinus septum is absent and the coronary sinus terminates in the left atrium (see Fig. 7.20).

Ventricular Septal Defects

Surgical Anatomy of Ventricular Septal Defects

When faced with a clinically significant ventricular septal defect, the primary concern of the surgeon is whether he can effect a safe and secure closure. The important anatomical considerations relate to the location of the defect within the ventricular septum, as this determines its proximity to the atrioventricular conduction axis and to the leaflets of the atrioventricular and arterial valves.

The categorization of ventricular septal defects proposed by Soto and co-workers[16] is invaluable in that it focuses the attention of the surgeon on these pertinent features. In short, Soto and his colleagues suggested that defects could be defined according to whether they were embedded in the musculature of the septum, were bordered directly by fibrous continuity between the atrioventricular valves and an arterial valve (perimembranous defects), or were bordered directly by fibrous continuity between the leaflets of the aortic and pulmonary valves (Fig. 7.36). Defects in the third group, described as being doubly committed and juxtaarterial, are located, of necessity, within the outflow tract of the right ventricle. The other groups of defects, however, can be further described according to whether they open primarily to the inlet, to the apical trabecular, or to the outlet component of the right ventricle.

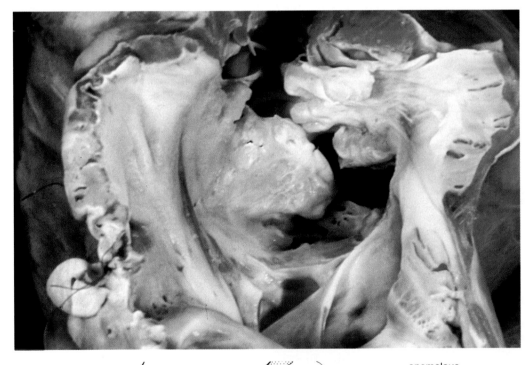

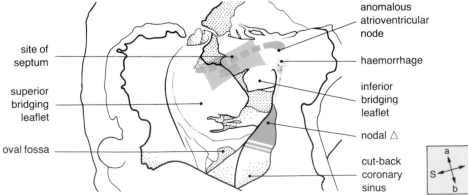

Fig. 7.35 *In this specimen, viewed in surgical orientation, there is gross malalignment between the muscular ventricular septum and the atrial septum. As a consequence, the atrioventricular conduction axis originates from an anomalous node in the posterior aspect of the atrioventricular junction rather than from the apex of the nodal triangle.*

Perimembranous Defects
The essence of the largest group of defects, termed perimembranous, is that a part of the central fibrous body, the area of fibrous continuity between the leaflets of the mitral, aortic, and tricuspid valves, forms a direct part of the rim of the defect. The defects are termed 'perimembranous', rather than 'membranous', because the atrioventricular component of the membranous septum is always represented in the area of fibrous continuity as part of the central fibrous body (Fig. 7.37). Furthermore, a remnant of the interventricular component is frequently found as a fold of fibrous tissue in the postero–inferior margin (Fig. 7.38).

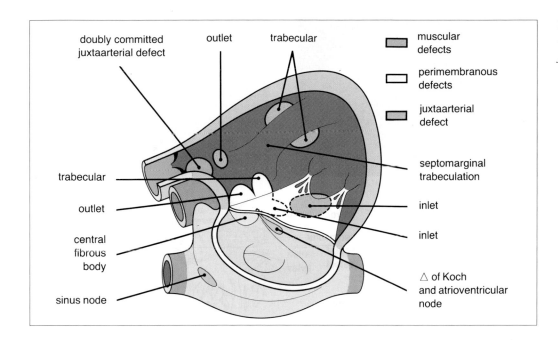

Fig. 7.36 *This diagram, shown in surgical orientation, illustrates the categorization used for differentiation of the various types of ventricular septal defect.*

Labels in Fig. 7.36: doubly committed juxtaarterial defect; outlet; trabecular; muscular defects; perimembranous defects; juxtaarterial defect; trabecular; outlet; central fibrous body; sinus node; septomarginal trabeculation; inlet; inlet; △ of Koch and atrioventricular node

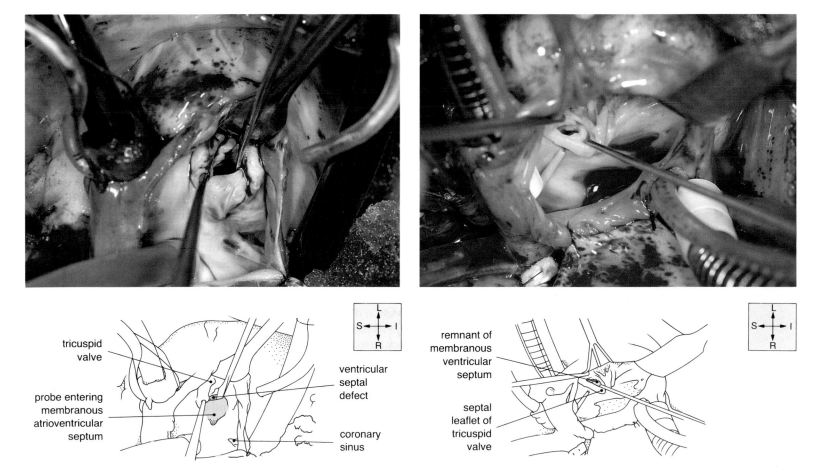

Fig. 7.37 *This view, through a right atriotomy with retraction of the leaflets of the tricuspid valve, shows the fibrous tissue of the atrio-ventricular septum lifted by the nerve hook that forms a direct border of those defects we categorize as being perimembranous.*

Labels in Fig. 7.37: tricuspid valve; probe entering membranous atrioventricular septum; ventricular septal defect; coronary sinus

Fig. 7.38 *In this heart, viewed through a right atriotomy and through the orifice of the tricuspid valve, there is a remnant of the interventricular membranous septum in the postero-inferior margin of the perimembranous defect.*

Labels in Fig. 7.38: remnant of membranous ventricular septum; septal leaflet of tricuspid valve

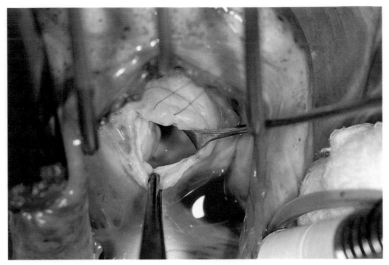

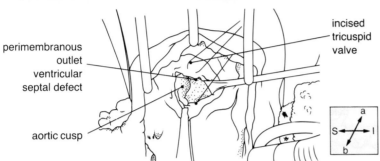

perimembranous outlet ventricular septal defect

incised tricuspid valve

aortic cusp

Fig. 7.43 *This view is through a right atriotomy and the incised junction of the septal and anterior leaves of the tricuspid valve. It shows a perimembranous defect opening to the outlet of the right ventricle. Note the relationship of the leaflets of the aortic valve to the left hand margin of the defect.*

ventricular septum. The non–coronary and right coronary leaflets of the aortic valve are much more closely related to the left–hand margin (Fig. 7.43).

Muscular Defects
The essential feature of muscular defects is that they are entirely enclosed within the muscular part of the ventricular septum. As with perimembranous defects, they can be located so as to open within the inlet, trabecular or outlet components of the septum, but will be separated by the musculature of the septum from the attachments of the valvar leaflets.

Inlet Muscular Defects. The significant feature of a muscular defect opening to the inlet is that its position is inferior to the conduction tissue axis. Thus, when viewed by the surgeon through the tricuspid valve (Fig. 7.44), the axis is located on the left–hand margin of the defect. The proximity of the axis to the edge depends upon how

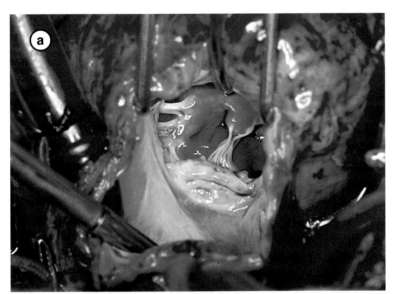

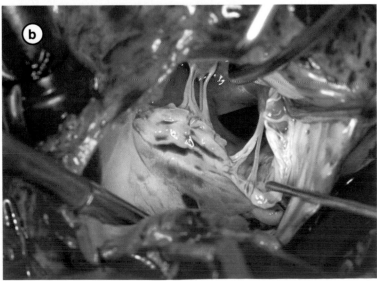

Fig. 7.44 *These views through a right atriotomy and across the orifice of the tricuspid valve show a muscular defect opening to the inlet of the right ventricle. (a) The course of the atrioventricular conduction axis, shaded green, is to the left hand of the surgeon. (b) Reflection of the septal leaflet of the tricuspid valve shows the muscle bar separating the upper margin of the defect from the attachment of the valve.*

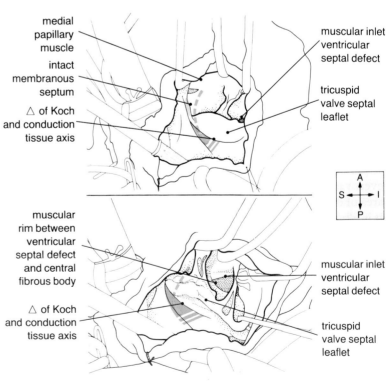

medial papillary muscle

intact membranous septum

△ of Koch and conduction tissue axis

muscular inlet ventricular septal defect

tricuspid valve septal leaflet

muscular rim between ventricular septal defect and central fibrous body

△ of Koch and conduction tissue axis

muscular inlet ventricular septal defect

tricuspid valve septal leaflet

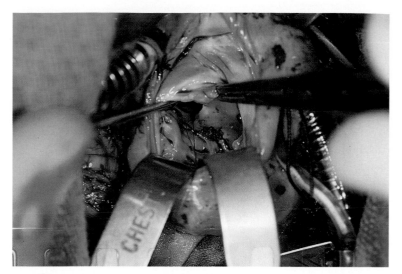

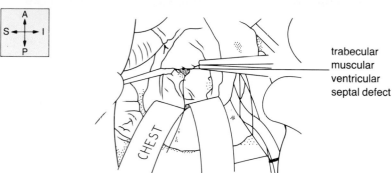

Fig. 7.45 *This view through a right atriotomy and the tricuspid valve shows a muscular defect opening into the apical trabecular component of the right ventricle.*

trabecular
muscular
ventricular
septal defect

close the defect is to the area of the intact membranous septum. The upper margin of the muscular septum separates the septal leaflet of the tricuspid valve from the mitral valve, and its size will determine whether it is suitable to be an anchorage for sutures.

Trabecular Muscular Defects. Defects opening through the apical trabecular part of the septum can be single and large (Fig. 7.45), double and large, or multiple (Fig. 7.46a). They are unrelated to the proximal parts of the conduction tissue axis but may be related to ramifications of the distal bundle branches. The right ventricular aspect of these defects is frequently obscured by the coarse apical trabeculations. Indeed, multiple small defects may not be visible through a right ventriculotomy. In some instances, the openings may be more readily identified from the left ventricular aspect, where there is often a solitary hole (Fig. 7.46b).

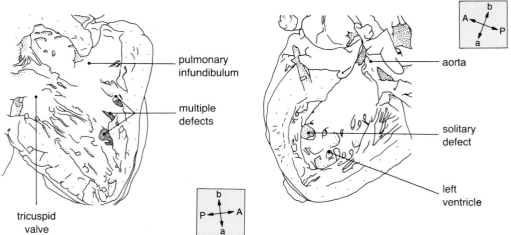

Fig. 7.46 *(a) In this heart, viewed in surgical orientation, three defects are seen anteriorly within the apical trabecular component of the right ventricle. (b) The left ventricular view, seen in anatomical orientation, illustrates the solitary opening on the left of the multiple defects visible from the right ventricular aspect.*

pulmonary
infundibulum

multiple
defects

tricuspid
valve

aorta

solitary
defect

left
ventricle

Outlet Muscular Defects. Muscular defects opening to the outlet of the right ventricle are relatively rare in the heart with concordant atrioventricular and ventriculo–arterial connexions and, when found, are often small (Fig. 7.47). On initial inspection, the endocardium may appear to be heaped up at the edges to produce a fibrous rim. Close inspection will show whether the posterior limb of the septomarginal trabeculation is fused with the ventriculo–infundibular fold to form a muscular postero-inferior rim to the defect. When present, the fusion of these muscle bars separates the edge of the defect from the axis of atrioventricular conduction tissue. The superior rim is the muscular outlet septum, which separates the leaflets of the pulmonary valve from the right coronary leaflet of the aortic valve, the latter attached to its left ventricular surface. If this superior rim is attenuated, then the leaflet of the aortic valve may prolapse through the defect (Fig. 7.48).

Doubly Committed Defect

The final type of ventricular septal defect is the doubly committed and juxtaarterial (or 'supracristal') defect. The feature of this defect is absence of both the muscular outlet septum and the posterior aspect of the subpulmonary infundibulum. Because of the absence of these structures, the facing leaflets of the aortic and pulmonary valves are in fibrous continuity in the superior rim of the defect (Fig. 7.49). There may be a firm fibrous raphe between the leaflets, so that they are attached at the same level, or else part of the aortic sinus may interpose between them, producing valvar offsetting. In either event, sutures can be secured in the region of fibrous continuity. The inferior rim of the defect is often similar to that found in a right ventricular muscular defect which opens to the outlet component, in that the posterior limb of the septomarginal trabeculation fuses with the ventriculo–infundibular fold (Fig. 7.49). This muscular rim again

buttresses the atrioventricular conduction tissue axis away from the edge of the defect. Occasionally, however, a doubly committed and juxtaarterial defect may extend to be bordered by the fibrous continuity between the leaflets of the aortic and tricuspid valves (perimembranous). The conduction axis is then much closer to its inferior corner (Fig. 7.50).

Concordant Atrioventricular Connexion

Although the descriptions thus far relate to ventricular septal defects in hearts with concordant atrioventricular and ventriculo–arterial connexions, this typology, and the guidance it gives to the site of the conduction axis, is also valid for hearts with a concordant atrioventricular connexion but with abnormal ventriculo–arterial connexions (see Chapter 8, p.000). The only exception is the defect found in the presence of an overriding and straddling tricuspid valve (see below).

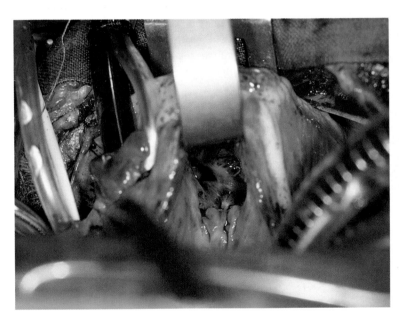

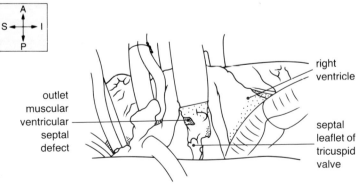

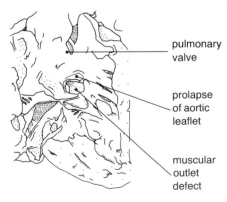

Fig. 7.47 *This defect is seen through a right atriotomy with the tricuspid valve retracted. It shows a muscular defect opening into the outlet of the right ventricle.*

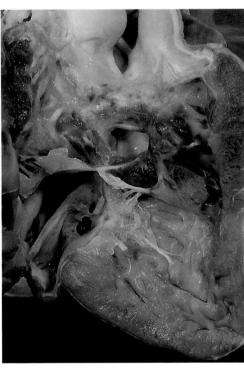

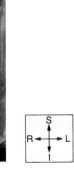

Fig. 7.48 *In this heart, viewed in anatomical orientation, the right coronary leaflet of the aortic valve prolapses through a muscular defect opening to the right ventricle.*

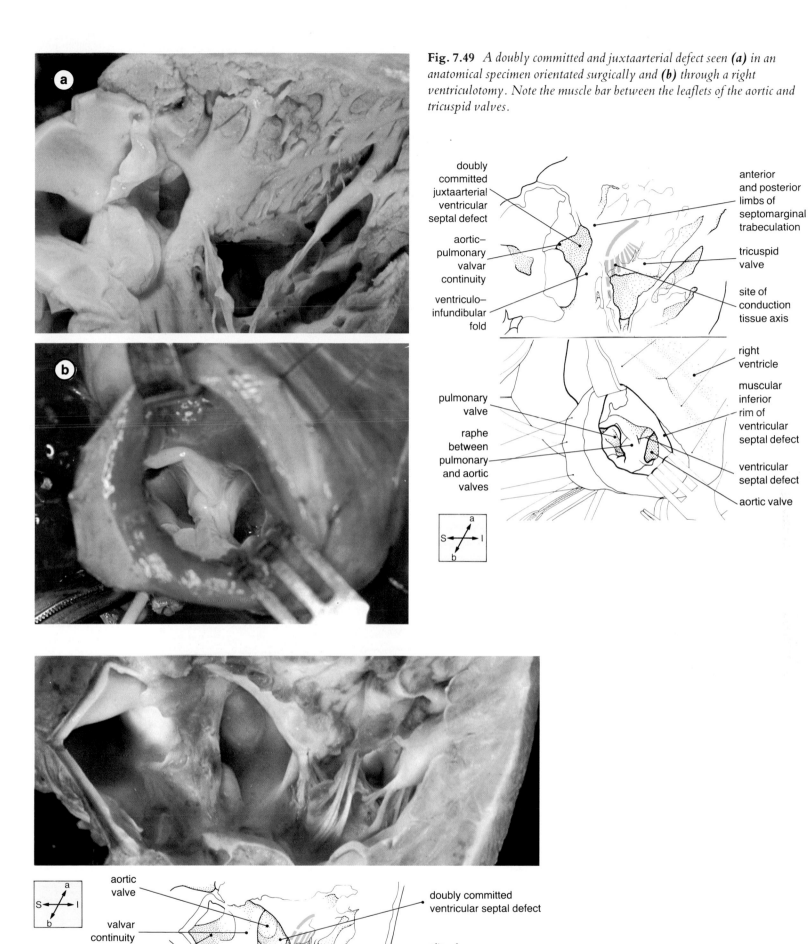

Fig. 7.49 *A doubly committed and juxtaarterial defect seen **(a)** in an anatomical specimen orientated surgically and **(b)** through a right ventriculotomy. Note the muscle bar between the leaflets of the aortic and tricuspid valves.*

doubly committed juxtaarterial ventricular septal defect

aortic–pulmonary valvar continuity

ventriculo–infundibular fold

anterior and posterior limbs of septomarginal trabeculation

tricuspid valve

site of conduction tissue axis

pulmonary valve

raphe between pulmonary and aortic valves

right ventricle

muscular inferior rim of ventricular septal defect

ventricular septal defect

aortic valve

aortic valve

valvar continuity

pulmonary valve

doubly committed ventricular septal defect

site of penetrating bundle

aortic–tricuspid valvar continuity

Fig. 7.50 *This doubly committed and juxtaarterial ventricular septal defect, viewed in surgical orientation, extends so that its postero-inferior margin is formed by fibrous continuity between the leaflets of the aortic and tricuspid valves (perimembranous). Note the proximity of the conduction axis to the margin of the defect.*

Malformations of the Atrioventricular Valves

Introduction

The pathological lesions which affect atrioventricular valves, both acquired and congenital, are legion. Not all are amenable to surgical repair. Those interested in the overall pathology are referred to recent reviews[19,20]. This section will concentrate on features of immediate surgical relevance.

Surgical Anatomy of Valve Malformations

The anatomy of atrioventricular valves indicates that problems may be encountered at the atrioventricular junction (the 'annulus'), in the leaflets, or in the tension apparatus. Sometimes the components of the valve, along with the entire atrioventricular connexion, are totally absent (valvar 'atresia'). This entity will be discussed in Chapter 8. The lesions to be considered in this section can affect either the morphologically tricuspid or mitral valves but, because the tricuspid valve usually functions in a low pressure environment, the lesions are more frequently manifest when affecting the mitral valve. Each lesion will be dealt with in turn, indicating its proclivity towards one or the other valve.

Overriding of the Atrioventricular Junction

Of considerable surgical significance is overriding of the atrioventricular junction, in other words, the valvar orifice is connected to both ventricles astride a septal defect. Almost always this is associated with straddling of the valvar tension apparatus, that is, with the tendinous cords attached across the defect (Fig. 7.51).

Although it is the site of insertion of the tension apparatus across the septum that determines the surgical options, the degree of override is also important. Overriding usually indicates septal malalignment, with major consequences in terms of the arrangement of the conduction tissues. Straddling and overriding can affect either valve and can occur in various segmental combinations. (For straddling in the setting of double inlet ventricle and discordant atrioventricular connexion, see Chapter 8.) This section is concerned with straddling valves and a concordant atrioventricular connexion.

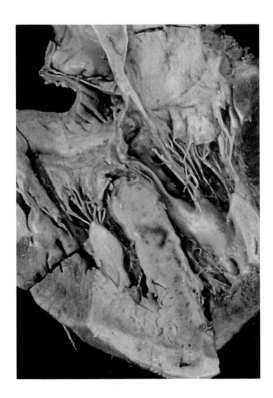

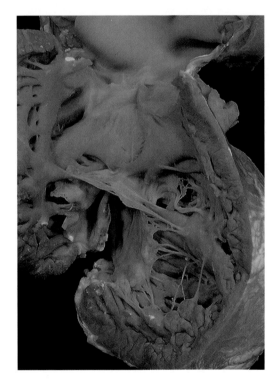

Fig. 7.51 *This 'four-chamber' section, viewed in anatomical orientation, shows a heart with a concordant atrioventricular connexion in which there is overriding of the orifice of the tricuspid valve and straddling of its tension apparatus.*

Fig. 7.52 *This heart with a concordant atrioventricular and discordant ventriculo–arterial connexion (complete transposition), viewed in anatomical orientation, has straddling of the mitral valvar leaflets through a defect opening to the outlet of the right ventricle.*

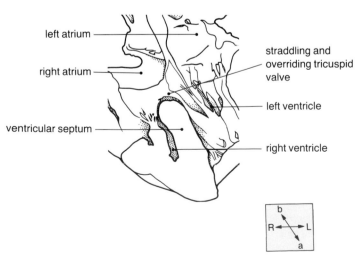

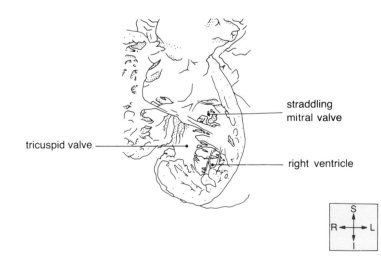

Straddling of the Mitral Valve

When the mitral valve straddles, it does so through a ventricular septal defect that opens to the outlet of the right ventricle, with the muscular ventricular septum normally related to the atrial septum at the crux (Fig. 7.52). With this arrangement, the conduction tissue is normally disposed. Usually, the anterolateral papillary muscle of the mitral valve is abnormally attached within the right ventricle, arising from the septomarginal trabeculation alongside, but separate from, the anterior papillary muscle of the tricuspid valve. This arrangement, seen with either complete transposition or double outlet right ventricle

with subpulmonary defect (Taussig–Bing malformation), can seriously compromise surgical repair.

Straddling of the Tricuspid Valve

Straddling of the tricuspid valve is found more frequently with isolated ventricular septal defects (Fig. 7.53) or with tetralogy, but it may also exist with abnormal ventriculo–arterial connexions. The salient feature is that the muscular ventricular septum does not extend to the crux (Fig. 7.53c). The ventricular septal defect reflects malalignment between the atrial and ventricular septal structures. The conduction axis originates not from the normal atrio-

ventricular node, but from an anomalous node in the postero-lateral margin of the right atrioventricular junction (Fig. 7.53). This node is formed where the muscular septum comes into contact with the junction. The septal leaflet of the tricuspid valve is usually tethered to the enlarged posteromedial papillary muscle of the mitral valve. A 'mini-septation' procedure is often necessary for complete ventricular repair, which carries a high risk of producing heart block[21]. Alternatively, a patch can be placed by sewing the stitches exclusively in the straddling leaflet of the tricuspid valve.

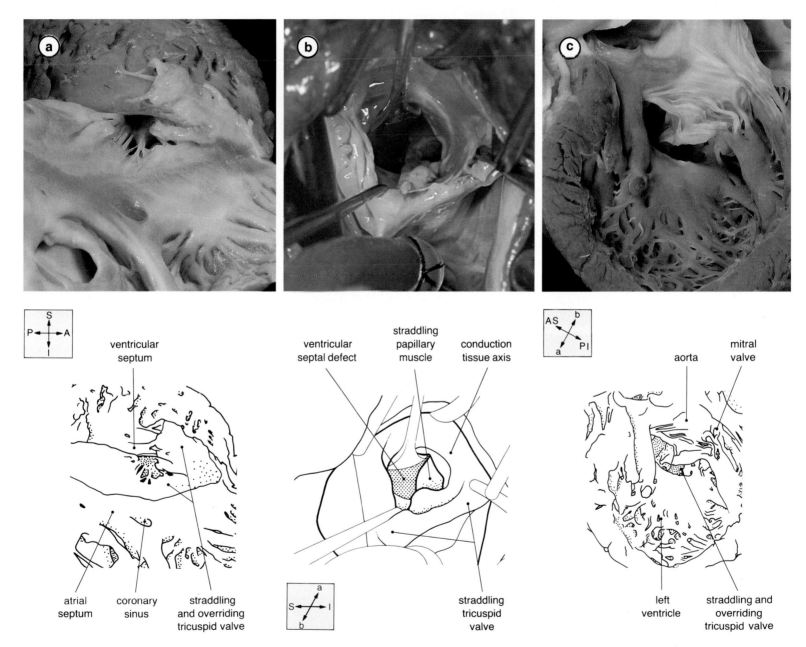

Fig. 7.53 *These (a) anatomical and (b) surgical views arranged in comparable orientation, show the right atrial aspect of straddling and overriding of the tricuspid valve with a basically concordant atrioventricular connexion. Note the anomalous location of the atrioventricular node and* *the axis of conduction tissue. (c) The view of the left ventricle of the heart shown in (a), seen in anatomical orientation, shows the malalignment of the ventricular septum relative to the crux (juxtacrux defect).*

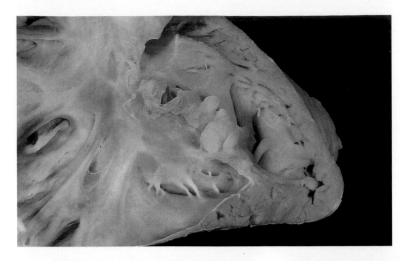

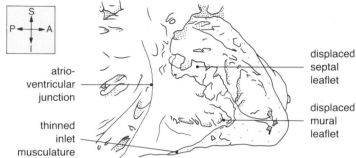

Fig. 7.54 *This anatomical orientation of the opened right atrioventricular junction shows the origin of the hinge point of the septal and mural leaflets of the tricuspid valve within the ventricle. This feature, usually described as 'downwards displacement', is the hallmark of Ebstein's malformation.*

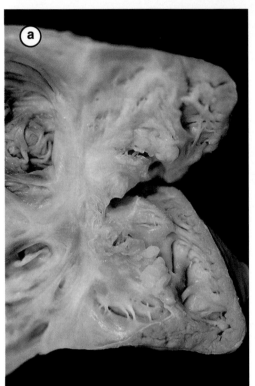

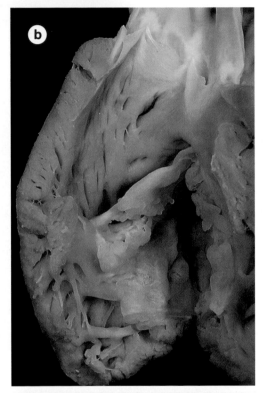

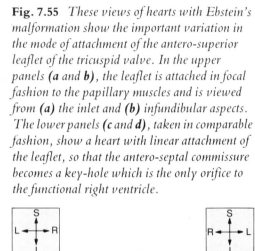

Fig. 7.55 *These views of hearts with Ebstein's malformation show the important variation in the mode of attachment of the antero-superior leaflet of the tricuspid valve. In the upper panels (**a** and **b**), the leaflet is attached in focal fashion to the papillary muscles and is viewed from (**a**) the inlet and (**b**) infundibular aspects. The lower panels (**c** and **d**), taken in comparable fashion, show a heart with linear attachment of the leaflet, so that the antero-septal commissure becomes a key-hole which is the only orifice to the functional right ventricle.*

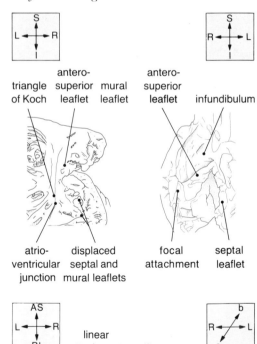

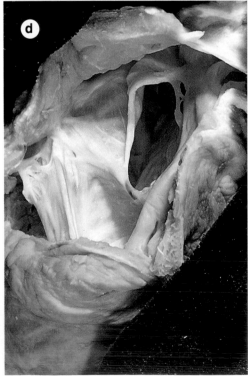

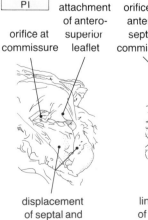

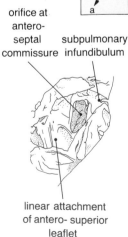

Dilatation of the Atrioventricular Junction

Dilatation of the atrioventricular junction occurs almost exclusively as an acquired lesion. A dilated mitral orifice is most frequently secondary to myocarditis. When surgical narrowing of the orifice is indicated, often it can be accomplished using various annuloplasty techniques without resorting to replacement of the valve. Dilatation of the tricuspid orifice is seen most frequently as a result of right heart failure.

Ebstein's Malformation
More of a challenge surgically is the dilatation that accompanies Ebstein's malformation. The crucial feature of this anomaly is that the hinge point of the septal and mural leaflets of the tricuspid valve is towards the junction of the inlet and apical trabecular components of the right ventricle, rather than at the atrioventricular junction (Fig. 7.54). The antero-superior leaflet is less affected in terms of its junctional attachment, but shows important variations in its distal attachments[22]. These can be focal (Fig. 7.55a and b) but, in more severe cases, the leading edge of the leaflet is attached in a linear fashion, severely restricting antegrade flow into the pulmonary trunk (Fig. 7.55c and d). In the most severe form, the antero-superior leaflet completely blocks this junction, producing an imperforate Ebstein's malformation which presents as tricuspid atresia (see Chapter 8).

Ebstein's malformation requires surgical treatment when there is significant dilatation of the true atrioventricular junction, and the wall of the inlet component of the right ventricle is both dilated and thinned. Reparative operations require placing the sutures in the area of thinning, and particular care should be taken to avoid the right coronary artery and its branches. In the septal area, the triangle of Koch remains the guide to the atrioventricular conduction axis (Fig. 7.56). Ebstein's malformation involving the left-sided morphologically tricuspid valve in congenitally corrected transposition is discussed in Chapter 8. It should be remembered, nonetheless, that, rarely, an Ebstein-like lesion can involve the normally located morphologically mitral valve[23,24].

Leaflet Malformation

Malformations of the leaflets can be summarized in terms of dysplasia, prolapse and clefts.

Dysplasia
The morphology of the dysplastic process is thickening and 'heaping up' of the substance of the leaflet, usually with obliteration of the intercordal spaces. A dysplastic valve may pose a significant surgical problem. It is frequently seen with atresia of the outflow tract and as an integral part of Ebstein's malformation[25]. Isolated dysplasia is exceedingly rare except in neonatal life, when it is usually a fatal lesion.

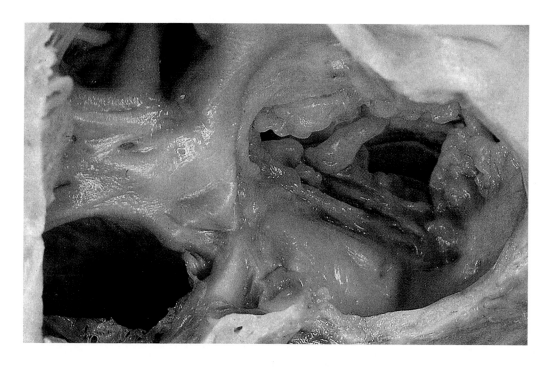

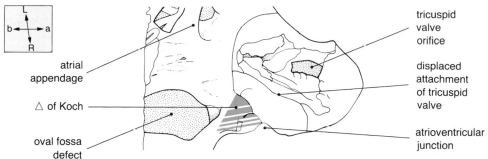

Fig. 7.56 *This heart, viewed in surgical orientation, shows how the triangle of Koch remains the guide to the atrial components of the atrioventricular conduction tissue axis despite the abnormal attachments of the septal leaflet of the tricuspid valve in Ebstein's malformation.*

Prolapse

Prolapse occurs more frequently, and is usually associated with deficiency of the tension apparatus (Fig. 7.57). It can be repaired by valvar replacement or by various valvoplasty techniques (Fig. 7.58a and b), including cordal shortening.

Isolated Clefts

The isolated cleft can be repaired by reconstituting its edges. Isolated clefts of the aortic leaflet of the mitral valve (Fig. 7.59) should be distinguished from so-called 'clefts' in atrioventricular septal defects (Fig. 7.22). The latter structure, as has been discussed, is a functional commissure in a valve with three leaflets.

Malformations of the Tension Apparatus

Some of the abnormalities of the tension apparatus that accompany malformations of the junction or leaflets, such as straddling papillary muscles, have also been discussed. The so-called 'parachute' deformity is the most worrisome lesion of the tension apparatus, apart from exceptionally rare anomalies such as so-called arcade lesions[26]. Some confusion exists about the definition of a 'parachute' valve. Some would define it as fusion of the papillary muscle groups so that all the cords insert into a common muscle mass[27]. Others, following the original description of Shone et al.[28], define a parachute lesion of the mitral valve as absence or gross hypoplasia of one commissure together with absence of its supporting papillary muscle. Either way, surgical reconstruction is difficult and replacement is likely to be necessary. Parachute deformity of the mitral valve may be further complicated by other lesions, such as supravalvar left atrial stenosing ring and coarctation of the aorta. Parachute malformation of the tricuspid valve can occur, but is rarely of clinical significance.

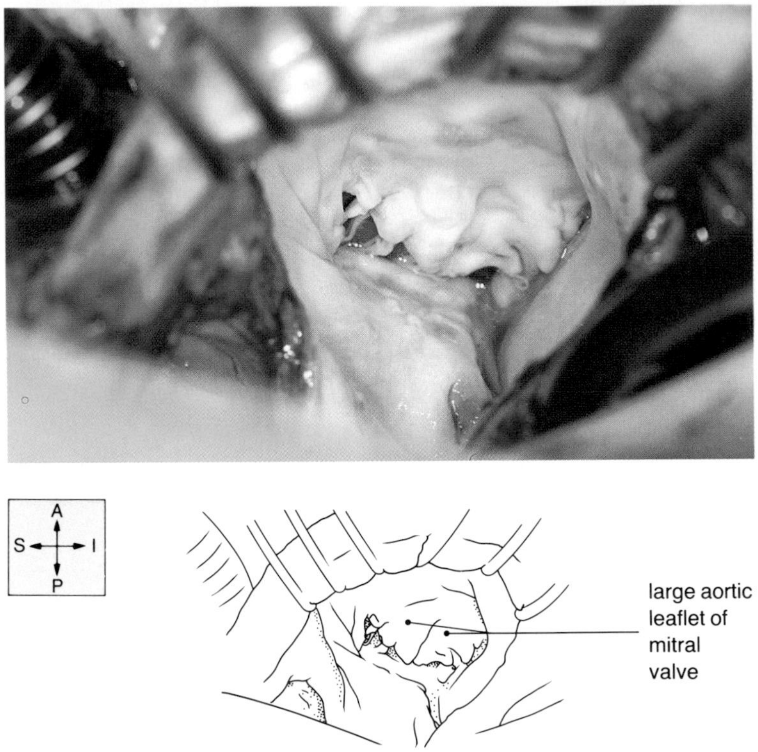

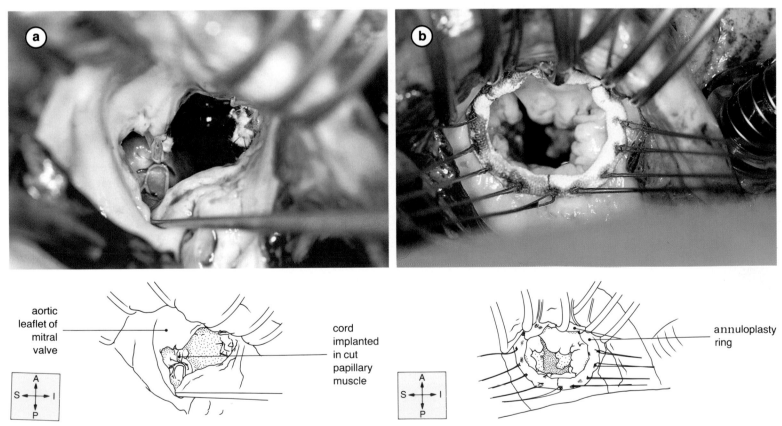

Fig. 7.57 *These surgical views of the mitral valve show prolapse of its aortic leaflet.*

large aortic leaflet of mitral valve

aortic leaflet of mitral valve

cord implanted in cut papillary muscle

annuloplasty ring

Fig. 7.58 *When the leaflets of the mitral valve are prolapsed, then the cords supporting them are usually elongated. As shown in these surgical views, repair consists of* **(a)** *cordal shortening and* **(b)** *valvoplasty.*

Malformations of the arterial valves and outflow tracts

Introduction

In this section, the surgical aspects of obstruction of the ventricular outflow tracts, valvar stenosis, and atresia of the outflow tracts are described. In the normally connected heart, obstruction in the left ventricular outflow tract produces sub-aortic stenosis. It must then be remembered that the same anatomic lesions will produce subpulmonary obstruction in the patient with complete transposition. Similarly, obstruction of the right ventricular outflow tract produces subpulmonary obstruction in the heart with normal segmental connexions, but sub-aortic stenosis in hearts with a discordant ventriculo–arterial connexion. When both outflow tracts are connected to the same ventricle, the anatomical problems are more discrete. These are considered separately in Chapter 8.

Aortic Valvar Stenosis

Stenosis of the aortic valve can be discussed as occurring at valvar, subvalvar, and supravalvar levels. Aortic regurgitation is ultimately a valvar problem and the perivalvar anatomy is often of great importance. To understand fully the substrates for stenosis and regurgitation across the arterial valves, it is essential to have a firm grasp of the arrangement of the valvar leaflets at the ventriculo–arterial junction. As described in Chapters 2 and 3, the arterial valves do not possess an 'annulus' in the sense of a circular ring of collagen that supports the leaflets. The only ring within the valvar complex is the circular area over which the fibrous wall of the great arterial trunk is supported by the underlying ventricular structures, which are partly muscular and partly fibrous in the left ventricle, but exclusively muscular at the right ventriculo–arterial junction. So the leaflet attachments are arranged as half moons, with the bases of the leaflets attached to ventricular muscle, but the apices of the commissures to the fibrous wall of the arterial trunk. When seen in closed position, the three leaflets then coapt snugly along the commissures extending from the circumferential margins of the arterial wall to the centre of the valve (Fig. 7.60). It is on the basis of malformations of coaptation under pressure of the diastolic column of blood that stenosis or regurgitation occurs within the valvar complex.

Valvar aortic stenosis may occur with unicuspid, bicuspid, tricuspid and, rarely, even quadricuspid valves. Dysplastic lesions are also seen in the aortic valve, but only rarely can surgery provide the answer to this problem.

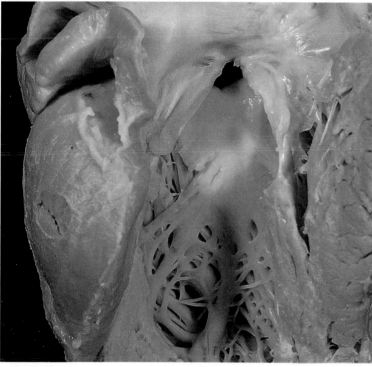

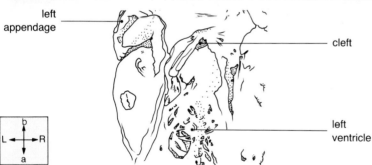

left appendage — cleft

left ventricle

Fig. 7.59 *This specimen, seen from the inlet aspect of the left ventricle in anatomical orientation, has a cleft in the aortic leaflet of an otherwise normally structured mitral valve. This lesion should be distinguished from the so-called 'cleft', which is in fact a functional commissure, found in the left atrioventricular valve of hearts with deficient atrioventricular septation (Fig. 7.23a).*

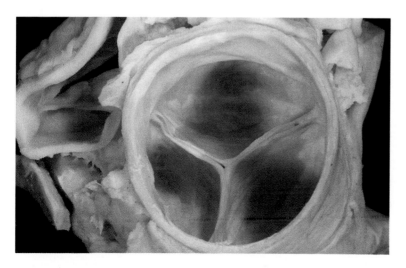

Fig. 7.60 *This view of the aortic valve, seen from above in its closed position, shows how the three commissures extend from the periphery to the centre of the valvar orifice and are closed by the hydrostatic pressure of the column of blood they support.*

Unicuspid Valve

The unicuspid valve usually has one or two abortive commissural raphes (Fig. 7.61). The leaflets are also abnormally attached in a linear rather than a semilunar fashion. Little can be done other than an attempt to open the valve as much as possible, short of producing severe regurgitation. Attempts to open the rudimentary raphe invariably result in prolapse of the leaflets and regurgitation.

Bicuspid Valve

A valve with two effective leaflets is most frequently seen in the adult patient. Perhaps this is because a bicuspid valve may not, in itself, be intrinsically stenotic. Usually it is only with the effects of time and turbulence that these valves become manifestly obstructive.

If the valvar morphology has not been totally obscured by calcific deposits, a bicuspid valve seen at operation will take one of two forms. Occasionally the two leaflets are of equal size, the commissures bisecting the aortic root (Fig. 7.62a). This type is frequently found in patients with coarctation of the aorta. In the other form, the leaflets are unequal, with the large, or conjoined, leaflet often exhibiting an eccentrically placed raphe (Fig. 7.62b). Both coronary arteries may arise from the sinuses of the conjoined leaflet, but they may also be positioned so that one coronary artery arises from the conjoined sinuses and the other from the third sinus[29]. If valves with two effective leaflets are seen before they become rigid and distorted by calcification, some relief from the stenosis can be obtained by careful enlargement of the ends of the single commissure.

Tricuspid Valve

Aortic stenosis does occur in patients presenting with valves having three leaflets, but this is rather rare. A possible cause of such stenoses is the unequal size of the leaflets in the normal aortic valve which, coupled with the high pressure in the aortic root, may lead to the development of calcification and stenosis in the elderly[30].

Subvalvar Stenosis

Subvalvar stenosis may be fibrous, fibro-muscular or muscular, reflecting the fact that the left ventricular outflow tract is partly muscular and partly fibrous. The muscular portion comprises the ventriculo–infundibular fold anterolaterally, the outlet septum anteriorly and the upper edge of the trabecular septum posteriorly. The fibrous part comprises the central fibrous body, the area of continuity between the leaflets of the aortic and mitral valves and the left fibrous trigone. Subvalvar stenoses may also be either fixed or dynamic in nature.

Fixed Stenosis

Of the variants producing fixed stenosis, a subvalvar fibrous shelf is perhaps most easily approached surgically. Though it appears circular when viewed through the usually normal aortic valve, and indeed it can be circular (Fig. 7.63), this is not always the case. A relatively thin shelf of tissue sometimes runs from beneath the

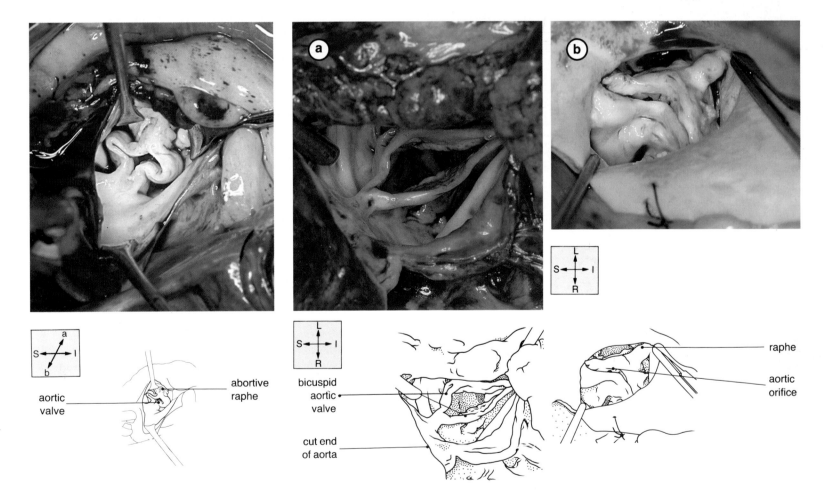

Fig. 7.61 *This view of an abnormal aortic valve seen through an aortotomy shows the so-called unicuspid, unicommissural arrangement, due to fusion of commissures during development.*

Fig. 7.62 *These views, taken through an aortotomy, show (**a**) a valve with two leaflets of comparable size and (**b**) a bicuspid aortic valve with a raphe in one of the leaflets.*

non-coronary leaflet of the aortic valve, over the site of the penetrating bundle, to the septal musculature, finally coursing over the ventriculo–infundibular fold to involve the aortic leaflet of the mitral valve. If dissection is performed prudently[31], a circumferential lesion can be completely removed (Fig. 7.63b), taking particular care where the shelf intimately overlies the conduction tissues. Too vigorous an attack on the side of the mitral valve may lead to detachment of that structure. In cases where the ventricular septum appears to be playing a part in causing the stenosis, it may be prudent to remove a segment of muscle (Fig. 7.64).

In cases where complete removal proves difficult, interruption of the fibrous shelf in the safe area over the ventriculo–infundibular fold will result in a safe and satisfactory relief of the stenosis. The same rules apply when resecting the variant of aortic stenosis producing a fibromuscular tunnel. Surgical correction, however, may be less successful than with a simple shelf, since the tunnel extends farther into the left ventricle, making the obstruction it produces more difficult to relieve.

A rather rare form of fixed sub-aortic obstruction is produced by hypertrophy of the usually inconspicuous anterolateral muscle bundle[32]. This muscle runs down the outflow tract from the ventriculo–infundibular fold to the ventricular septum. In its course over the parietal wall it would not be expected to involve the conduction tissues.

Anomalous attachment of the mitral valve can also cause fixed obstruction, as can a deviated muscular outlet septum. The former is usually seen with atrio-ventricular septal defect, while the latter occurs only, but not always, in the presence of a ventricular septal defect (Fig. 7.65).

The final fixed type of sub-aortic obstruction is produced by so-called 'tissue tags'. These herniate from any adjacent fibrous tissue structure, but are exceedingly rare as an isolated lesion in the normally connected heart[33]. They can produce significant obstruction of the left ventricular outflow tract in hearts with an atrioventricular septal defect or complete transposition.

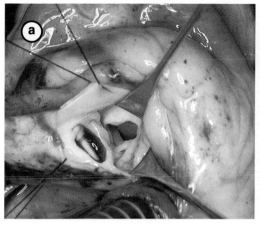

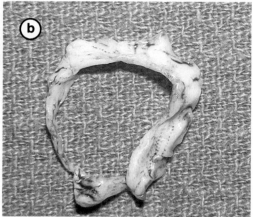

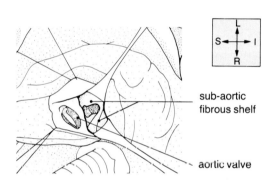

sub-aortic
fibrous shelf

aortic valve

Fig. 7.63 *(a) This view, taken through the aortic valve, shows a circular fibrous shelf producing sub-aortic stenosis, while (b) shows the shelf subsequent to its surgical removal.*

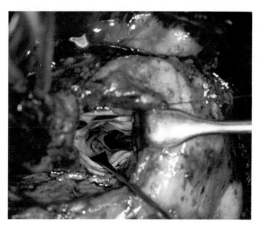

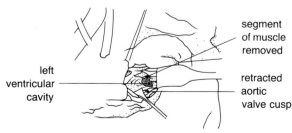

Fig. 7.64 *This operative view shows how a segment of ventricular muscle can safely be removed to relieve shelf-like fibrous obstruction of the left ventricular outflow tract.*

left
ventricular
cavity

segment
of muscle
removed

retracted
aortic
valve cusp

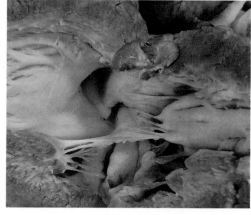

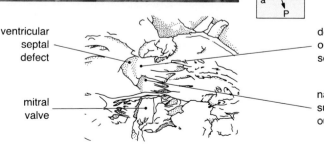

Fig. 7.65 *This view of the left ventricular outflow tract seen in anatomical orientation shows fixed obstruction produced by the posterior deviation of the muscular outlet septum through a ventricular septal defect.*

ventricular
septal
defect

mitral
valve

detailed
outlet
septum

narrowed
sub-aortic
outlet

Dynamic Stenosis

Dynamic subvalvar obstruction is a result of septal musculature thickening abutting the aortic leaflet of the mitral valve during ventricular systole. This usually creates a ridge of thickened endocardium easily seen through the aortic valve. If an operation becomes necessary, resection of this muscle bundle, as advocated by Morrow.[34], offers satisfactory relief of the obstruction. Again the surgeon must scrupulously avoid the conduction tissue as it emerges beneath the commissure between the right and non-coronary leaflets and descends on the interventricular septum (Fig. 7.66).

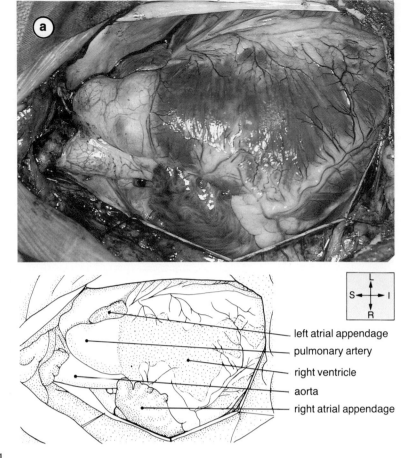

left atrial appendage
pulmonary artery
right ventricle
aorta
right atrial appendage

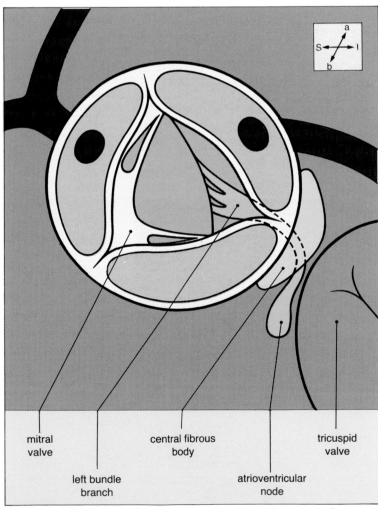

mitral valve

central fibrous body

tricuspid valve

left bundle branch

atrioventricular node

Fig. 7.66 *This diagram illustrates the view of the sub-aortic outflow tract obtained by the surgeon working through the aortic valve, and shows the location of the axis of atrioventricular conduction tissue.*

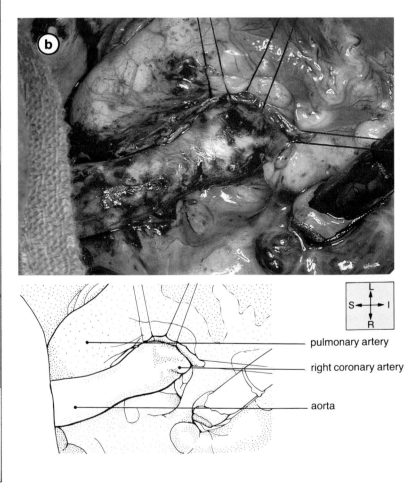

pulmonary artery
right coronary artery
aorta

Fig. 7.67 *(a) An operative view of a heart with supravalvar aortic stenosis shows a small aortic root in comparison with the normal sized pulmonary artery. (b) Further dissection reveals the supravalvar constriction.*

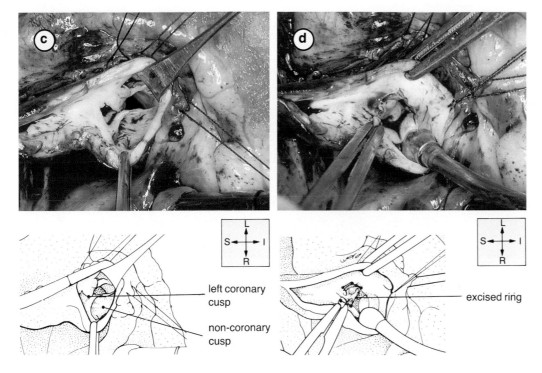

left coronary cusp

non-coronary cusp

excised ring

(c) An extensive vertical excision into the non-coronary sinus shows a markedly constricted ring with a particularly narrow left coronary sinus. (d) The bar of tissue, resembling an exaggeration of the aortic bar, is excised within the aorta, releasing the attachments of the left coronary leaflet to allow full excursion.

Supravalvar Stenosis

Supravalvar aortic stenosis is said to occur as one of three types: an hourglass, a membranous and a more diffuse tubular deformity. All forms are rare and, fortunately, the severe tubular type is extremely unusual. Two problems are shared by all three varieties because of the narrowing of the aorta at the junction of the sinuses with the ascending tubular aorta. First, the aortic sinuses, which usually contain the coronary arteries, may be converted into a high pressure zone in which the arteries provide the only run-off other than through the distal stenosis. This can produce marked dilatation of both the sinuses and the coronary arteries. Second, the circumferential narrowing at the sinutubular junction ('aortic bar') tends to tether the three aortic leaflets at the apices of their commissures in such a way that it is rarely enough to perform a simple 'aortoplasty'[35]. If possible, all three sinuses should be opened to release the tethering of the cusps. This can be accomplished by resecting the thickened aortic 'bar' and inserting a pericardial patch (Fig. 7.67).

(e) Resecting the bar and inserting a helical pericardial patch enlarges the aorta, (f) so that the aorta is now approximately the same size as the pulmonary artery (compare with parts (a) and (b)).

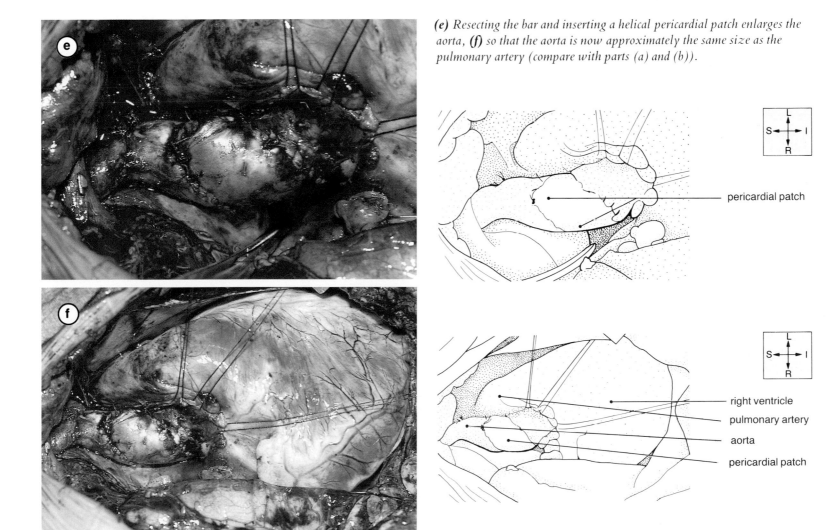

pericardial patch

right ventricle

pulmonary artery

aorta

pericardial patch

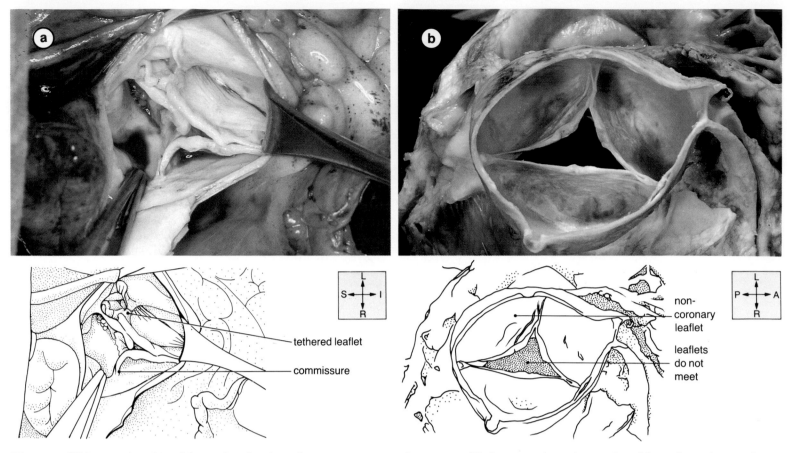

Fig. 7.68 *This operative view of the aortic valve through an aortotomy (a) shows a regurgitant valve as the consequence of tethering of one of its leaflets.*

In contrast, (b) the anatomic specimen, viewed from above, is regurgitant because of dilatation of the ventriculo–arterial junction.

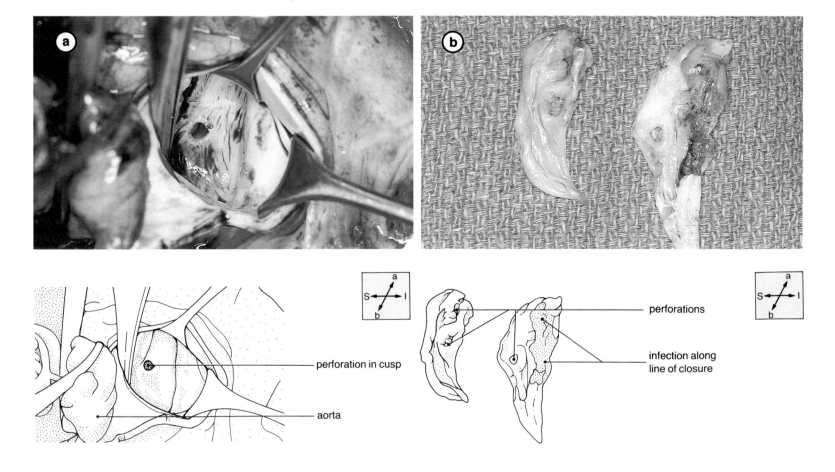

Fig. 7.69 *(a) This operative view, taken through an aortotomy, shows a perforation in one leaflet of a bicuspid valve due to infective endocarditis.*

(b) Removal of the leaflets showed that both were perforated by the infective process.

Causes of Aortic Valvar Insufficiency

Aortic valvar insufficiency may be due to congenital malformation of the valve (Fig. 7.68a), its supporting structures (Fig. 7.68b), or both, or it may be secondary to an infectious process in the aortic root (Fig. 7.69) or to 'degenerative' disease. Occasionally, aortic insufficiency may be due to trauma. Its frequent association with the doubly committed and juxta-arterial ventricular septal defect suggests that a deficiency in the structures support-ing the leaflets plays some role in these problems. Prolapse of the leaflets and insufficiency may occur with other types of ventricular septal defect (Fig. 7.70) or, even when the ventricular septum is intact, the latter situation usually being associated with a bicuspid aortic valve.

Surgical Management of the Aortic Valve

The critical importance of the anatomy of this region is perhaps best demonstrated by the problems exhibited by patients with endocarditis of the aortic valve. Because the valve is the 'keystone' to all the other valves and chambers of the heart, an eroding abscess in the aortic root may lead to the formation of a fistula involving any of these adjacent structures. Thus, the patient may present with findings of left heart failure, left-to-right shunting, complete heart block or any combination of these, in addition to the usual signs of sepsis. Surgical management clearly requires a detailed knowledge of this area, since one may be faced with virtual disruption of the ventriculo–arterial connexion[36]. A very

similar problem can occur when the aortic root, or the fibrous 'coronet', is severely damaged by dissection or marked degene-ration of its fibrous structure.

Obstruction of the Right Ventricular Outflow Tract

As with aortic stenosis, stenosis of the right ventricular outflow can occur at the valvar, supravalvar or subvalvar levels. The latter is discussed in association with tetralogy of Fallot (see below). Dysplasia of the valvar leaflets is most often seen as marked distortion and thickening, although three 'leaflets' can sometimes be recognized (Fig. 7.71). It can be associated with insufficiency as well as stenosis.

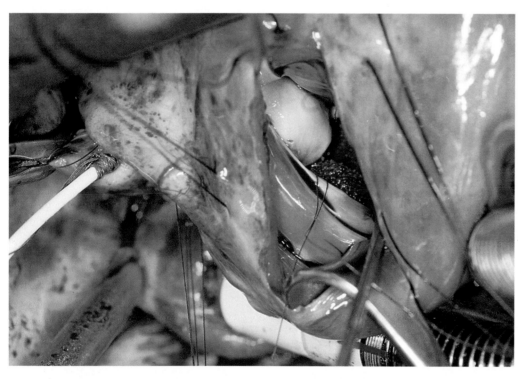

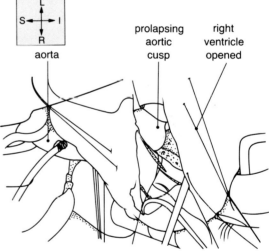

Fig. 7.70 *This operative view, seen through a right ventriculotomy, shows prolapse of the leaflets of the aortic valve in the setting of a perimembranous ventricular septal defect opening to the outlet of the right ventricle.*

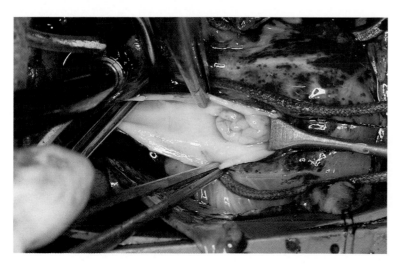

Fig. 7.71 *This operative view through an incision in the pulmonary trunk shows gross dysplasia of the leaflets of the pulmonary valve.*

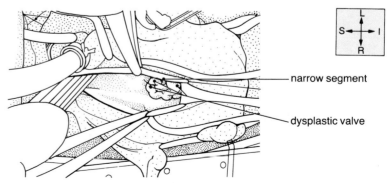

Pulmonary Valvar Stenosis

Isolated pulmonary stenosis is often found in the form of a dome-shaped valve with three well developed but fused commissures (Fig. 7.72). In some cases, the leaflets are attached to the wall of the pulmonary trunk along the commissural lines, leaving only a restricted opening (Fig. 7.73) and a narrowed arterial root. These areas of tethering can be dissected from the arterial wall and incised, resulting in a more satisfactory relief of the obstruction (Fig. 7.74).

The effectiveness of surgery is best measured six to nine months after operation, since significant secondary obstruction at the subvalvar level may maintain a pressure gradient across the outflow tract. This muscular hypertrophy will amost always regress with time[37].

Supravalvar Stenosis

Supravalvar stenosis usually takes the form of a waist-like narrowing of the pulmonary trunk just distal to the valve (Fig. 7.75), though it may occur at the sinutubular junction or anywhere at one or more locations within the pulmonary arterial tree. Narrowing has also been reported within collateral vessels directly supplying the lung from the aorta in cases of tetralogy with pulmonary atresia[38]. Very rarely, the obstructions may be membrane-like, but the usual lesion is more akin to a segment of tubular hypoplasia. These lesions, if anatomically accessible, are amenable to enlargement using a simple patch.

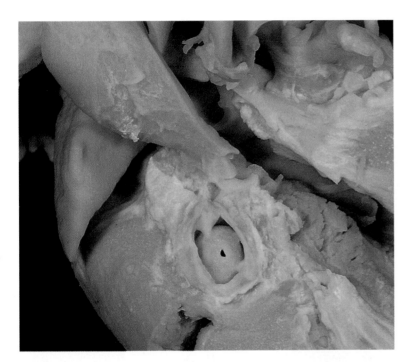

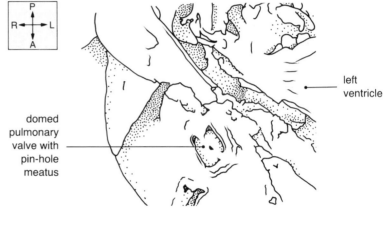

Fig. 7.72 *This pulmonary valve is viewed from above in anatomic orientation. There is gross fusion of the commissures, leaving a dome with a central meatus the size of a pin-hole.*

domed pulmonary valve with pin-hole meatus

left ventricle

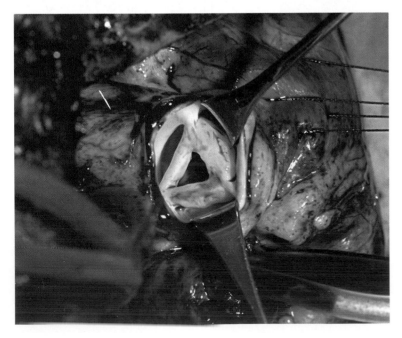

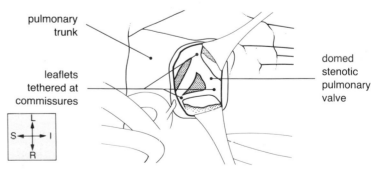

Fig. 7.73 *This pulmonary valve, seen through an incision in the pulmonary trunk, has fusion of its commissures and tethering of the commissures to the wall of the pulmonary trunk.*

pulmonary trunk

leaflets tethered at commissures

domed stenotic pulmonary valve

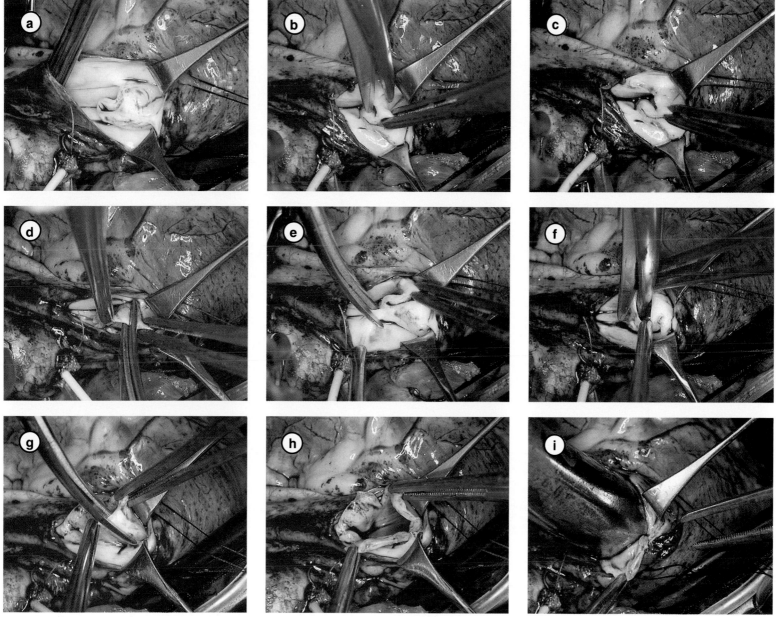

Fig. 7.74 *This series of panels taken through an incision in the pulmonary trunk shows how the commissural fusion and tethering, such as shown in Fig. 7.73, can be relieved by surgery.*

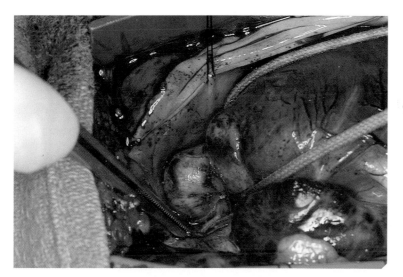

Fig. 7.75 *This view through a median sternotomy shows waist-like narrowing of the pulmonary trunk at the level of the sinutubular bar, that is so-called supravalvar narrowing. The abnormal valve in this heart was shown in Fig. 7.71.*

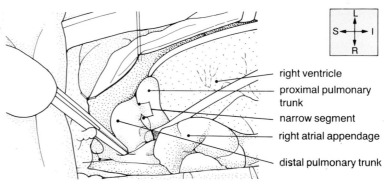

right ventricle

proximal pulmonary trunk

narrow segment

right atrial appendage

distal pulmonary trunk

Tetralogy of Fallot

One form of obstruction of the right ventricular outflow tract is so clearly demarcated that it constitutes an entity in its own right, namely tetralogy of Fallot. Its anatomical hallmark is antero-superior deviation of the insertion of the outlet septum combined with muscular sub-pulmonary obstruction[39]. In the normal heart, the outlet septum is an inconspicuous structure which is firmly anchored to the muscular septum between the limbs of the septomarginal trabeculation and is fused with the extensive ventriculo–infundibular fold. It is the alignment of these three structures (outlet septum, ventriculo–infundibular fold and septomarginal trabeculation) which produces the normal supraventricular crest in continuity with the so-called 'septal band'.

In tetralogy of Fallot, the insertion of the outlet septum into the muscular ventricular septum occurs along or superior to the anterior limb of the septomarginal trabe-culation. In a single stroke, this deviation divorces the outlet septum from the ventriculo–infundibular fold, this, combined with hypertrophied septoparietal trabe-culations narrows the subpulmonary out-flow tract, opens up a ventricular septal defect, and results in a biventricular connexion of the leaflets of the aortic valve (Fig. 7.76).

Ventricular Septal Defect

The ventricular defect opens beneath the ventricular outlets with a malalignment of the outlet septum. It may have fibrous continuity at its border between the leaflets of the aortic and tricuspid valves (peri-membranous) (Fig. 7.77) or else have a muscular postero-inferior rim[40] (Fig. 7.78). These features have the same implications on the disposition of the atrioventricular conduction tissue axis as they do in isolated ventricular septal defects (see p. 7.00). When the postero-inferior margin is the area of continuity between the leaflets of the aortic, tricuspid, and mitral valves (peri-membranous defect), the atrioventricular conduction axis penetrates beneath the atrioventricular membranous component of this fibrous area (Fig. 7.79). Often this is overlain by the so-called membranous flap, or pseudoflaps derived from the tri-cuspid valve[41]. Usually, in tetralogy the non-branching bundle and the branching bundle are carried down the left ventricular side of the septum some distance from the septal crest. In a minority of cases the bundle can branch directly astride the septum[42,43] and can then be traumatized by

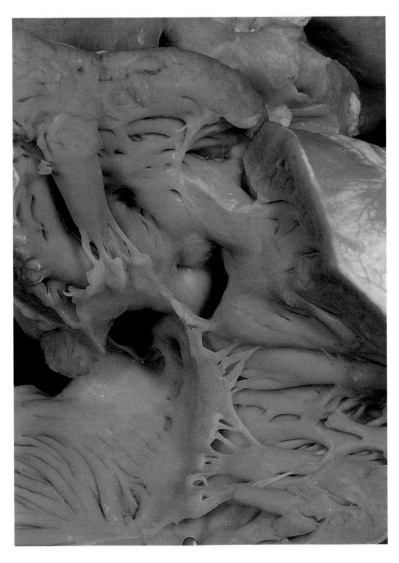

Fig. 7.76 *This view of the outlet of the right ventricle in tetralogy of Fallot, in anatomic orientation to, shows the divorce of the various muscular structures making up the normal outflow tract.*

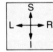

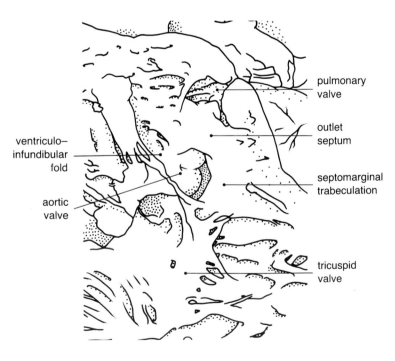

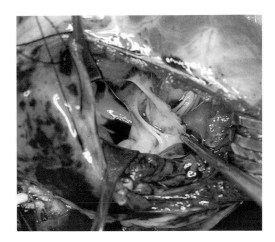

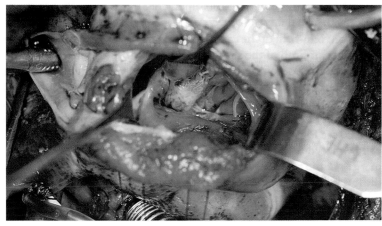

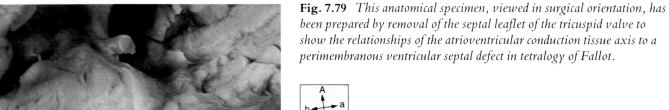

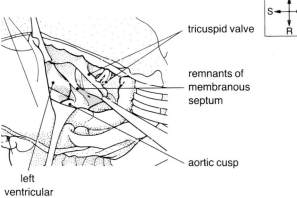

Fig. 7.77 This view through a right infundibulotomy shows a ventricular septal defect in tetralogy of Fallot that is bordered directly by fibrous continuity between the leaflets of the aortic and tricuspid valves (perimembranous defect).

tricuspid valve

remnants of membranous septum

aortic cusp

left ventricular cavity

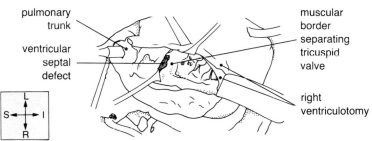

pulmonary trunk

ventricular septal defect

muscular border separating tricuspid valve

right ventriculotomy

Fig. 7.78 In this patient with tetralogy of Fallot, again viewed through a right infundibulotomy, the defect as seen from the right ventricle has exclusively muscular borders.

Fig. 7.79 This anatomical specimen, viewed in surgical orientation, has been prepared by removal of the septal leaflet of the tricuspid valve to show the relationships of the atrioventricular conduction tissue axis to a perimembranous ventricular septal defect in tetralogy of Fallot.

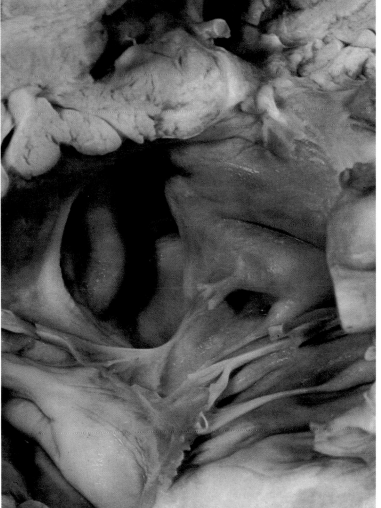

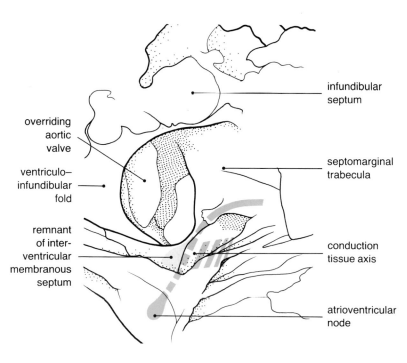

overriding aortic valve

ventriculo–infundibular fold

remnant of inter-ventricular membranous septum

infundibular septum

septomarginal trabecula

conduction tissue axis

atrioventricular node

A constrictive muscular ring is certainly formed, but its parietal segment is produced by hypertrophy of free-standing septoparietal trabeculations. This is important to the surgeon when deciding which muscle to resect in order to widen the narrowed outflow tract (Fig. 7.84).

The major limiting structure is always the hypertrophied septal insertion of the outlet septum, which can be dissected without fear of damaging vital structures. At the same time, any free-standing septoparietal trabeculations should certainly be identified and removed since they, too, never contain vital structures. The body of the outlet septum usually contributes to

the obstruction and ideally should be resected. Excessive resection of this structure, however, may lead to damage to the aortic valvar leaflets arising from the left ventricular aspect (Fig. 7.85).

It is also usual to resect the parietal insertion of the outlet septum (Fig. 7.84c). This fuses with the ventriculo–infundibular fold, which is the inner curvature of the heart. Care must be taken in this area not to perforate through to the right-sided atrioventricular groove. Dissection or injudicious placement of sutures in this region can damage the right coronary artery[50]. It is very unusual for the septo-

marginal trabeculation itself (the 'septal band') to contribute to the subpulmonary obstruction and, therefore, it is usually unnecessary to resect its limbs. Nonetheless, its body and the moderator band may be hypertrophied, particularly when the latter structure has a high take-off. Severe hypertrophy produces a two-chambered right ventricle and the intervening 'septum' may require resection. The anterior papillary muscle of the tricuspid valve often arises from the inlet aspect of the obstructing shelf. Care must be taken, therefore, not to damage this muscle during resection.

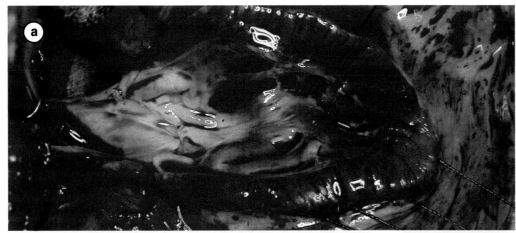

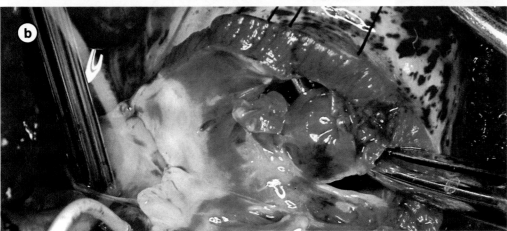

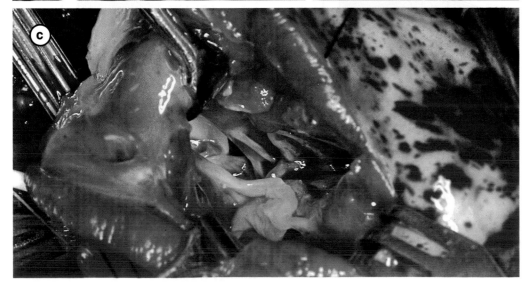

Fig. 7.84 *These operative views are taken through a right infundibulotomy.* **(a)** *The surgical view of how the stenotic orifice of the infundibular chamber is formed in part by the hypertrophied outlet septum but to the other side by septoparietal trabeculations.* **(b)** *The septoparietal trabeculations can be excised and* **(c)** *the obstruction is completely relieved by the resection of the parietal extension of the outlet septum.*

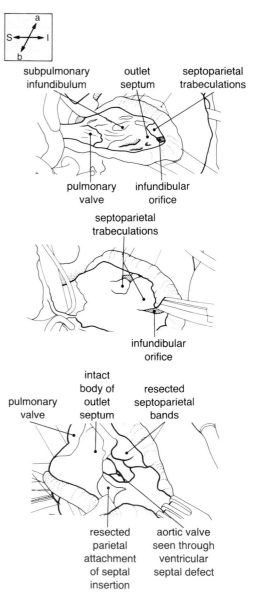

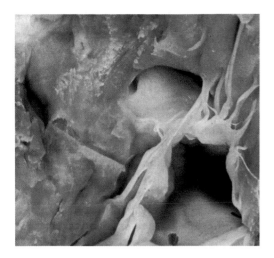

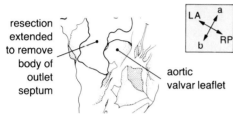

Fig. 7.85 *In this anatomical specimen with tetralogy of Fallot, viewed in surgical orientation, the outlet septum has been resected to show the proximity of the leaflets of the aortic valve on its left ventricular aspect.*

Connexion of the Aortic Valvar Leaflets
The final variable in tetralogy of Fallot is the connexion of the leaflets of the overriding aortic valve. This varies from the aorta being connected mostly to the left ventricle (concordant ventriculo–arterial connexion) to its being connected mostly to the right ventricle (double outlet connexion). The degree of override should not markedly affect the surgical procedure although, with greater commitment of the aorta to the right ventricle, the placement of the ventricular septal patch becomes more important. The 'internal conduit' constructed from the left ventricle to the aorta may further complicate relief of the right ventricular outflow obstruction, while it is always necessary to ensure an adequate outlet from the left ventricle.

Pulmonary Stenosis
Although the primary obstruction in tetralogy is at the infundibular level, the pulmonary valve is frequently stenotic. This must be relieved during operative repair. The sequels of postoperative pulmonary regurgitation are not yet clearly established, but they would certainly appear to be less troublesome than those of residual pulmonary stenosis.

Pulmonary Atresia

Tetralogy of Fallot
The most common type of pulmonary atresia with ventricular septal defect is, in essence, tetralogy of Fallot with infundibular pulmonary atresia. This is the most appropriate descriptor[51].

The ventricular anatomy includes deviation of the outlet septum sufficient to block completely the subpulmonary infundibulum. The anatomy of the ventricular septal defect can vary as in tetralogy, but the intracardiac anatomy is of relatively minor surgical significance.

Morphology of the Pulmonary Arteries
The feature which dominates the surgical options is the morphology of the pulmonary arteries. Although exceedingly rarely the pulmonary arteries may be supplied through a persistent fifth arch[52], an aortopulmonary window or coronary arterial fistulas[53]; in essence the lungs are supplied either through a persistent arterial duct or through major aortopulmonary collateral arteries. Rarely, a duct and collateral arteries can supply the same lung.

When a duct is present and the pulmonary arteries are confluent (Fig. 7.86), the

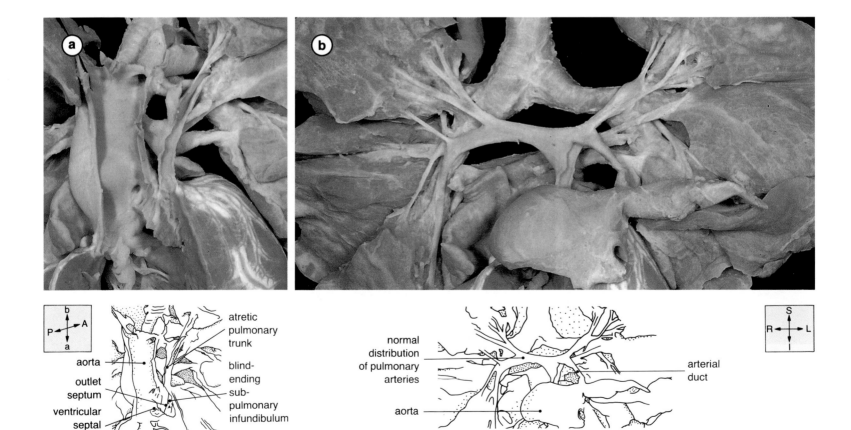

Fig. 7.86 *(a) This specimen of tetralogy with pulmonary atresia, viewed in anatomical orientation, has confluent pulmonary arteries supplied by an arterial duct. (b) In this case the pulmonary arteries have a normal segmental distribution.*

Whatever the intracardiac anatomy, it is rare that one finds the thread-like pulmonary arteries seen so frequently with tetralogy and pulmonary atresia. Furthermore, the flow of pulmonary blood is almost always duct-dependent. With prostaglandins now available to improve ductal flow, the pulmonary arteries are almost always of sufficient size to permit construction of a systemic–pulmonary shunt. Other options, such as the need for pulmonary valvotomy, should be decided after assessment of the precise anatomy of the individual case[58].

Causes of Pulmonary Valvar Insufficiency

Pulmonary valvar insufficiency may be congenital or acquired, the latter usually secondary to surgical intervention or pulmonary hypertension. Congenital pulmonary valvar insufficiency may be

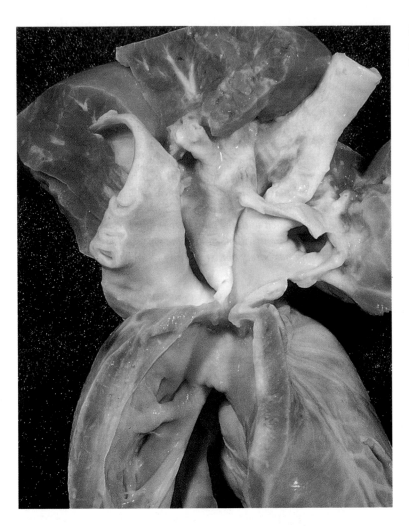

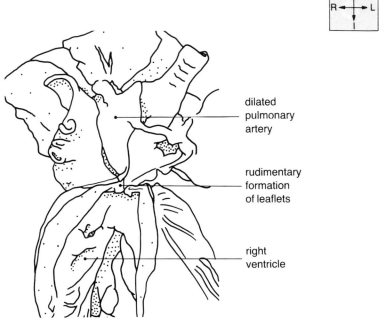

Fig. 7.91 *In this specimen, seen in anatomical orientation, with tetralogy of Fallot and rudimentary formation of the leaflets of the pulmonary valve, there is gross dilatation of the pulmonary trunk and arteries.*

dilated pulmonary artery

rudimentary formation of leaflets

right ventricle

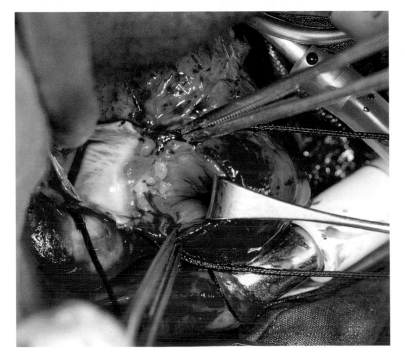

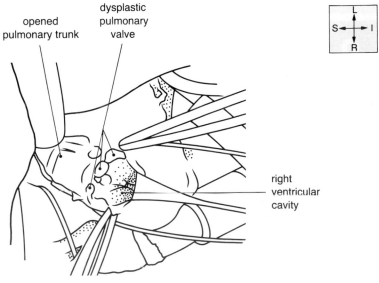

Fig. 7.92 *This operative view shows the right ventriculo–pulmonary arterial junction with the markedly malformed pulmonary valve tissue in a patient with tetralogy of Fallot.*

opened pulmonary trunk

dysplastic pulmonary valve

right ventricular cavity

associated with marked deformity of the valvar tissue, as in valvar dysplasia, or with the absence of valvar tissue altogether. Rudimentary leaflets may be seen with an intact ventricular septum[60] or in combination with ventricular septal defect (Fig. 7.91). Absence of the leaflets of the pulmonary valve is also found in combination with tetralogy of Fallot[61] (Fig. 7.92).

While gross pulmonary valvar insufficiency may be relatively well tolerated by the right heart, it can result in marked enlargment of the pulmonary trunk and arteries and is usually associated with the absence of the arterial duct[62] (Fig. 7.93). Indeed, compromise of the tracheo-bronchial tree by these grossly enlarged

vessels (Fig. 7.94) results in most patients presenting with symptoms of respiratory distress. Because only a limited number of cases have come to surgical correction, the efficacy of valvar replacement with or without arterial plication has not been proved[63]. Fortunately, this is a rare condition.

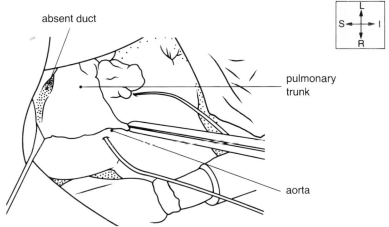

Fig. 7.93 *Operative view of the grossly enlarged pulmonary trunk of the patient illustrated in Fig. 7.92. Note the absence of an arterial duct or ligament.*

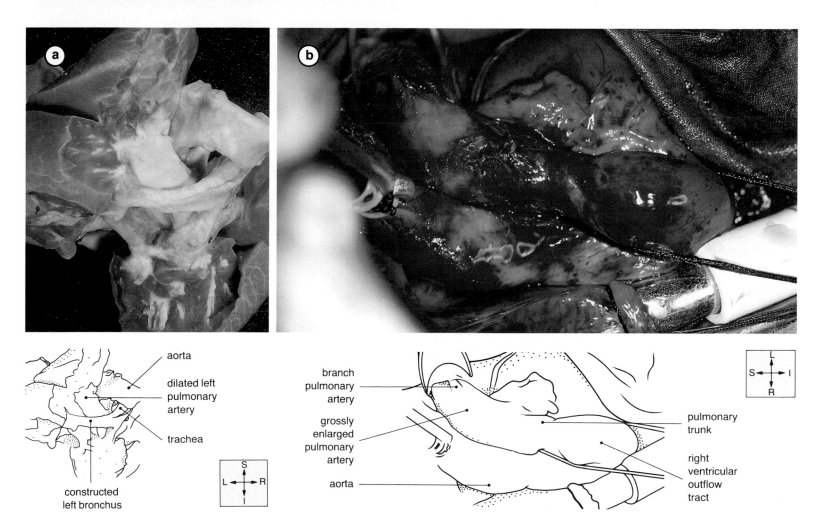

Fig. 7.94 *(a) This view of the hilum of the left lung of the patient seen in Fig. 7.91, viewed from behind, shows the obstruction produced by the gross dilatation of the left pulmonary artery as it crosses the bronchus.*

(b) This operative view of the patient shown in Figs 7.92 and 7.93 shows the grossly enlarged left pulmonary artery. On bypass the left pulmonary artery is seen to be as large as the aorta.

References

1. Ettedgui, J.A., Siewers, R.D., Anderson, R.H. & Zuberbuhler, J.R. (1990) The diagnostic echocardiographic features of the superior caval ('sinus venosus') interatrial communication. *British Heart Journal*, **64**, 329–331.

2. Quaegebeur, J., Kirklin, J.W., Pacifico, A.D. & Bargeron, I.M. Jr. (1979) Surgical experience with unroofed coronary sinus. *Annals of Thoracic Surgery*, **27**, 418–425.

3. Becker, A.E. & Anderson, R.H. (1982) Atrioventricular septal defects. What's in a name? *Journal of Thoracic and Cardiovascular Surgery*, **83**, 461–469.

4. Penkoske, P.A., Neches, W.H., Anderson, R.H. & Zuberbuher, J.R. (1985) Further observations on the morphology of atrioventricular septal defects. *Journal of Thoracic and Cardiovascular Surgery*, **90**, 611–622.

5. Wilcox, B.R., Mattos, S.S., Anderson, R.H. & Henry, G.W. (1990) Unusual termination of the coronary sinus with septal malalignment in atrioventricular septal defects. *Annals of Thoracic Surgery*, **50**, 767–770.

6. Anderson, R.H. & Ho, S.Y. (1989) The surgical anatomy of atrioventricular septal defect. In *Perspectives in Pediatric Cardiology Volume 2. Pediatric Cardiac Surgery Part 1*. Edited by G. Crupi, L. Parenzan & R.H. Anderson. Mount Kisco, New York: Futura Publishing Company, Inc., pp. 81–85.

7. McGoon, D.C., Puga, F.T. & Danielson, G.K. (1983) Atrioventricular canal. In *Gibbon's Surgery of the Heart*. Edited by D.C. Sabiston & F.C. Spencer. Philadelphia: J.B. Lippincott, pp. 81–85.

8. Rastelli, G.C., Kirklin, J.W. & Titus, J.L. (1966) Anatomic observations on complete form of persistent common atrioventricular canal with special reference to atrioventricular valves. *Mayo Clinic Proceedings*, **41**, 296–308.

9. Piccoli, G.P., Wilkinson, J.L., Macartney, F.J., Gerlis, I.M. & Anderson, R.H. (1979) Morphology and classification of complete atrioventricular defects. *British Heart Journal*, **42**, 633–639.

10. Carpentier, A. (1977) Surgical anatomy and management of the mitral component of atrioventricular canal defects. In *Paediatric Cardiology*. Edited by R.H. Anderson & E.A. Shinebourne. Edinburgh: Churchill Livingstone, pp. 477–486.

11. Anderson, R.H., Zuberbuhler, J.R., Penkoske, P.A. & Neches, W.H. (1985) Of clefts, commissures and things. *Journal of Thoracic and Cardiovascular Surgery*, **90**, 605–610.

12. Ebels, T.J., Anderson, R.H., Devine, W.A., Debich, D.E., Penkoske, P.A. & Zuberbuhler, J.R. (1990) Anomalies of the left atrioventricular valve and related ventricular septal morphology in atrioventricular septal defects. *Journal of Thoracic and Cardiovascular Surgery*, **99**, 299–307.

13. Piccoli, G.P., Ho, S.Y., Wilkinson, J.L., Macartney, F.J., Gerlis, I.M. & Anderson, R.H. (1982) Left sided obstructive lesions in atrioventricular septal defects. *Journal of Thoracic and Cardiovascular Surgery*, **83**, 453–460.

14. Ebels, T., Ho, S.Y., Anderson, R.H., Meijboom, E.J. & Eilgelaar, A. (1986) The surgical anatomy of the left ventricular outflow tract in atrioventricular septal defect. *Annals of Thoracic Surgery*, **41**, 483–488.

15. Pillai, R., Ho, S.Y., Anderson, R.H., Shinebourne, E.A. & Lincoln, C. (1984) Malalignment of the interventricular septum with atrioventricular septal defect: its implications cncerning conduction tissue disposition. *Thoracic Cardiovascular Surgeon*, **32**, 1–3.

16. Soto, B., Becker, A.E., Moulaert, A.J., Lie, J.T. & Anderson, R.H. (1980) Classification of ventricular septal defects. *British Heart Journal*, **43**, 332–343.

17. Milo, S., Ho, S.Y., Wilkinson, J.L. & Anderson, R.H. (1980) The surgical anatomy and atrioventricular conduction tissues of hearts with isolated ventricular septal defects. *Journal of Thoracic and Cardiovascular Surgery*, **79**, 244–255.

18. Gerbode, F., Hultgren, H., Melrose, D. & Osborn, J. (1958) Syndrome of left ventricular–right atrial shunt, successful surgical repair of defect in five cases with observation of bradycardia on closure. *Annals of Surgery*, **148**, 433–446.

19. Becker, A.E. (1983) Valve pathology in the paediatric age group. In *Paediatric Cardiology Volume 5*. Edited by R.H. Anderson, F.J. Macartney, E.A. Shinebourne & M. Tynan. Edinburgh: Churchill Livingstone, pp. 345–360.

20. Thiene, G., Frescura, C. & Daliento, L. (1986) The pathology of the congenitally malformed mitral valve. In *Paediatric Cardiology Volume 6*. Edited by C. Marcelletti, R.H. Anderson, A.E. Becker, A. Corno, D. di Carlo & E. Mazzera. Edinburgh: Churchill Livingstone, pp. 225–239.

21. Pacifico, A.D., Soto, B. & Bargeron, I.M. Jr. (1979) Surgical treatment of straddling tricuspid valves. *Circulation*, **60**, 655–664.

22. Leung, M.P., Baker, E.J., Anderson, R.H. & Zuberbuhler, J.R. (1988) Cineangiographic spectrum of Ebstein's malformation: its relevance to clinical presentation and outcome. *American Journal of Cardiology*, **11**, 154–161.

23. Ruschhaupt, D.G., Bharati, S. & Lev, M. (1976) Mitral valve malformation of Ebstein type in absence of corrected transposition. *American Journal of Cardiology*, **38**, 109–112.

24. Leung, M., Rigby, M.L., Anderson, R.H., Wyse, R.K.H. & Macartney, F.J. (1987) Reversed off-setting of the septal attachments of the atrioventricular valves and Ebstein's malformation of the morphologically mitral valve. *British Heart Journal*, **57**, 184–187.

25. Becker, A.E., Becker, M.J. & Edwards, J.E. (1971) Pathologic spectrum of dysplasia of the tricuspid valve, features in common with Ebstein's malformation. *Archives of Pathology*, **91**, 167–178.

26. Layman, T.E. & Edwards, J.E. (1967) Anomalous mitral arcade: A type of congenital mitral insufficiency. *Circulation*, **35**, 389–395.

27. Rosenquist, G.C. (1974) Congenital mitral valve disease associated with coarctation of the aorta. A spectrum that includes parachute deformity of the mitral valve. *Circulation*, **49**, 985–993.

28. Shone, J., Sellers, R., Anderson, R.H., Adams, P., Lillehei, C.W. & Edwards, J.E. (1963) The developmental complex of parachute mitral valve. *American Journal of Cardiology*, **11**, 714–725.

29. Angelini, A., Ho, S.Y., Anderson, R.H., Devine, W.E., Zuberbuhler, J.R., Becker, A.E. & Davies, M.J. (1989) The morphology of the normal aortic valve as compared with the aortic valve having two leaflets. *Journal of Thoracic and Cardiovascular Surgery*, **98**, 362–367.

30. Vollebergh, F.E.M.G. & Becker, A.E. (1977) Minor congenital variations in cusp size in tricuspid aortic valves. Possible link with isolated aortic stenosis. *British Heart Journal*, **39**, 1006–1011.

31. McKay, R. & Ross, D.N. (1982) Technique for the relief of discrete subaortic stenosis. *Journal of Thoracic and Cardiovascular Surgery*, **84**, 917–920.

32. Moulaert, A.J. & Oppenheimer-Dekker, A. (1976) Anterolateral muscle bundle of the left ventricle, bulboventricular flange and subaortic stenosis. *American Journal of Cardiology*, **37**, 78–81.

33. Anderson, R.H., Lenox, C.C. & Zuberbuhler, J.R. (1983) Morphology of ventricular septal defect associated with coarctation of the aorta. *British Heart Journal*, **50**, 176–181.

34. Morrow, A.G. (1978) Hypertrophic subaortic stenosis: operative methods utilized to relieve left ventricular outflow obstruction. *Journal of Thoracic and Cardiovascular Surgery*, **76**, 423–430.

35. Doty, D.B., Polansky, D.B. & Jenson, C.B. (1977) Supravalvular aortic stenosis. Repair by extended aortoplasty. *Journal of Thoracic and Cardiovascular Surgery*, **74**, 362–371.

36. Frantz, P.J., Murray, G.F. & Wilcox, B.R. (1980) Surgical management of left ventricular–aortic discontinuity complicating bacterial endocarditis. *Annals of Thoracic Surgery*, **29**, 1–7.

37. Gilbert, J.W., Morrow, A.G. & Talbert, J.W. (1963) The surgical significance of hypertrophic infundibular obstruction accompanying valvar pulmonary stenosis. *Journal of Thoracic and Cardiovascular Surgery*, **46**, 457–467.

38. Haworth, S.G. & Macartney, F.J. (1980) Growth and development of pulmonary circulation in pulmonary atresia with ventricular septal defect and major aortopulmonary collateral arteries. *British Heart Journal*, **44**, 14–24.

39. Anderson, R.H. & Tynan, M. (1988) Tetralogy of Fallot — a centennial review. *International Journal of Cardiology*, **21**, 219–232.

40. Anderson, R.H., Allwork, S.P., Ho, S.Y., Lenox, C.C. & Zuberbuhler, J.R. (1981) Surgical anatomy of tetralogy of Fallot. *Journal of Thoracic and Cardiovascular Surgery*, **81**, 887–896.

41. Susuki, A., Ho, S.Y., Anderson, R.H. & Deanfield, J.E. (1990) Further morphologic studies on tetralogy of Fallot with particular emphasis on the prevalence and structure of the membranous flap. *Journal of Thoracic and Cardiovascular Surgery*, **99**, 528–535.

42. Titus, J.L., Daugherty, G.W. & Edwards, J.E. (1963) Anatomy of the atrioventricular conduction system in ventricular septal defect. *Circulation*, **28**, 72–81.

43. Anderson, R.H., Monro, J.L., Ho, S.Y., Smith, A. & Deverall, P.B. (1977) Les voies de conduction auriculo-ventriculaires dans le tetralogie de Fallot. *Coeur*, **8**, 793–807.

44. Ando, M. (1974) Subpulmonary ventricular septal defect with pulmonary stenosis. Letter to Editor. *Circulation*, **50**, 412.

45. Neirotti, R., Galindez, E., Kreutzer, G., Coronel, A.R., Pedrini, M. & Becu, L. (1978) Tetralogy of Fallot with sub-pulmonary ventricular septal defect. *Annals of Thoracic Surgery*, **25**, 51–56.

46. Blackstone, E.H., Kirklin, J.W., Bertranou, E.G., Labrosse, C.J., Soto, B. & Bargeron, I.M. Jr. (1979) Preoperative prediction from cineangiograms of post-repair right ventricular pressure in tetralogy of Fallot. *Journal of Thoracic and Cardiovascular Surgery*, **78**, 542–552.

47. Kirklin, J.W., Blackstone, E.H., Pacifico, A.D., Brown, R.N. & Bargeron, I.M. Jr. (1979) Routine primary repair vs two-stage repair of tetralogy of Fallot. *Circulation*, **60**, 373–385.

48. Van Praagh, R. (1968) What is the Taussig–Bing malformation? *Circulation*, **38**, 445–449.

49. Kjellberg, S.R., Mannheimer, E., Rudhe, U. & Jonsson, B. (1959) *Diagnosis of Congenital Heart Disease*. 2nd Edition. Chicago: Year Book Medical Publishers.

50. McFadden, P.M., Culpepper, W.S. III & Ochsner, J.L. (1982) Iatrogenic right ventricular failure in tetralogy of Fallot repairs: reappraisal of a distressing problem. *Annals of Thoracic Surgery*, **33**, 400–402.

51. Alfieri, O., Blackstone, E.H., Kirklin, J.W., Pacifico, A.D. & Bargeron, I.M. Jr. (1978) Surgical treatment of tetralogy of Fallot with pulmonary atresia. *Journal of Thoracic and Cardiovascular Surgery*, **76**, 321–335.

52. Macartney, F.J., Scott, O. & Deverall, P.B. (1974) Haemodynamic and anatomical characteristics of pulmonary blood supply in pulmonary atresia with ventricular septal defect — including a case of persistent fifth aortic arch. *British Heart Journal*, **36**, 1049–1060.

53. Pahl, E., Fong, L., Anderson, R.H., Park, S.C. & Zuberbuhler, J.R. (1989) Fistulous communications between a solitary coronary artery and the pulmonary arteries as the primary source of pulmonary blood supply in tetralogy of Fallot with pulmonary valve atresia. *American Journal of Cardiology*, **63**, 140–143.

54. Dobell, A.R.C. & Grignon, A. (1977) Early and late results in pulmonary atresia. *Annals of Thoracic Surgery*, **24**, 264–274.

55. Moulton, A.L., Bowman, F.O., Edie, R.N., Hayes, C.J., Ellis, K., Gersony, W.M. & Malm, J. (1979) Pulmonary atresia with intact ventricular septum. Sixteen-year experience. *Journal of Thoracic and Cardiovascular Surgery*, **78**, 527–536.

56. Freedom, R.M., Dische, M.R. & Rowe, R.D. (1978) The tricuspid valve in pulmonary atresia with intact ventricular septum. A morphological study of 60 cases. *Archives of Pathology and Laboratory Medicine*, **102**, 28–31.

57. Zuberbuhler, J.R. & Anderson, R.H. (1979) Morphological variations in pulmonary atresia with intact ventricular septum. *British Heart Journal*, **41**, 281–288.

58. de Leval, M., Bull, C., Stark, J., Anderson, R.H., Taylor, J.F.N. & Macartney, F.J. (1982) Pulmonary atresia and intact ventricular septum: surgical management based on a revised classification. *Circulation*, **66**, 272–280.

59. Bull, C., de Leval, M.R., Mercanti, C., Macartney, F.J. & Anderson, R.H. (1982) Pulmonary atresia with intact ventricular septum: a revised classification. *Circulation*, **66**, 266–271.

60. Smith, R.D., DuShane, J.W. & Edwards, J.E. (1959) Congenital insufficiency of the pulmonary valve: including a case of fetal cardiac failure. *Circulation*, **20**, 554–560.

61. Macartney, F.J. & Miller, G.A.H. (1970) Congenital absence of the pulmonary valve. *British Heart Journal*, **32**, 483–490.

62. Emmanouilides, G.C., Thanopoulos, B., Siassi, B. & Fishbein, M. (1976) Agenesis of ductus arteriosus associated with the syndrome of tetralogy of Fallot and absent pulmonary valve. *American Journal of Cardiology*, **37**, 403–409.

63. Goor, D.A. & Lillehei, C.W. (1975) Pulmonary valvular insufficiency. In *Congenital Malformations of the Heart*. New York: Grune and Stratton, pp. 336–339.

LESIONS IN ABNORMALLY CONNECTED HEARTS

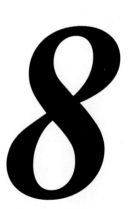

Double Inlet Ventricle

Introduction

Over the years, hearts with double inlet ventricle have represented one of the greater challenges to surgical correction, and have also posed the greatest problems in adequate description and categorization. Thus, even now, the lesions are often described in terms of 'single ventricles' or 'univentricular hearts', despite the fact that most hearts with a double inlet atrioventricular connexion have two chambers within the ventricular mass — one large and the other small[1-3].

This section will describe the relevant anatomic characteristics of all those hearts unified by the presence of the double inlet *connexion*, irrespective of whether or not they have one or two ventricles, and avoiding any controversies of whether a chamber within the ventricular mass does or does not deserve ventricular status. Pointless arguments regarding definitions of a ventricular chamber have tended to obscure many of the important morpho-

logical features of the hearts to be discussed. With our approach, as discussed in Chapter 6, a heart has a double inlet atrioventricular connexion whenever the greater part of both atrioventricular junctions (those of the right-sided and left-sided atrial chambers) are connected to the same ventricle. Usually, such a connexion is guarded by two separate atrioventricular valves, one for each atrium (Fig. 8.1). It can also exist when the two atrial chambers are connected to the same ventricle through a common valve (Fig. 8.2), or in the presence of overriding and straddling atrioventricular valves when the precise arrangement of the overriding junctions is such as to leave the majority connected to the same ventricle (Fig. 8.3). It is these atrioventricular connexions that determine the surgical options since, whenever hearts are found with double inlet ventricle as defined above, either there must be a solitary ventricle present or else, in those hearts with two ventricles, one of them must be incomplete or rudimentary, lacking a complete inlet component.

Surgical Anatomy of Double Inlet Ventricle

Although the surgical options will be the same, the hearts qualifying for this category can show marked anatomic variation. They can exist with any arrangement of the atrial chambers, with one of three ventricular morphologies, with the variations in valvar morphology discussed above, with any ventriculo–arterial connexion, and with varied associated malformations[1-3]. From the surgical viewpoint, the most important differentiating feature is the morphology of the ventricular mass. Three subsets can be distinguished: those with the atrial chambers connected to a dominant left ventricle in the presence of a rudimentary and incomplete right ventricle; those with a dominant right and an incomplete and rudimentary left ventricle; and those with a solitary ventricle of indeterminate morphology. These three variants must then be distinguished from other hearts that, in essence, have a huge ventricular septal defect.

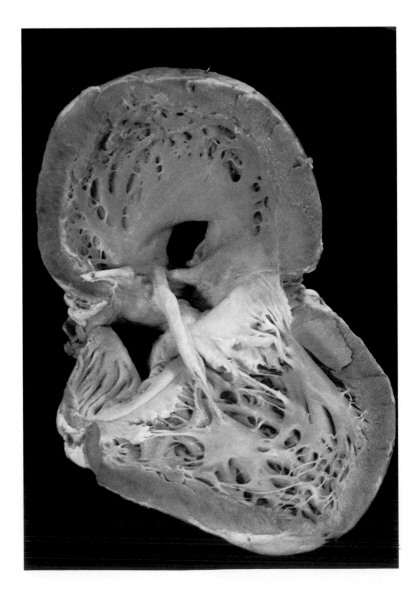

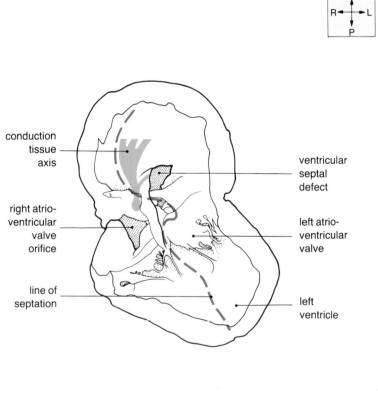

Fig. 8.1 *This specimen, shown in anatomic orientation, has been opened like a clam to show double inlet through two atrioventricular valves to a dominant left ventricle. There is a discordant ventriculo–arterial connexion. The site of the anomalous axis for atrioventricular conduction has been superimposed.*

conduction tissue axis

ventricular septal defect

right atrio-ventricular valve orifice

left atrio-ventricular valve

line of septation

left ventricle

An obvious way of surgically correcting these hearts with double inlet is to septate the dominant or solitary ventricle. The overall morphologic arrangement, however, usually conspires to defeat this option, so that the most frequent surgical tactic is to use the Fontan procedure or one of its modifications[4-8]. In this section, therefore, we will concentrate on those features influencing the Fontan procedure, although we will discuss those morphologies that lend themselves to septation, since this approach is still favoured by some surgeons[9], having fallen from grace in those centres that initially pioneered its use[10-11].

Double Inlet Left Ventricle

The most frequent variant of double inlet ventricle is seen when the atrial chambers are connected to a dominant left ventricle (Fig. 8.1). Often termed a 'single ventricle with outlet chamber', the other chamber

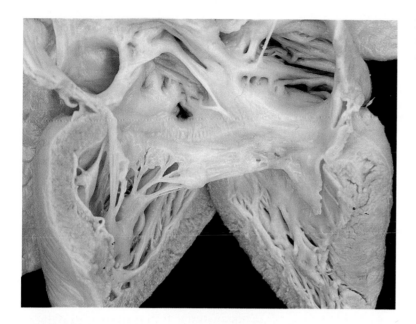

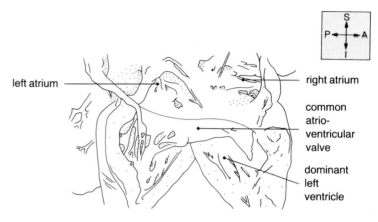

Fig. 8.2 *This specimen, viewed from the right side in anatomic orientation, has a double inlet to a dominant left ventricle with both atrioventricular junctions guarded by a common valve.*

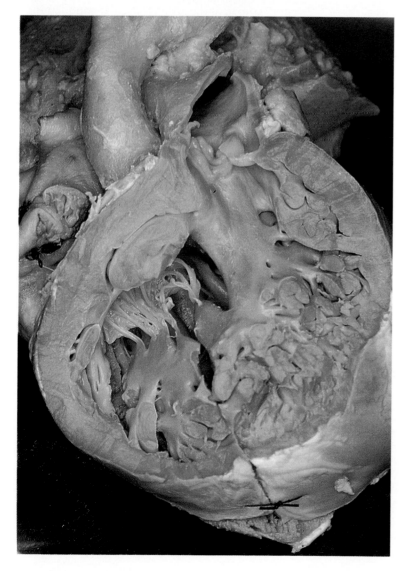

Fig. 8.3 *In this specimen with double inlet left ventricle, the right atrioventricular valve straddles and overrides such that its greater part is connected to the dominant left ventricle.*

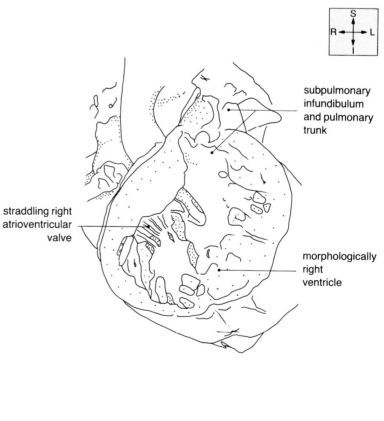

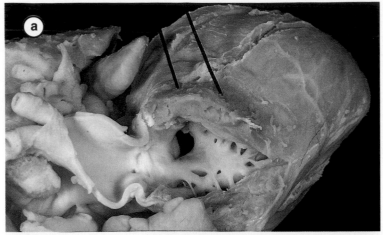

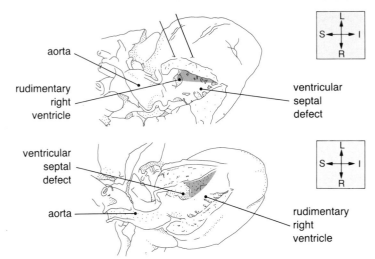

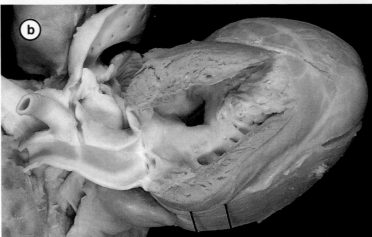

Fig. 8.4 *These rudimentary right ventricles from hearts with a double inlet left ventricle are seen in surgical orientation: (a) a right-sided rudimentary ventricle; (b) a rudimentary ventricle in left-sided location. Both figures have been marked to show the area of septum that can safely be removed to enlarge the septal defect.*

is, in reality, an incomplete and rudimentary right ventricle. It lacks its inlet component, either completely when the atrial chambers are exclusively connected to the dominant left ventricle, or for the greater part when there is overriding of one (or rarely both) atrioventricular junction(s) (Fig. 8.3). The relationship of the incomplete right ventricle can vary in that it may be to the right or left of the dominant left ventricle. It is always located in an antero-superior position (Fig. 8.4).

Indeed, the morphology of the incomplete ventricle is affected to a greater extent by the ventriculo–arterial connexion than by its position, and this connexion also dictates the surgical options. Usually, the ventriculo–arterial connexion is discordant, that is to say the aorta arises from the rudimentary and incomplete right ventricle, while the pulmonary trunk is connected to the dominant ventricle. The crucial feature is then the dimensions of the ventricular septal defect, since this must be of adequate size to support the systemic circulation irrespective of the surgical tactics to be adopted. Often it is restrictive, and may then require surgical enlargement. The major anatomic feature of concern is the course of the atrioventricular conduction tissue axis. Originating from an anomalously located atrioventricular node (see below), irrespective of the location of the rudimentary right ventricle, the axis always runs postero-inferior to the defect when viewed from the right ventricle and is carried on the left ventricular aspect of the septal crest (Figs 8.4 and 8.5). When the ventriculo–arterial connexion is discordant, the rudimentary ventricle usually has a very short outlet portion and a more extensive apical trabecular component. So the safest way to enlarge the defect surgically[12] is to remove a wedge of the muscular septum

Fig. 8.5 *This diagram, drawn in surgical orientation, shows the relationship of the axis of atrioventricular conduction tissue to the ventricular septal defect in double inlet left ventricle when viewed from the rudimentary and incomplete right ventricle.*

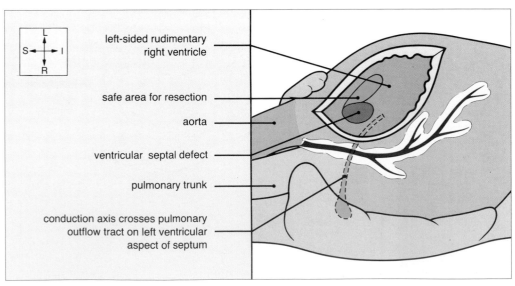

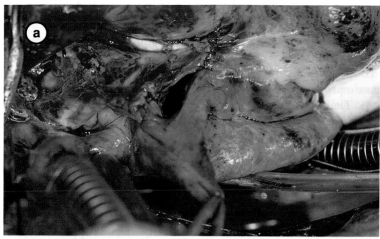

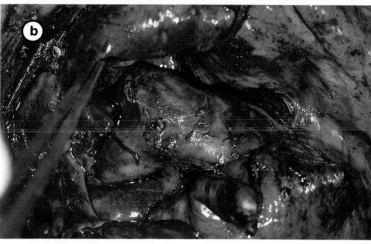

pulmonary trunk

incision in roof
of right atrium

right atrial
appendage

aorta

left pulmonary
artery

pulmonary trunk

right atrium

Fig. 8.6 *(a)* An
operative view
showing the incision in
the right atrial roof at
its junction with the
appendage. *(b)* This
view shows the
completed anastomosis
of the pulmonary
trunk to the right
atrium.

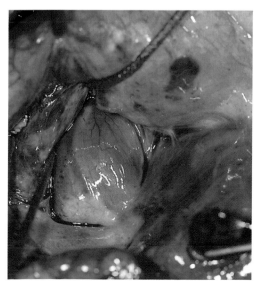

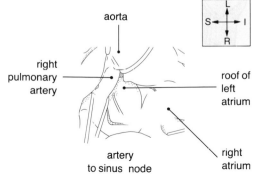

aorta

right
pulmonary
artery

roof of
left
atrium

artery
to sinus node

right
atrium

Fig. 8.7 *This view of the same heart as seen
in Fig. 8.6 shows the artery to the sinus node
coursing across the roof of the left atrium near the
interatrial groove at the base of the right atrial
appendage.*

closest to the obtuse margin of the heart as
marked by the left-sided delimiting
coronary artery (Figs 8.4 and 8.5).

Holmes Heart
Less frequently in hearts with double inlet
left ventricle, the ventriculo–arterial
connexion may be concordant or a double
outlet from the dominant or rudimentary
ventricle. The variant with a concordant
connexion is of most interest. Often
described as the 'Holmes Heart'[13], the
rudimentary right ventricle in this anomaly
is markedly different from the variant with
a discordant ventriculo–arterial connexion.
The outlet component is much longer
when the pulmonary trunk arises from the
incomplete right ventricle, and the chamber
is virtually indistinguishable from the
rudimentary right ventricle seen in hearts
with tricuspid atresia. The ventricular
septal defect is often restrictive in this form
of double inlet left ventricle, and the same
rules pertain should it require surgical
enlargement. This is unlikely to be performed, however, unless a septation is also
attempted. The more likely approach will
be to perform a Fontan procedure by
means of an atriopulmonary connexion
(see below). The rudimentary right
ventricle will then be excluded from the
circulation.

Fontan Procedure
Taken overall, the Fontan procedure (or
one of its modifications) will be the most
likely operation for hearts with double
inlet left ventricle. It can successfully be
used for all the various anatomic variants
whenever the haemodynamic criteria are
satisfactory[14]. Today, the procedure
almost always includes connecting the
right atrium directly, in one way or
another, to the pulmonary arteries. There
were vogues for the use of aortic homo-
grafts for this procedure[15], along with the
insertion of valves at the orifices of the
caval veins[16], these manoeuvres being
designed to preserve the pumping function
of the right atrium. Now, it is much more
usual to anastomose directly the atrial roof
at its junction with the appendage to the
pulmonary trunk (Fig. 8.6). Juxtaposition
of the atrial appendages, a not infrequent
associated malformation with double inlet
left ventricle, makes this anastomosis even
simpler.
   The important structures to be avoided
when connecting the atrium to the
pulmonary arteries are the sinus node and
its arterial supply. In this respect, the
crucial area is the interatrial groove through
which the artery to the sinus node courses
irrespective of its arterial origin (Fig. 8.7).

ventricular valve. The rudimentary and incomplete left ventricle, usually found in a left-sided position, although sometimes found to the right, is then nothing more than a trabeculated pouch (Fig. 8.11).

The Fontan procedure is the most likely surgical option, in which case the landmarks within the atrial chambers, together with the surgical caveats, are as discussed for double inlet left ventricle.

Sometimes, double inlet right ventricle can be found with a concordant atrioventricular connexion, often with a common valve guarding the atrioventricular junctions. Should the ventricular septal defect between dominant right and rudimentary left ventricle require enlargement in this situation (Fig. 8.12), the axis of

atrioventricular conduction descends from a node within its usual position in the triangle of Koch except when the rudimentary ventricle is right-sided[21]. Other than with this very rare occurrence, therefore, it is the antero-cephalad margin of the ventricular septum that can be resected (Fig. 8.12). Those rare hearts with double inlet to a solitary and indeterminate ventricle usually co-exist with isomerism of the atrial appendages, when the multiple associated malformations dominate the picture. Even in examples occurring with a usual arrangement of the atrial chambers, the crossing of tension apparatus from the atrioventricular valves along with particularly coarse apical trabeculations tends to conspire against septation (Fig. 8.13).

Therefore, these hearts are also most likely to attract repair by means of the Fontan option, and the same rules apply as discussed above.

It is those hearts with huge ventricular septal defects that may be confused with double inlet to a solitary ventricle (Fig. 8.14). Septation in these rare anomalies can also be a formidable undertaking, but the presence of a rim of muscular septum separating the apical trabecular components, together with the inlet septum rising to the crux, provide the anatomic landmarks. The axis of conduction tissue descends from the regular atrioventricular node when the atrioventricular connexion is concordant in this setting (Fig. 8.14).

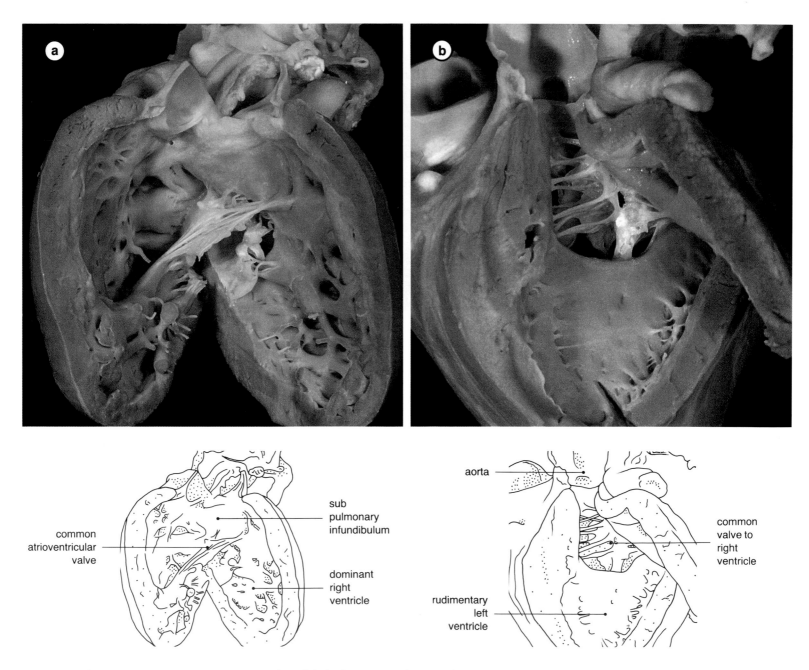

Fig. 8.12 *These views, in anatomic orientation, show* **(a)** *the dominant right ventricle in a specimen with double inlet through a common atrioventricular valve with concordant ventriculo–arterial connexion. and* **(b)** *the incomplete and rudimentary left-sided left ventricle that gives rise to the aorta.*

Tricuspid and Mitral Atresia

Introduction

The essence of most examples of tricuspid atresia is complete absence of the right atrioventricular connexion (see Chapter 6, Fig. 6.2). In similar fashion, a good proportion of cases of mitral atresia exist because of the absence of the left atrio-ventricular connexion (see Fig. 6.9). The ventricular morphology in these hearts is directly comparable to those with double inlet, with the obvious proviso that only one valve enters the dominant ventricle when one connexion is absent, since the atrioventricular junctions connect to only

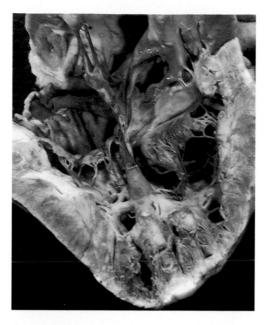

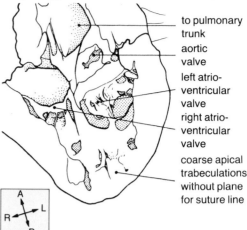

Fig. 8.13 *This specimen, seen in anatomic orientation, has double inlet to and double outlet from a solitary ventricle of indeterminate morphology.*

to pulmonary trunk
aortic valve
left atrio-ventricular valve
right atrio-ventricular valve
coarse apical trabeculations without plane for suture line

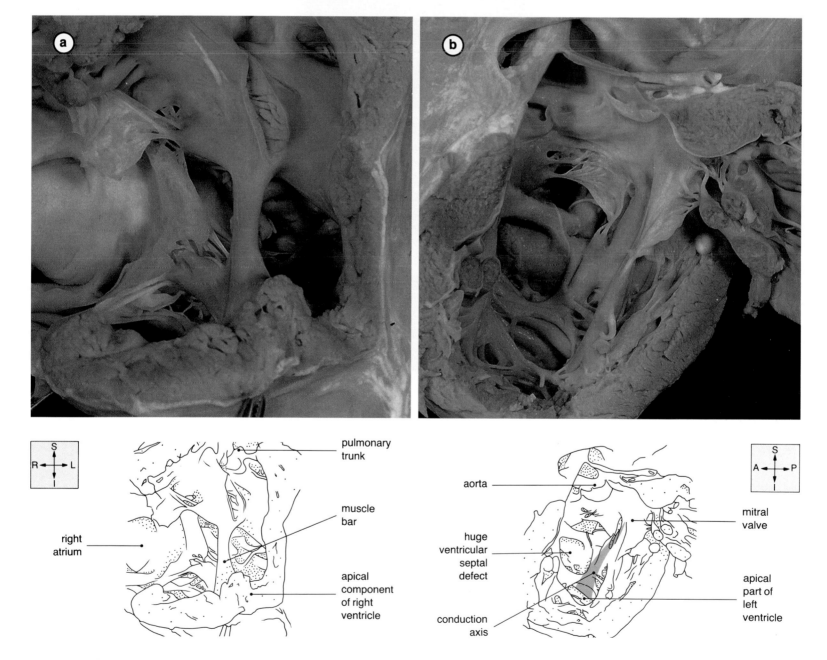

pulmonary trunk

muscle bar

apical component of right ventricle

right atrium

aorta

huge ventricular septal defect

conduction axis

mitral valve

apical part of left ventricle

Fig. 8.14 *These views, in anatomic orientation, show (a) the right and (b) left ventricles in a heart with a concordant atrioventricular connexion and a huge ventricular septal defect. The site of the axis of atrioventricular conduction tissue has been marked on the left ventricular aspect of the septum.*

one ventricle. The possible segmental combinations are just as great when one atrioventricular connexion is absent as is the case for double inlet ventricle. By far the greatest number of cases encountered, however, have what are recognized as 'classical' types of valvar atresia. It is on these that attention will be concentrated.

Surgical Anatomy of Tricuspid Atresia

In tricuspid atresia, the morphologically right atrium is usually blind-ending with no vestige of the tissues of the tricuspid valve in its floor (Fig. 8.15). Because of the absent connexion, the right ventricle is rudimentary and incomplete (Fig. 8.16), completely lacking its inlet component. The apical trabecular part of the incomplete ventricle is separated from the left ventricle by the apical trabecular septum which, as in double inlet left ventricle, does not extend to the crux.

Concordant Ventriculo–Arterial Connexion

The surgical procedure for 'correction' is again the Fontan operation or one of its modifications. Initially, in hearts with a concordant ventriculo–arterial connexion, attempts were often made to incorporate the rudimentary right ventricle into the pulmonary circulation[22]. Presently, most if not all surgeons use an atriopulmonary connexion. When preparing the right atrium, the muscle bundles and the arterial supply should be disturbed as little as possible. Preservation of the sinus node and its blood supply is particularly important, as atrial arrhythmia is a recognized life-threatening postoperative complication. The rules for avoidance of these structures are as described above for double inlet ventricle. Whenever a well-formed Eustachian valve is encountered (a frequent occurrence), it should be preserved. The atrium can be connected to the pulmonary arteries using a valved aortic homograft, but it is much more usual for the surgeon to make a direct, wide connexion between the right atrium and the pulmonary arteries. The artery to the sinus node may

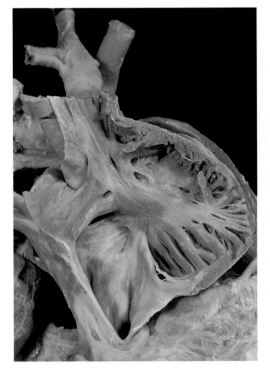

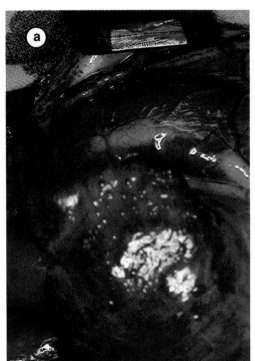

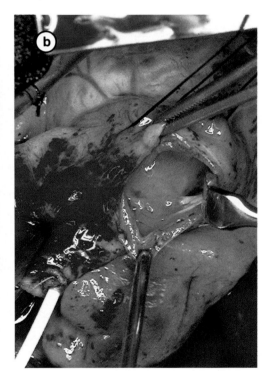

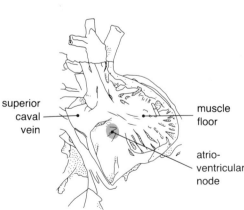

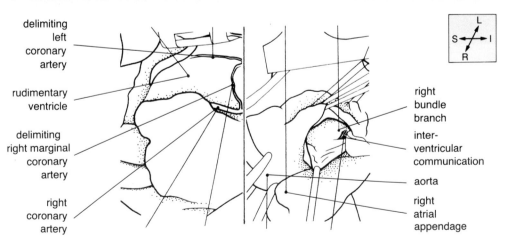

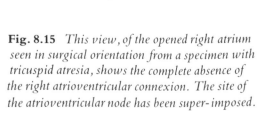

Fig. 8.15 *This view, of the opened right atrium seen in surgical orientation from a specimen with tricuspid atresia, shows the complete absence of the right atrioventricular connexion. The site of the atrioventricular node has been super-imposed.*

Fig. 8.16 *These operative views through a median sternotomy in a patient with tricuspid atresia show (a) the site of the rudimentary right ventricle and (b) the view through an incision within the rudimentary ventricle.*

be particularly at risk during this procedure as the artery traverses the interatrial groove. Another alternative, as for double inlet left ventricle, is to construct a cavopulmonary anastomosis[19]. In this case, the suture lines must be kept well away from the conduction tissues and their blood supply.

Discordant Ventriculo–Arterial Connexion

When the Fontan procedure is performed in hearts with a discordant ventriculo–arterial connexion, it may be necessary to resect the margins of the ventricular septal defect should it be restrictive. This must be done in a way that avoids the atrioven-tricular conduction axis on the left ventricular aspect of the septum. When seen from the right ventricle, this runs postero-inferior to the septal defect as in double inlet left ventricle, except in those rare cases where the communication is atretic and an apical trabecular defect is present (Fig. 8.17).

Imperforate Valvar Membrane

In very rare cases, tricuspid atresia may be due to an imperforate valvar membrane interposed between the right atrium and ventricle[23]. It will be exceptional if the membrane is of a size sufficient to permit its resection and replacement with a prosthesis.

Surgical Anatomy of Mitral Atresia

Operative treatment of mitral atresia is complicated because of its usual association with aortic atresia. Direct surgical correction involves reconstruction of the arterial pathways as an initial procedure followed by a subsequent modified Fontan procedure[24–26]. The options in these procedures are dictated by the arterial rather than the ventricular morphology (Fig. 8.18). In some cases of 'mitral' atresia, however, the aortic outflow tract is patent. 'Mitral atresia' may not be the best description of all these hearts since, in many, the embryological considerations suggest that the left connexion, had it formed, would have been guarded by a tricuspid valve.

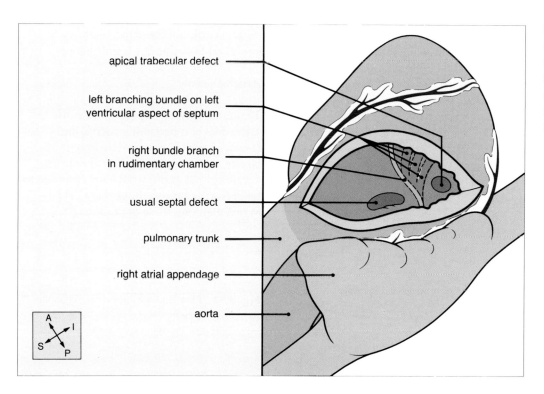

apical trabecular defect

left branching bundle on left ventricular aspect of septum

right bundle branch in rudimentary chamber

usual septal defect

pulmonary trunk

right atrial appendage

aorta

Fig. 8.17 *This diagram, viewed in surgical orientation, shows the route of the atrio-ventricular conduction tissue axis relative to the usual ventricular septal defect in tricuspid atresia, and to a defect within the apical trabecular component of the incomplete and rudimentary right ventricle.*

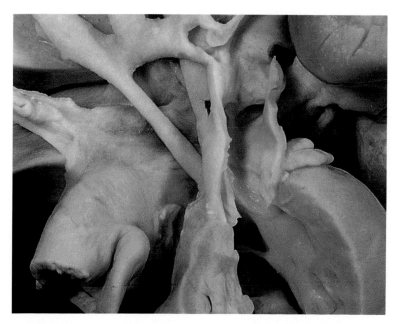

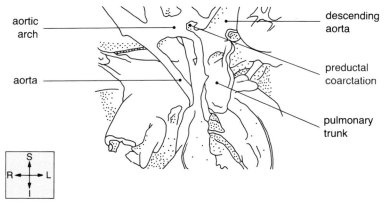

aortic arch

aorta

descending aorta

preductal coarctation

pulmonary trunk

Fig. 8.18 *This specimen, viewed in anatomic orientation, shows the typical arrangement of the arterial trunks in combined aortic and mitral atresia that provides the challenge to surgical repair by the Norwood procedure. Note the preductal aortic coarctation and the arterial duct feeding the descending aorta.*

Irrespective of such speculation, all cases have absence of the left-sided atrioventricular connexion so that pulmonary venous return has no route to the ventricles other than by way of an atrial septal defect and the right atrioventricular valve. Initial survival in these cases, therefore, depends on the state of the atrial septum. The operation of choice is likely to be a Blalock–Hanlon septostomy, after which some sort of modified Fontan procedure may be possible, particularly if it is possible to construct a cavopulmonary connexion.

Complete Transposition

Introduction

This malformation is characterized by the atrial chambers being connected to their appropriate ventricles but with inappropriate ventriculo–arterial connexions. The result is a concordant atrioventricular connexion combined with a discordant ventriculo–arterial connexion. Most refer to this combination simply as 'transposition' or 'TGA'. This usage is less than precise.

In the past there has been disagreement as to whether the term 'transposition' should be used only to describe a discordant ventriculo–arterial connexion[27], or could be used to describe any heart with an anterior aorta[28]. More significantly, those using the term 'TGA' to describe a discordant ventriculo–arterial connexion do not restrict it to the setting of a concordant atrioventricular connexion. 'Transposition', when defined simply as a discordant ventriculo–arterial connexion, can coexist with a discordant atrioventricular connexion, with double inlet ventricle, or with the absence of one atrioventricular connexion. It is these latter anomalies that then become the dominant features. There is, therefore, a need for a term that describes only the chamber combinations of a concordant atrioventricular connexion and a discordant ventriculo–arterial connexion (Fig. 8.19). The preferred term is 'complete transposition'.

Some still use 'd-transposition' to the same end, but this convention does not accurately describe those cases with the usual atrial arrangement, a concordant atrioventricular connexion and a discordant ventriculo–arterial connexion, and a left-sided aorta. Neither does 'd-transposition' describe the majority of patients presenting with the chamber combinations which produce complete transposition along with a mirror-image atrial arrangement.

It should also be noted that complete transposition, as here defined, refers only to patients with usual and mirror-image arrangements. When a discordant ventriculo–arterial connexion occurs in the setting of isomerism of the atrial appendages, it is the anomalies at the venoatrial and atrioventricular junctions which usually dominate the anatomical and clinical considerations. These cases are, therefore, excluded from the category of complete transposition described here.

Surgical Anatomy of Complete Transposition

From the surgical standpoint, the two major subgroups of complete transposition are those without any major additional complicating lesions (simple complete transposition) and those with additional malformations (complex complete transposition). The morphological aspects of the complicating anomalies will be dealt with in turn, but the atrial anatomy is comparable within the whole group.

Atrial Anatomy

Though a corrective procedure at the arterial level is becoming increasingly favoured as the operative treatment of choice, operations designed to redirect venous blood at the atrial level continue to be performed throughout the world. When planning these operations (the

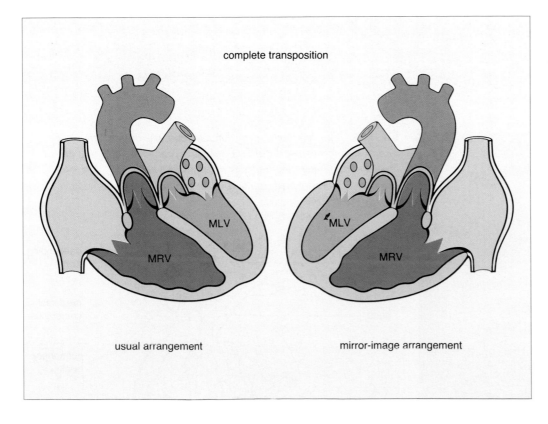

complete transposition

MLV
MRV

usual arrangement

MLV
MRV

mirror-image arrangement

Fig. 8.19 *This diagram shows the segmental combinations that produce the lesion described, preferably, as complete transposition.*

Mustard and Senning procedures), the disposition of the cardiac nodes and their blood supply is an important factor.

Sinus Node

The presence of a discordant ventriculo–arterial connexion does not in any way affect the position of the sinus node, so the rules enunciated in Chapter 2 for avoidance of this node are equally applicable in the case of complete transposition. The entire terminal groove should be avoided as the sinus node may occupy a 'horseshoe' position over the crest of the junction of the superior caval vein with the right atrium, although it is usually in a lateral position (see Fig. 2.10). The nodal artery may enter the groove across the crest of the appendage or after it has taken a retrocaval course (see Fig. 2.16b). Of more importance is the course taken by the nodal artery as it ascends the interatrial groove. The artery frequently burrows into the atrial musculature, running within the superior border of the oval fossa (Fig. 8.20). It is at risk in this position when incising the septum for either a Senning or Mustard procedure, or during a Blalock–Hanlon septostomy.

Certain considerations are crucial when carrying out a venous switch procedure. Cannulation of the superior caval vein should be performed a good distance from the cavoatrial junction, incising the right atrium well clear of the terminal groove and avoiding traction, suction or suturing in the area of the superior border of the groove. If an incision is required across the groove to widen the newly constructed pulmonary venous atrium in Mustard's operation, it can be made between the right pulmonary veins without fear of damaging the sinus node or its artery.

Arrhythmias. This discussion is pertinent to the genesis of arrhythmias after Mustard's operation or the Senning procedure. It has been suggested that the arrhythmias are due to the damage to the so-called 'specialized internodal pathways'. As explained in Chapter 2, there are no such pathways composed of histologically specialized tissue. Instead, the atrioventricular impulse is preferentially conducted from the sinus node through the thicker muscles of the right atrial wall and septum. It is advantageous, therefore, to preserve at least one of these routes. If the terminal crest is to be divided to enlarge the new pulmonary venous atrium, this is a further reason to preserve the superior border of the oval fossa. These procedures, together with scrupulous avoidance of the sinus node and its blood supply, mean that arrhythmias can be considerably reduced after atrial redirection procedures.

Atrioventricular Node

It is always important to avoid the atrioventricular node. The landmarks to this vital structure are the same as in the normal heart (Fig. 8.21). Providing all surgery is performed outside the triangle of Koch, injury to the node will be avoided. The technique of cutting back the coronary sinus should be carefully considered. It is possible to perform this procedure without damaging the node and its zones of transitional cells, but the incision will undoubtedly cross one of the preferential routes of conduction. For this reason, it is safer to place the inferior suture line so as to avoid completely the triangle of Koch.

Ventricular Septal Defect

The major complicating lesion in complete transposition is the presence of a ventricular septal defect with or without obstruction of the left ventricular outflow tract. Any other lesion can coexist if anatomically possible and the anatomy will then be as described for the lesion in isolation.

A ventricular septal defect in complete transposition can be as variable in morphology as those found in isolation (see Chapter 7, p.7.18). The majority of defects open between the outlet components of the ventricular mass and have their own peculiar characteristics. They can either be

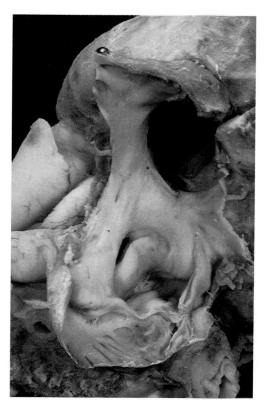

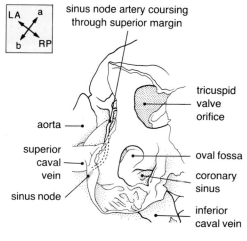

Fig. 8.20 *This dissection of a specimen of completion transposition seen in surgical orientation shows the relationship of the artery to the sinus node to the superior rim of the oval fossa.*

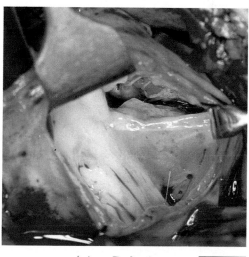

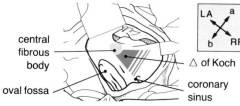

Fig. 8.21 *This view through a right atriotomy shows the landmarks of the triangle of Koch.*

perimembranous (Fig. 8.22a) or have a muscular postero–inferior rim (Fig. 8.22b). The distinguishing feature, as in tetralogy of Fallot, is whether or not the posterior limb of the septomarginal trabeculation fuses with the ventriculo–infundibular fold. If there is fusion (Fig. 8.22b), the resultant muscle will buttress the conduction axis and there will be valvar discontinuity between the leaflets of the tricuspid and pulmonary valves. If there is no fusion, the defect will be perimembranous and there will be fibrous continuity between the valvar leaflets. The penetrating bundle will be at risk in this area of fibrous continuity (Fig. 8.22a).

These defects have other features of surgical significance. The tension apparatus of the tricuspid valve tends to course over the defect and attach to the outlet septum or to the ventriculo–infundibular fold. This makes closure of the defect difficult without causing damage to the tricuspid

valve. Also, the borders of the defect diverge towards the parietal and anterior heart walls. In hearts with a concordant ventriculo–arterial connexion, the anterior margin of a ventricular septal defect is usually well circumscribed. In the setting of complete transposition, the outlet septum becomes malaligned in relation to the rest of the muscular ventricular septum as it inserts into the anterior wall of the right ventricular outflow tract. The defect is, therefore, more difficult to close at this anterior margin.

Defects opening to the inlet of the right ventricle, be they perimembranous or muscular, also have surgical significance, as do those opening centrally (Fig. 8.23). Should a Rastelli procedure be considered for a patient with this type of defect and with coexisting pulmonary stenosis, there will be difficulty in connecting the defect to the aorta. Apical or multiple muscular defects also present this disadvantage for

intraventricular redirection to the aorta. Defects opening to the ventricular inlet which are also perimembranous are the harbingers of a straddling tricuspid valve. This should always be suspected when the right ventricle is hypoplastic. A straddling valve markedly increases the risks of surgery, not least because of the abnormal disposition of the conduction tissues (see Chapter 7, Fig. 7.39).

Pulmonary Stenosis

Subpulmonary obstruction in complete transposition can be produced by any lesion which would be produced by sub-aortic obstruction in the normal heart. Rarer lesions, such as anomalous insertion of the tension apparatus of the atrioventricular valve, are probably beyond surgical repair. Aneurysm of the membranous septum or similar fibrous tissue 'tags' (Fig. 8.24) should be readily amenable to

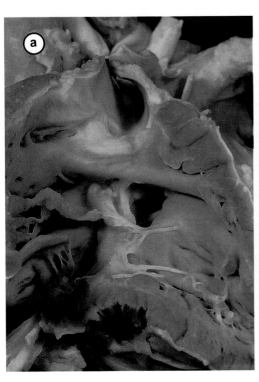
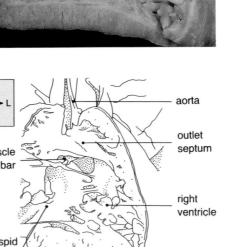
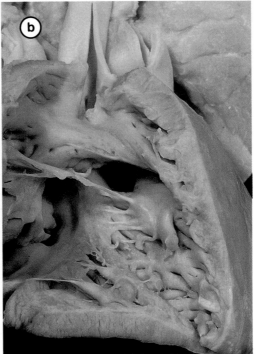

Fig. 8.22 *(a) This anatomic orientation of a specimen with complete transposition shows the right ventricular aspect of a perimembranous defect opening to the sub-aortic outlet with malalignment of the outlet septum and overriding of the pulmonary valvar leaflets. (b) This specimen, also in anatomic orientation, has a ventricular septal defect opening to the right ventricular outlet with a muscular postero-inferior rim. Note the malalignment of the outlet septum.*

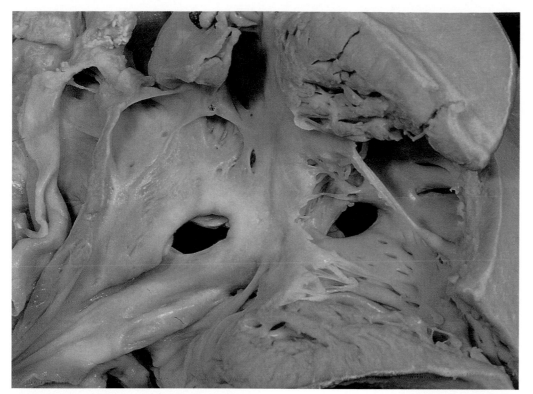

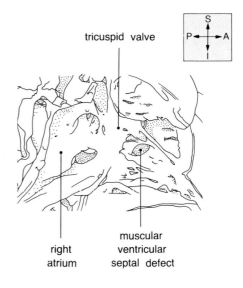

Fig. 8.23 *This anatomic orientation of the right ventricular aspect of a midmuscular ventricular septal defect in a specimen with complete transposition, illustrates the difficulty that would be encountered in trying to connect such a defect to the aorta.*

tricuspid valve

right atrium

muscular ventricular septal defect

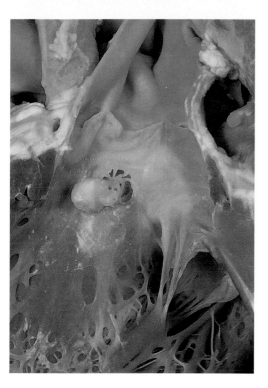

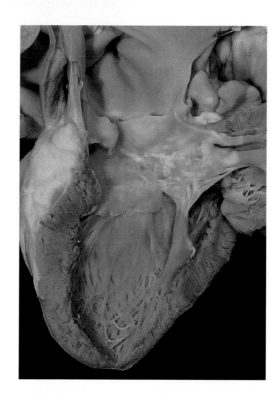

Fig. 8.24 *This anatomic orientation of the left ventricle from a specimen with complete transposition, shows a tissue tag from the septal leaflet of the tricuspid valve herniating through a perimembranous ventricular septal defect.*

Fig. 8.25 *In this anatomic orientation of the left ventricular outflow tract of a specimen with complete transposition there is obstruction due to a fibrous shelf that extends onto the leaflet of the mitral valve.*

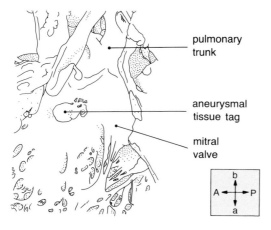

pulmonary trunk

aneurysmal tissue tag

mitral valve

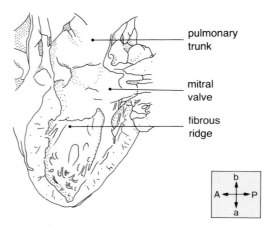

pulmonary trunk

mitral valve

fibrous ridge

removal, although a subpulmonary fibrous diaphragm poses more problems as it directly overlies the left bundle branch (Fig. 8.25). The difficulties are compounded when the fibrous obstruction is more extensive, because then it can form a subvalvar tunnel. The other quadrants of the outflow tract are also vulnerable because of their proximity to the left coronary artery or because they are formed by leaflets of the mitral valve. The safest area for resection is beneath the remnant of the left margin of the ventriculo–infundibular fold[29].

When subpulmonary obstruction coexists with a ventricular septal defect, there is almost always posterior deviation and insertion of the outlet septum into the left ventricle. This usually means that the aortic valve overrides the septum and there is a substantial septal deficiency, which is favourable for a Rastelli procedure (Fig. 8.26). Should the defect be restrictive, and a Rastelli operation is still desirable, it is possible to resect safely the outlet septum,

which never harbours conduction tissue. Should the defect be situated other than between the ventricular outlets, the chances of successfully accomplishing a Rastelli procedure are considerably reduced. Valvar pulmonary stenosis also frequently accompanies subvalvar stenosis.

Variation in Arterial and Infundibular Anatomy

Thus far, we have devoted attention exclusively to the segmental anatomy of complete transposition. There is, of course, further variation in terms of both arterial relationships and infundibular anatomy. These variations do not alter the intracardiac anatomy and are of relatively minor surgical significance. For example, the aorta is usually anterior and to the right in complete transposition but, in some cases, the aorta may be anterior and to the left (Fig. 8.27). In even rarer cases, it may be posterior and to the right of the pulmonary trunk (Fig. 8.28). As suggested, these

different relationships do not alter the basic anatomy. They do show why it is inadvisable to use the term 'd-transposition' for the group as a whole, since it makes little sense to use this term for a patient with a left-sided aorta.

There are some clues to associated lesions to be drawn from these unexpected arterial relationships. With a left-sided aorta, there is a high incidence of septal defects which are doubly committed and juxtaarterial (Fig. 8.29). This arrangement is convenient for direct connexion of the aorta to the left ventricle and Rastelli's procedure. When the aorta is posterior, there is usually a subpulmonary infundibulum with the aortic valve in fibrous continuity with the mitral valve through the roof of a perimembranous septal defect. This unusual anatomy can create difficulty both at initial diagnosis and at subsequent surgery. More recently, cases with a posterior aorta have been observed with an intact ventricular septum[30].

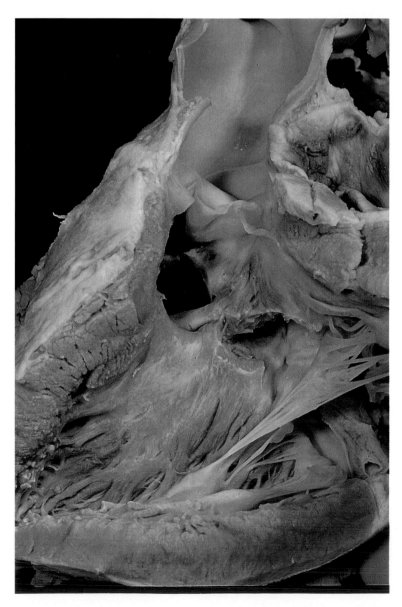

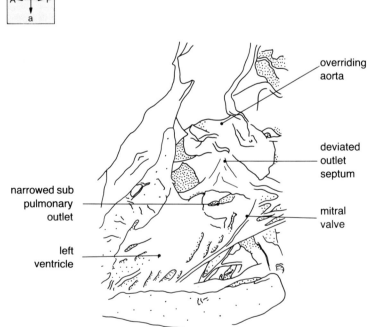

Fig. 8.26 *This specimen of complete transposition, seen from the left ventricle in anatomic orientation, displays a posterior deviation of the outlet septum that is most suitable for the Rastelli procedure.*

overriding aorta

deviated outlet septum

mitral valve

narrowed sub pulmonary outlet

left ventricle

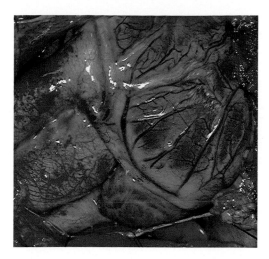

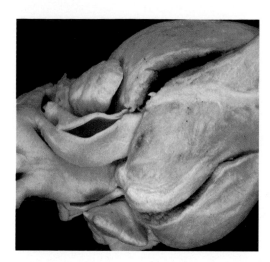

Fig. 8.27 *This surgical view through a median sternotomy shows a heart with complete transposition with the usual atrial arrangement in which the aorta is anterior and leftward relative to the pulmonary trunk.*

Fig. 8.28 *This specimen of complete transposition, shown in surgical orientation, has the aorta in a posterior and rightward position relative to the pulmonary trunk ('normal relations').*

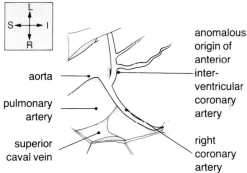

anomalous origin of anterior interventricular coronary artery

aorta

pulmonary artery

superior caval vein

right coronary artery

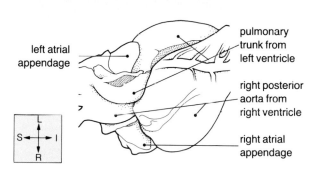

left atrial appendage

pulmonary trunk from left ventricle

right posterior aorta from right ventricle

right atrial appendage

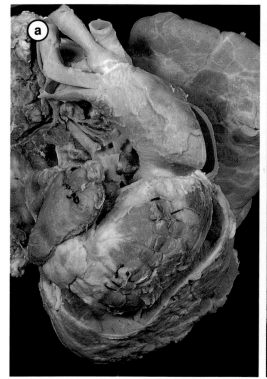

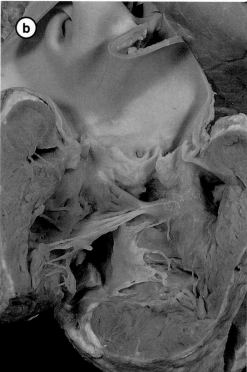

Fig. 8.29 *These anatomical orientations of a specimen with complete transposition and usual atrial arrangement illustrate (a) a left-sided aorta relative to the pulmonary trunk, the heart being in the right chest and (b) the doubly committed and juxtaarterial defect found in this heart. Note the presence of an additional muscular outlet defect.*

pulmonary trunk

left-sided aorta

apex to right

aortic–pulmonary continuity

doubly committed ventricular septal defect

right ventricle

aorta

muscle bar

muscular outlet ventricular septal defect

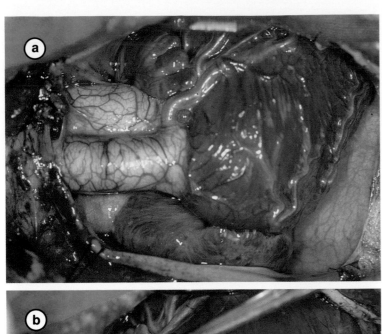

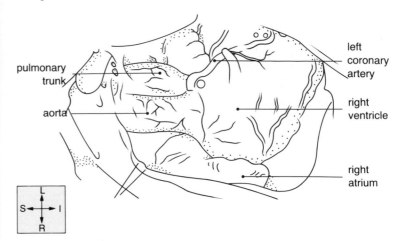

Fig. 8.30 *These are operative views of a heart with complete transposition. The* **(a)** *left and*

(b) *right coronary arteries arise from the aorta facing the pulmonary artery.*

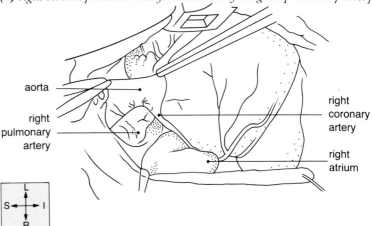

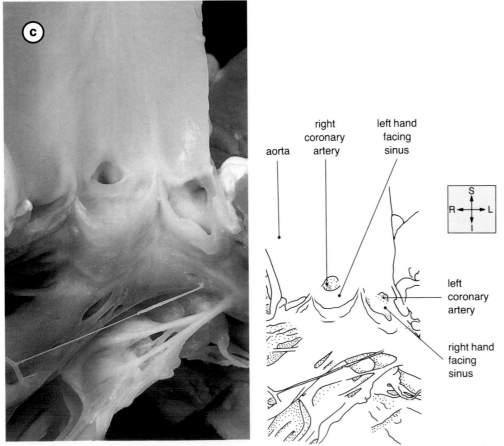

(c) This view of the opened aortic root, shown in anatomical orientation, reveals the origins of the coronary arteries from the aortic sinuses that face the pulmonary trunk. Note that the artery arising from the left hand sinus, the right coronary artery in this specimen, arises above the sinutubular bar.

Variations in infundibular morphology are unlikely to give problems. The expected sub-aortic muscular infundibulum in the right ventricle is most frequently encountered with pulmonary–mitral fibrous continuity in the left ventricle. Rarely, there may be a complete muscular infundibulum in both ventricles. Even more rarely, as described above, there may be a subpulmonary infundibulum with continuity between the leaflets of the aortic and mitral valve, particularly when the discordantly connected aorta is in posterior position.

Morphology of the Coronary Arteries and the Arterial Switch Procedure
A feature achieving increasing surgical importance in complete transposition, because of the burgeoning popularity of the arterial switch procedure, is the morphology of the coronary arteries. The operation involves transecting the ascending aorta and pulmonary trunk and reconnecting them to the appropriate ventricles. Some have advocated the ingenious construction of windows between the arterial trunks that allow the reconnexion of the arterial trunks without

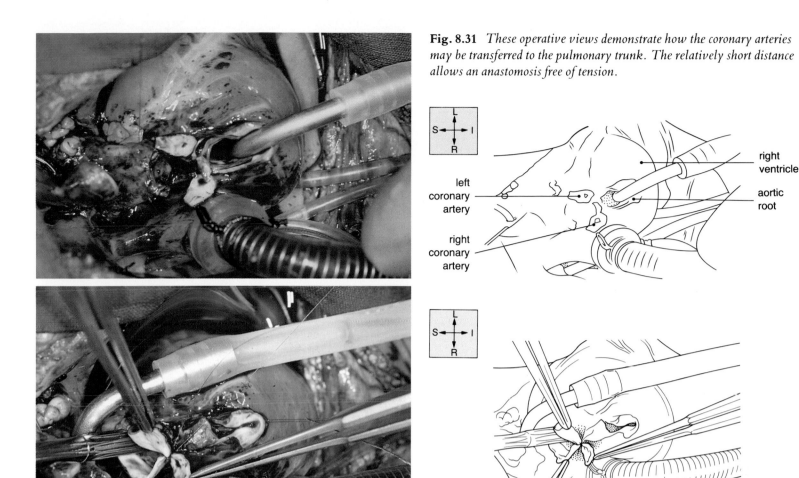

Fig. 8.31 *These operative views demonstrate how the coronary arteries may be transferred to the pulmonary trunk. The relatively short distance allows an anastomosis free of tension.*

right ventricle

aortic root

left coronary artery

right coronary artery

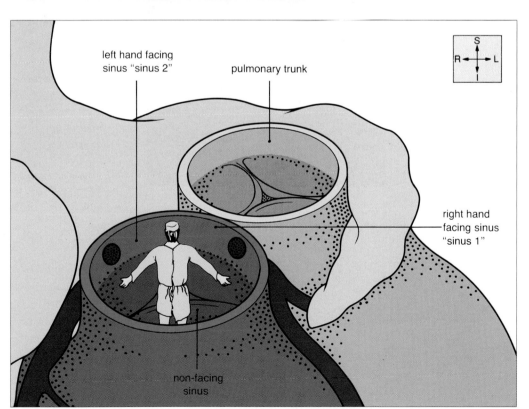

left hand facing sinus "sinus 2"

pulmonary trunk

right hand facing sinus "sinus 1"

non-facing sinus

Fig. 8.32 *This diagram shows how the two aortic sinuses that face the pulmonary trunk can always be described accurately as being to the surgeon's left hand or right hand, irrespective of the relationship of the arterial trunks, when the surgeon is considered to be standing in the non-facing sinus and looking towards the pulmonary trunk. Conventionally, the sinus to the right hand is described as 'number 1', while that to the left hand is 'number 2'.*

translocation of the coronary arteries[31]. Others have performed complicated manoeuvres involving the use of conduits[32-35]. Presently, however, translocation of the coronary arteries carries little hazard, particularly when the arteries originate from a favourable location from the aorta. Almost invariably, the coronary arteries arise from those aortic sinuses that face the pulmonary trunk (Fig. 8.30)[36]. In the arterial switch, therefore, the origins of the coronary arteries are transferred across a relatively short distance (Fig. 8.31). This holds true irrespective of the relationship of the aorta to the pulmonary trunk.

The variable relationships of the arterial trunks, however, can produce problems in naming the aortic sinuses and, hence, the origin of the coronary arteries. Truly formidable conventions are created if attempts are made to catalogue each and every pattern, while use of simple alpha-numeric codes is self-evidently procrustean. As suggested by the group from Leiden[37], it is best to name the aortic sinuses from the stance of the observer standing in the non-facing sinus and looking towards the pulmonary trunk (Fig. 8.32). One sinus is then always to the observer's right hand (often called sinus number 1), while the other sinus is left-handed (sinus number 2). The coronary arteries can then arise from either of these sinuses in any possible combination, although certain limited patterns predominate[37].

Unusual features which may compromise surgical transfer of the arteries during the switch procedure are largely related to an anomalous course of the coronary arteries in relation to the vascular pedicle (Fig. 8.33) or else an intramural course of the origin of the coronary artery across a valvar commissure[38]. What may also be significant is that, sometimes, the origin of the sinus node artery is very close to the origin of one coronary artery from an aortic sinus (Fig. 8.34). In these circumstances, transfer of the coronary artery

itself may traumatize or destroy the artery to the sinus node. Otherwise, there is no evidence of postoperative rhythm problems subsequent to the arterial switch procedure.

Congenitally Corrected Transposition

Introduction

The term 'congenitally corrected transposition' is used to describe the combination of discordant atrioventricular and ventriculo–arterial connexions. As thus defined, congenitally corrected transposition can exist with the atrial chambers in their usual arrangement or in a mirror-image position (Fig. 8.35). It cannot, by

definition, be found when there is isomerism of the atrial appendages.

To comprehend fully the complexities of corrected transposition, it is important to note the malalignment between the inlet part of the ventricular septum and the atrial septum[39]. These two septal structures are in line at the crux but, when traced forwards, they diverge markedly. This produces a gap into which is wedged the subpulmonary outflow tract from the morphologically left ventricle. This abnormal anatomy accounts for the single most important surgical feature of congenitally corrected transposition, namely the unusual disposition of the atrioventricular conduction tissues. Because of the septal malalignment, it is not possible for

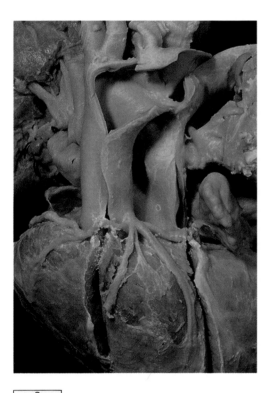

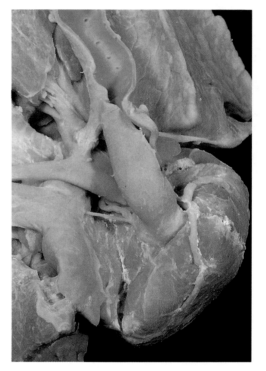

Fig. 8.33 *In this specimen with complete transposition, viewed in anatomic orientation, all the coronary arteries arise from the right hand facing sinus (number 1). The right coronary artery then crosses in front of the aorta to reach the right atrioventricular groove, while the circumflex artery crosses the subpulmonary outflow tract from the left ventricle. Note that the arterial trunks are orientated in a side-by-side relationship with the aorta to the right.*

Fig. 8.34 *In this specimen with complete transposition, seen in anatomic orientation, the right coronary artery is absent. The dominant circumflex artery arises from the left hand facing sinus (number 2) and runs a retropulmonary course. Note, however, the origin of the artery to the sinus node adjacent to the take-off of the artery from the aortic sinus. The anterior interventricular artery arises from the right hand sinus (number 1) and gives rise to a prominent infundibular artery.*

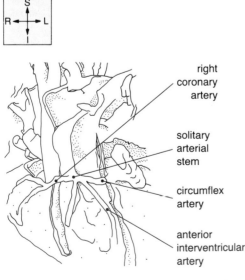

right coronary artery

solitary arterial stem

circumflex artery

anterior interventricular artery

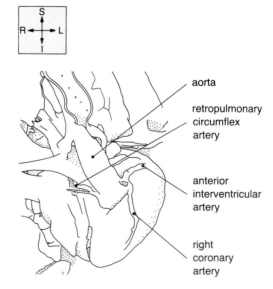

aorta

retropulmonary circumflex artery

anterior interventricular artery

right coronary artery

the normal atrioventricular node, at the apex of the triangle of Koch, to penetrate through the fibrous atrioventricular junction and make contact with the ventricular conduction tissues. Instead, an anomalous atrioventricular node, found in an antero-lateral position as occurs in double inlet left ventricle (see Fig. 8.8), gives rise to a penetrating atrioventricular bundle. This bundle penetrates the insulating plane of the atrioventricular junction lateral to the area of fibrous continuity between the leaflets of the pulmonary and mitral valves (Fig. 8.36). A long non-branching bundle then runs round the anterior quadrants of the subpulmonary outflow tract, crossing the characteristic anterior recess of the morphologically left

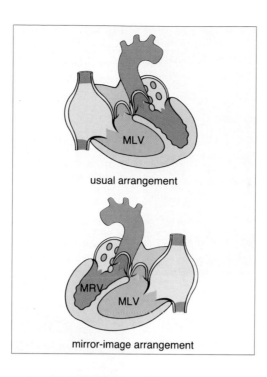

usual arrangement

mirror-image arrangement

Fig. 8.35 *This diagram shows the segmental combination that produces the lesion described, preferably, as a congenitally corrected transposition.*

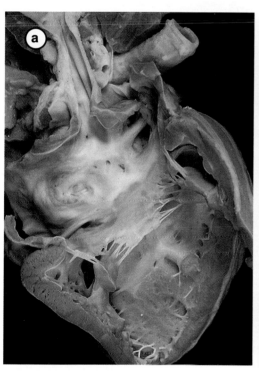

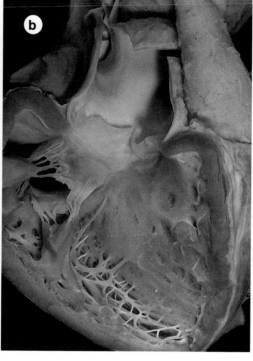

Fig. 8.36 *These anatomic orientations of a specimen with congenitally corrected transposition show the relationships of the atrioventricular conduction tissue axis to the mitral and pulmonary valves as seen (**a**) from the posterior aspect of the atrioventricular junction and (**b**) from the pulmonary outflow tract.*

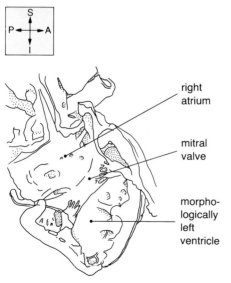

right atrium

mitral valve

morphologically left ventricle

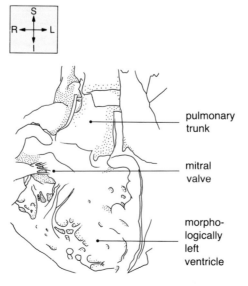

pulmonary trunk

mitral valve

morphologically left ventricle

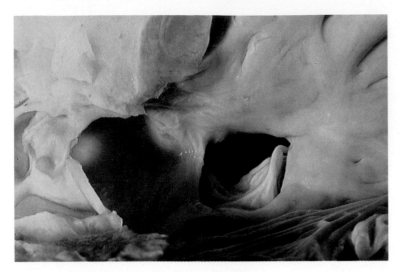

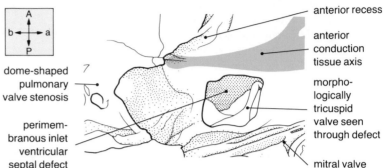

Fig. 8.37 *This surgical orientation of a specimen with congenitally corrected transposition illustrates the relationships of a perimembranous ventricular septal defect opening to the inlet of the morphologically left ventricle. Reproduced by kind permission of Prof. Anton E. Becker, University of Amsterdam.*

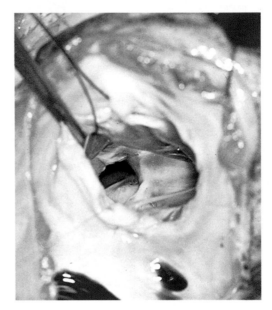

anterior recess

anterior conduction tissue axis

morphologically tricuspid valve seen through defect

dome-shaped pulmonary valve stenosis

perimembranous inlet ventricular septal defect

mitral valve

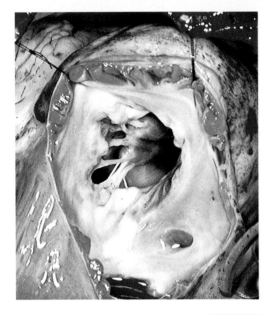

Fig. 8.38 *This surgical view of a perimembranous inlet ventricular septal defect in a congenitally corrected transposition, seen through the right-sided morphologically mitral valve, shows how the defect and the subpulmonary outflow tract are shielded behind the antero-septal commissure of the valve. Reproduced by kind permission of Dr. J. Quaegebeur, Columbia University, New York.*

right-sided mitral valve

anterior commissure

anomalous anterior node and bundle

regular node in △ of Koch (no contact)

coronary sinus

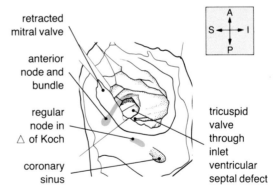

Fig. 8.39 *In this view, the defect shown in Fig. 8.38 has been revealed by retraction of the leaflets of the morphologically mitral valve. The location of the atrioventricular conduction axis has been superimposed.*

retracted mitral valve

anterior node and bundle

regular node in △ of Koch

coronary sinus

tricuspid valve through inlet ventricular septal defect

ventricle before descending onto the muscular ventricular septum and branching. The fan-like left branch of the bundle is distributed in the right-sided morphologically left ventricle, while the cord-like right branch of the bundle penetrates the septum to reach the left-sided morphologically right ventricle[40]. The discordantly connected aorta arises from this morphologically right ventricle, typically above a complete muscular infundibulum and usually in a left-sided position.

Surgical Anatomy of Associated Lesions

When congenitally corrected transposition exists without any other anomaly, the circulation of the blood is normal. Unfortunately, this situation is very much the exception[11]. Usually, one or more of three associated lesions are found. These are a ventricular septal defect, pulmonary stenosis, or anomalies of the left-sided atrioventricular valve. It is these lesions that require surgical treatment.

Ventricular Septal Defect

A ventricular septal defect is present in about 70% of cases. As in the heart with concordant atrioventricular connexions, it may be perimembranous, muscular, or doubly committed and juxtaarterial, but is usually of the perimembranous type and opens between the ventricular inlets. Then, because of the wedge position of the pulmonary valve, the pulmonary trunk tends to override the defect (Fig. 8.37).

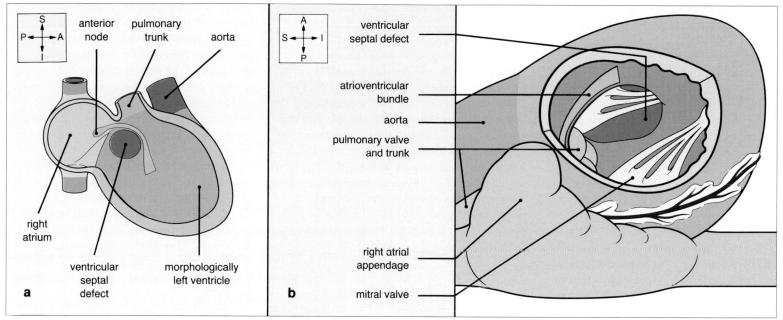

a — S / P ← → A — anterior node — pulmonary trunk — aorta — right atrium — ventricular septal defect — morphologically left ventricle

b — A / S ← → I / P — ventricular septal defect — atrioventricular bundle — aorta — pulmonary valve and trunk — right atrial appendage — mitral valve

Fig. 8.40 *These diagrams illustrate the difficulty in depicting the disposition of the atrioventricular conduction axis in congenitally corrected transposition.* **(a)** *In this case the depiction gives no depth and consequently suggests that the axis runs between the defect and the pulmonary trunk.*

(b) *When the drawing is made to give proper perspective, it is seen that the axis encircles the antero-cephalad quadrants of the subpulmonary outflow tract.*

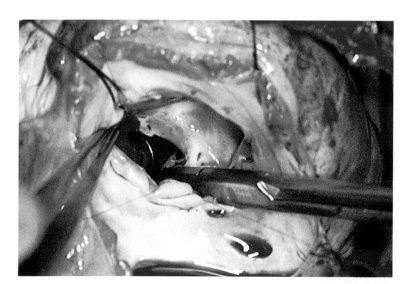

Fig. 8.41 *This further view of the heart shown in Fig. 8.38 illustrates how the conduction tissue axis can be avoided by placing sutures through the defect on its morphologically right ventricular aspect (left-sided). Reproduced by kind permission of Dr. J. Quaegebeur, Columbia University, New York.*

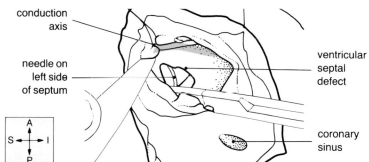

conduction axis — needle on left side of septum — ventricular septal defect — coronary sinus — A / S ← → I / P

When seen from the right atrium, it is shielded by the anterior commissure of the right-sided morphologically mitral valve (Fig. 8.38). The abnormal position of the atrioventricular node and the non-branching atrioventricular bundle must be borne in mind when closing the defect. A node at the apex of the triangle of Koch is also present, but hardly ever gives rise to a penetrating bundle. Instead, the bundle arises from the anomalous antero-lateral node, penetrates the arc of pulmonary–mitral valvar continuity, and then runs round the subpulmonary outflow tract to descend on the antero-superior margin of the defect (Fig. 8.39).

In the past, it was suggested that the bundle ran within the outlet septum between the pulmonary valve and the edge of the defect[42]. The axis of conduction tissue, so far as can be ascertained, has never been seen in this position. The reason why the bundle was shown in this site is probably one of perspective in the operating room. When the surgeon tries to put his observations onto paper in one dimension, it is difficult not to give the impression that the bundle passes between the valve and the defect (Fig. 8.40, left). Nonetheless, the true position of the bundle is anterior to the orifice of the pulmonary valve (Fig. 8.40, right).

Knowing the appropriate morphology, de Leval and his colleagues[43] have suggested that the safest way of closing the defect is to place sutures from the morphologically right ventricular (left-sided) aspect (Fig. 8.41). Although the defect opens mostly between the ventricular inlets, it can extend to become doubly committed and juxtaarterial. It is then roofed by the conjoined leaflets of the aortic and pulmonary valves (Fig. 8.42). When it is perimembranous and juxtaarterial, the conduction tissue remains in an anterior position. Cases have been described, particularly in the Far East[44], with so-called 'supracristal' defects. If such cases have a muscular inferior rim between the pulmonary and mitral valve, it is possible that the conduction tissue remains in anterior position to the defect. A comparable case has been seen with both a perimembranous and a muscular outlet defect. The conduction axis descended the muscle bar between them. If there is doubt, it is probably wise to map the disposition of the conduction tissue during the operation.

Pulmonary Stenosis

As with complete transposition, any of the lesions which produce obstruction of the left ventricular outflow tract will produce pulmonary stenosis in congenitally corrected transposition. Valvar stenosis in isolation is rare, but frequently coexists with subvalvar obstructive lesions. Particularly significant in this respect are fibrous tissue tags (Fig. 8.43). Fibrous diaphragmatic lesions (Fig. 8.44) or muscular obstruction are also encountered[45].

The overwhelming consideration in all of these types of stenosis is the presence of the non-branching bundle running round the anterior quadrants of the outflow tract. This makes it very difficult to resect these various lesions (apart from tags). Placement of a conduit is the safest means of avoiding postoperative heart block, although an ingenious method of avoiding the conduction tissues has been devised by Doty, Truesdell and Marvin[46].

Ebstein's Malformation

Ebstein's malformation is the lesion which most frequently afflicts the left-sided morphologically tricuspid valve. This involves the downward displacement of the septal and mural leaflets of the valve (Fig. 8.45). Only rarely is the inlet part of the ventricle dilated and thinned, as occurs so frequently in Ebstein's malformation

with a concordant atrioventricular connexion. Should replacement of the valve become necessary, the anterior position of the conduction tissues takes them out of the area of danger. In this respect, sometimes there is a normal node and bundle in congenitally corrected transposition, either in isolation or as part of a sling. An isolated posterior conduction system[47] is the rule when the atrial chambers are mirror-imaged and has been described in a case with the usual atrial arrangement[48]. In this particular case, there was better alignment than is usually expected between the inlet and atrial septal structures. Should there be a posterior node in a patient with Ebstein's malformation, the conduction system would then be at risk.

Straddling of the Tension Apparatus
The other anomaly that affects the left valve, and that can also affect the right valve, is straddling of the tension apparatus and overriding of the orifice. This does not alter the origin of the conduction tissues from an antero-lateral node but it will markedly increase the risks of surgery[49].

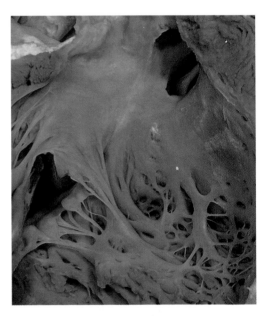

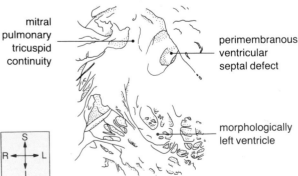

Fig. 8.42 *In this specimen, viewed in anatomic orientation, the perimembranous ventricular septal defect extends to become doubly committed and juxta-arterial, being roofed by the fibrous continuity between the leaflets of the aortic and pulmonary valves.*

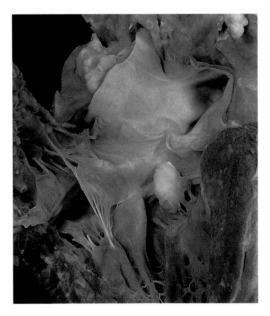

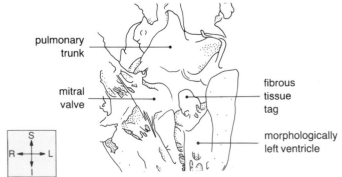

Fig. 8.43 *In this specimen, viewed in anatomic orientation, a fibrous tissue tag derived from the septal leaflet of the left-sided morphologically tricuspid valve herniates into the subpulmonary outflow tract.*

Double Outlet Ventricle

Introduction

When describing any specific ventriculo-arterial connexion, we have found it useful to apply the '50% law'. Thus, a double outlet ventricle can be described in terms of one that supports more than half of the circumference of the valvar leaflets of both great arteries. In the vast majority of cases, there is little question as to the anatomical assignment of an overriding valve, because only rarely does it appear to be equally committed to both chambers. Even then, if the decision is made according to the connexion of the leaflets as seen in short axis, there is little problem (Fig. 8.46). Making such designations on the basis of long axis views by means of angiography or echocardiography, however, can be misleading. Variations either in the angle of view or streaming of the angiographic material can make the appropriate assignment difficult. Nonetheless, if one accepts the '50% law' as a pragmatic convention for decision-making, the subject of double outlet ventricle becomes straightforward, if not even simple.

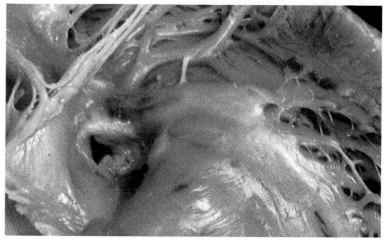

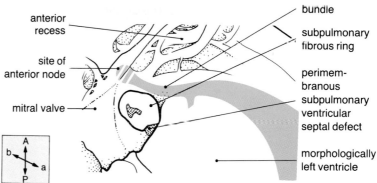

Fig. 8.44 *In this specimen with congenitally corrected transposition, seen in surgical orientation, a fibrous shelf produces subpulmonary obstruction in the presence of a perimembranous ventricular septal defect. The site of the atrioventricular conduction tissue axis has been superimposed.*

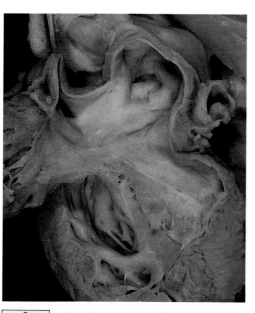

Fig. 8.45 *This specimen with congenitally corrected transposition, seen in anatomical orientation, shows Ebstein's malformation of the left-sided morphologically tricuspid valve. Thinning of the musculature of the inlet component of the morphologically right ventricle is seen.*

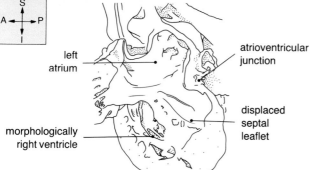

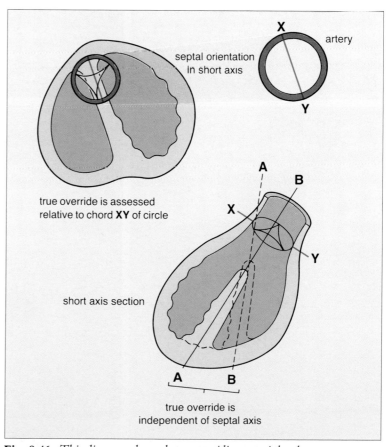

Fig. 8.46 *This diagram shows how overriding arterial valves are assigned to one or other ventricle on the basis of their connexion as judged in the short, rather than the long axis of the ventricular septum.*

Surgical Anatomy of Associated Cardiac Configurations

Because a double outlet ventriculo–arterial connexion can exist with such a wide variety of cardiac configurations, the possible combinations seem almost limitless. The cases most frequently encountered are those with both arteries arising from the right ventricle in the setting of a concordant atrioventricular connexion. Almost invariably a ventricular septal defect is present[50]. It is then the inter-relationships between the great arteries and the defect that is important to the surgeon (Fig. 8.47). Also of significance is the presence of other associated anomalies.

In the majority of cases, the aortic and pulmonary valves are related more or less 'normally'. In other words, the aortic valve is posterior and to the right of the pulmonary valve, and the pulmonary trunk spirals round the aorta towards its branching point (Fig. 8.48, left). In the remainder, the arterial trunks arise from the base of the heart in parallel, as anticipated for complete transposition. For a good proportion of these, the arterial valves are side by side; otherwise, the aortic valve is anterior (Fig. 8.48, middle). In a few cases the aorta is posteriorly located because the pulmonary trunk is enlarged. Almost always the aorta is to the right but, in a small number of cases, the aorta can be to the left (Fig. 8.48, right)[51].

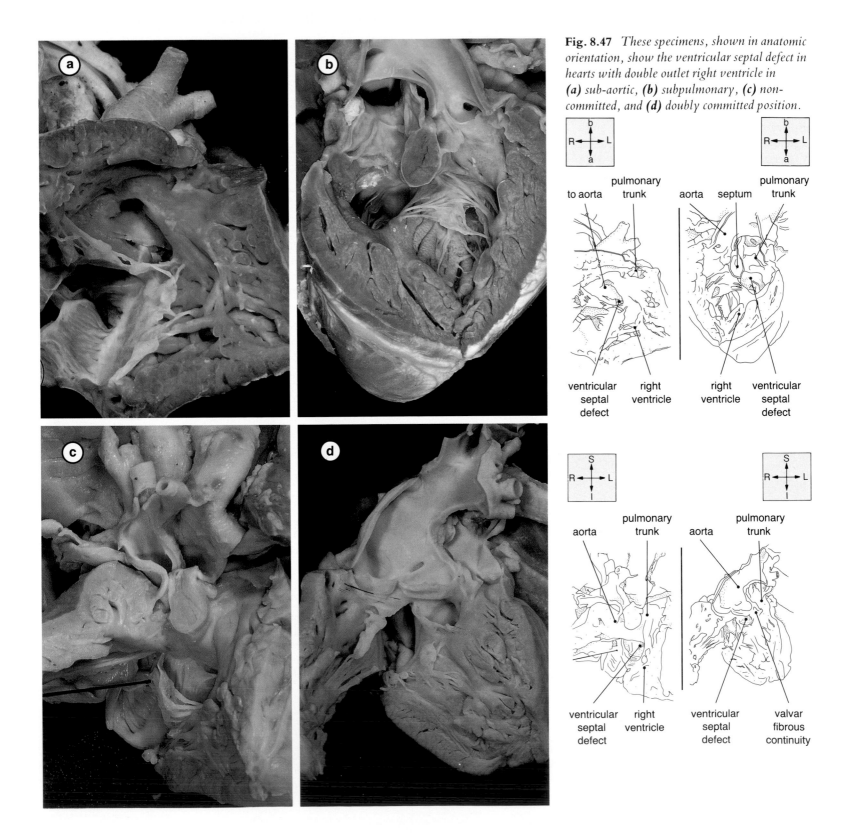

Fig. 8.47 *These specimens, shown in anatomic orientation, show the ventricular septal defect in hearts with double outlet right ventricle in* (**a**) *sub-aortic,* (**b**) *subpulmonary,* (**c**) *non-committed, and* (**d**) *doubly committed position.*

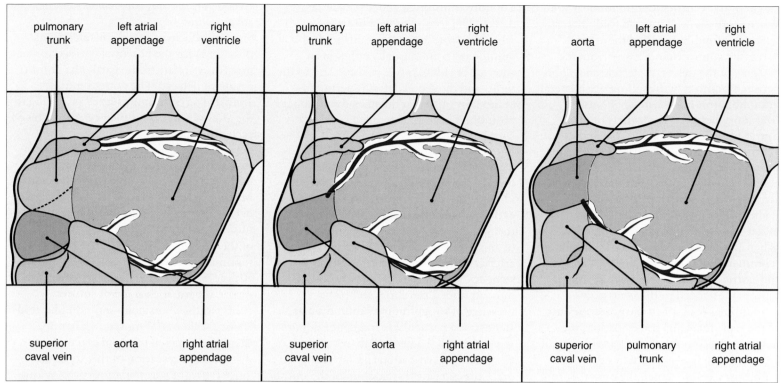

Fig. 8.48 *This diagram, drawn in surgical orientation, shows the three typical orientations of the arterial trunks to be found in hearts with double outlet right ventricle.*

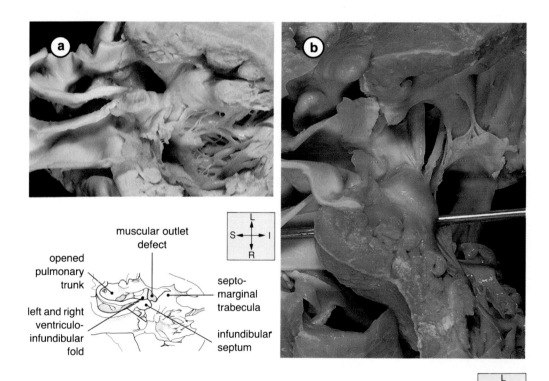

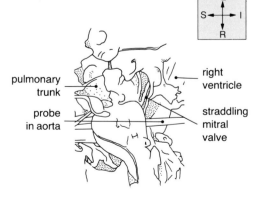

Fig. 8.49 *These specimens, seen in surgical orientation, show examples of double outlet right ventricle with subpulmonary ventricular septal defect in which the defect (a) has a muscular postero-inferior rim and (b) extends to become perimembranous, with fibrous continuity between the leaflets of the pulmonary and mitral valves. Note the straddling leaflet of the mitral valve that is attached to the outlet septum in the right ventricle. The probe is placed through the sub-aortic outflow tract.*

Ventricular Septal Defect

The most important associated anomaly is the ventricular septal defect, and its anatomy should be considered in two ways; first, with respect to its proximity to the great arteries[52] and second, with respect to its own intrinsic morphology[50]. When combining these two approaches, it must be remembered that, when there is double outlet from the right ventricle, the muscular septum itself separates only the inlet and apical trabecular components of the ventricles. The outlet septum is the muscular tissue, if present, between the two outlets from the right ventricle and is, therefore, exclusively a right ventricular structure.

The position of the defect in individual cases may vary in its relation to the great arteries but, almost invariably, the defect can be found cradled between the limbs of the septomarginal trabeculation. Its other borders vary depending on several features. The first is whether the septomarginal trabeculation fuses with the ventriculo–infundibular fold. If it does, there is a muscular inferior rim to the defect which protects the conduction tissue axis as in tetralogy or complete transposition (Fig. 8.49a). If it does not, there is continuity between the leaflets of the atrioventricular valves and the defect is perimembranous (Fig. 8.49b). The second feature is the extent of the ventriculo–infundibular fold. When there is a well formed fold, there is a bilateral infundibulum and the arterial valves are some distance away from the margins of the defect. A defect can still be perimembranous in the setting of a bilateral infundibulum, nonetheless, because of continuity between the leaflets of the mitral and tricuspid valves. When the ventriculo–infundibular fold is attenuated, the leaflets of one of the arterial valves are able to achieve fibrous continuity with an atrioventricular valve (Fig. 8.50).

The final feature is the relationship of the outlet septum to the other structures. When attached to the anterior limb of the septomarginal trabeculation, the defect is sub-aortic. When, in contrast, the outlet septum is attached to the ventriculo–infundibular fold, or to the posterior limb of the septomarginal trabeculation, the defect is placed beneath the left-sided great artery, which is almost always the pulmonary trunk. When the outlet septum is absent, the defect is doubly committed and juxtaarterial (Fig. 8.47c).

From this potential for variation, two 'typical' hearts with double outlet from the right ventricle stand out. The most frequent configuration is when the aortic valve is posterior and to the right of the pulmonary artery, with a perimembranous defect found in sub-aortic position. This arterial relationship can also be found with a doubly committed and juxtaarterial defect. The second type of heart is seen when the aorta ascends parallel to the pulmonary trunk, usually either in an anterior or side-by-side position and to the right, and the septal defect is perimembranous or muscular but in a subpulmonary position. This is the so-called 'Taussig–Bing' variant.

Identifying Further Abnormalities
It is also important for the surgeon to identify any other abnormalities in this extremely heterogeneous group of malformations. By far the most common set of anomalies relates to obstruction of the arterial outlets, such as infundibular stenosis, valvar stenosis, coarctation or interruption of the aortic arch. The presence of subpulmonary infundibular stenosis is a particularly frequent finding when the septal defect is sub-aortic (see Chapter 7). Coarctation and interrupted arch, together with straddling of the mitral valve, are frequent accompaniments of the 'Taussig–Bing' variant[53]. Common atrioventricular valves also occur in a significant number of cases. Unusual coronary arterial anatomy is found most frequently when the aorta is in an anterior or side-by-side position. In this situation, special consideration is needed when performing either a right ventriculotomy or an arterial switch procedure.

Considering the Surgical Anatomy of Other Abnormalities
Surgical and anatomical considerations (Fig. 8.51) for the potential corrective procedures relate to the particular combination of defects. The outlet septum, almost always present, serves as a guide to the arterial valves and their relationships to each other and to the ventricular septal defect. As described above, in cases with sub-aortic defects the septum usually inserts into the anterior limb of the septomarginal trabeculation. With subpulmonary defects, it usually inserts into the ventriculo–infundibular fold or into the posterior part of the ventricular septum. The outlet septum is always devoid of any vital structure, so it can be resected or used as a secure site for anchorage of sutures. In contrast, the ventriculo–infundibular fold is not a solid bar of muscle. Care must therefore be taken to avoid extensive dissection or resection of this structure, since the right coronary artery lies within the fold.

Knowledge of the type of ventricular septal defect will, as in isolated defects (see Chapter 7, Fig. 7.36), give accurate guidance to the disposition of the conduction tissue. Obstruction of the subpulmonary outflow tract requires the same attention to detail as when dealing with tetralogy of Fallot (see Chapter 7). Other cardiac anomalies will have to be

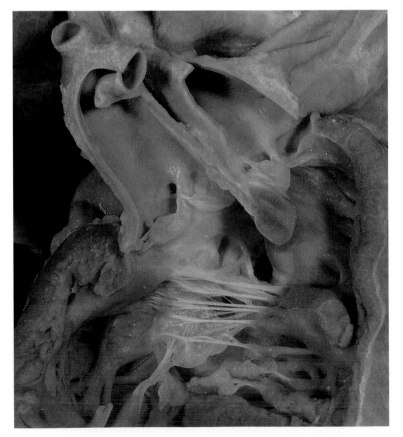

Fig. 8.50 *In this specimen, seen in anatomic orientation, there is unequivocal double outlet from the right ventricle with fibrous continuity between the leaflets of the aortic and the atrioventricular valves.*

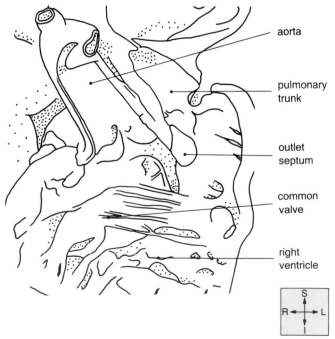

dealt with in the context of the particular cardiac configuration present.

'Bilateral Conus'

It may not have passed unnoticed that this anomaly has been discussed with little reference to the so-called 'bilateral conus'. This is because this feature is not taken to be an integral part of the anomaly. 'Double outlet' logically describes a ventriculo–arterial connexion, and that is what has been defined. The presence of a 'bilateral conus' depends simply on whether the ventriculo–infundibular fold separates the atrioventricular and arterial valves completely or is attenuated to permit fibrous continuity between the leaflets of the arterial and atrioventricular valves. Either arrangement can exist when the ventriculo–arterial connexion is one of double outlet.

Double Outlet Left Ventricle

Double outlet left ventricle can present with similar variations in arterial position and relationship to the ventricular septal defect as described for double outlet right ventricle. Though Otero Coto and co-workers[54] have pointed out that there have been no published descriptions of the conduction system in double outlet left ventricular connexion, studies from closely

related anomalies have been reported[55,56]. These studies suggest that the conduction axis is normally disposed when there are otherwise normal segmental connexions. It should also be remembered that, as with double outlet right ventricle, double outlet left ventricle can be found with any atrio-ventricular connexion. The rules for disposition of the conduction tissue will then change accordingly.

Common Arterial Trunk

Introduction

A common arterial trunk is one that directly supplies the systemic, pulmonary, and coronary arteries. In this way, the anomaly is distinguished from the other types of ventriculo–arterial connexion producing single outlet from the heart, namely a solitary aortic trunk with pulmonary atresia, a solitary pulmonary trunk with aortic atresia, or a solitary arterial trunk with an absence of the intra-pericardial pulmonary arteries (see Fig. 6.21, p.6.11). All of these arrangements are appropriately described as single outlet when it is not possible to determine the ventricular origin of an atretic great artery.

A common arterial trunk is guarded by a common arterial valve[57]. Some authori-ties[58,59] have suggested that common

trunks can have two discrete outflow tracts and separate aortic and pulmonary valves. From the surgical viewpoint, it is better to consider the latter lesions as large aorto-pulmonary windows. They pose far less severe problems for repair than do those malformations with a common outflow tract and valve that are the subject of this discussion.

It is also worthwhile to consider one anomaly already mentioned before leaving the vexatious realm of definitions. This is the lesion characterized by the presence of a solitary arterial trunk but with no evidence whatsoever of intrapericardial pulmonary arteries. The controversy as to whether the solitary great vessel is a common trunk ('truncus types IV') or an aorta is readily resolved by considering it to be a solitary arterial trunk. The supply to the pulmonary circulation is the key to surgical treatment of the malformation, as in tetralogy with pulmonary atresia (see p.7.45).

Surgical Anatomy of Common Arterial Trunk

The anatomical features that determine the success of surgical treatment for a common arterial trunk are its connexion to the ventricular mass, the state of the truncal valve, the morphology of the ventricular septal defect, the presence of associated

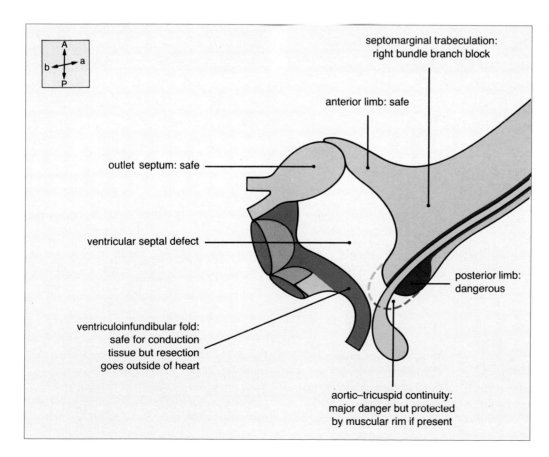

Fig. 8.51 *This diagram, shown in surgical orientation, illustrates the relationships of the ventricular septal defect in hearts with double outlet right ventricle.*

septomarginal trabeculation: right bundle branch block

anterior limb: safe

outlet septum: safe

ventricular septal defect

ventriculoinfundibular fold: safe for conduction tissue but resection goes outside of heart

posterior limb: dangerous

aortic–tricuspid continuity: major danger but protected by muscular rim if present

anomalies, and the arrangement of the great arteries arising from the trunk. Although a common trunk can exist with any atrioventricular connexion, it is very rarely found with other than a concordant atrioventricular connexion. The trunk usually overrides the ventricular septum and is connected more or less equally to the right and left ventricles (Fig. 8.52). The septal defect is present because of the complete lack of the outlet septum together with the septal components of the sleeves of infundibular muscle and, thus, is directly juxtaarterial. It is usually cradled between the limbs of the septomarginal trabeculation, with the posterior limb fusing with the ventriculo–infundibular fold (Fig. 8.53). As with other defects of

this type (see Chapter 7), the muscle bundle thus formed serves to buttress the axis of atrioventricular conduction tissue away from the septal crest. More rarely, there can be continuity between the truncal and tricuspid valves, which puts the conduction axis at great risk during closure when connecting the common trunk to the left ventricle (Fig. 8.54). In the rare instance that the defect is restrictive, it is usually because the common trunk is connected exclusively or predominantly to the right ventricle, often with a subtruncal infundibulum. If necessary, the defect may be enlarged along its antero-superior margins.

After surgical repair of a common trunk following the Rastelli technique[61], the

truncal valve effectively becomes the aortic valve. Valvar incompetence or stenosis, if present, is therefore of considerable significance. Although dysplastic truncal valves have been encountered with some frequency in autopsy studies of infant hearts[62], they do not seem to pose a major problem in surgical repair in infancy. The common trunk may also be predominantly connected to the left ventricle, but this variation works in the surgeon's favour and does not pose additional problems.

Morphology of the Great Arteries

Variation in morphology of the great arteries is found in both the pulmonary and aortic pathways.

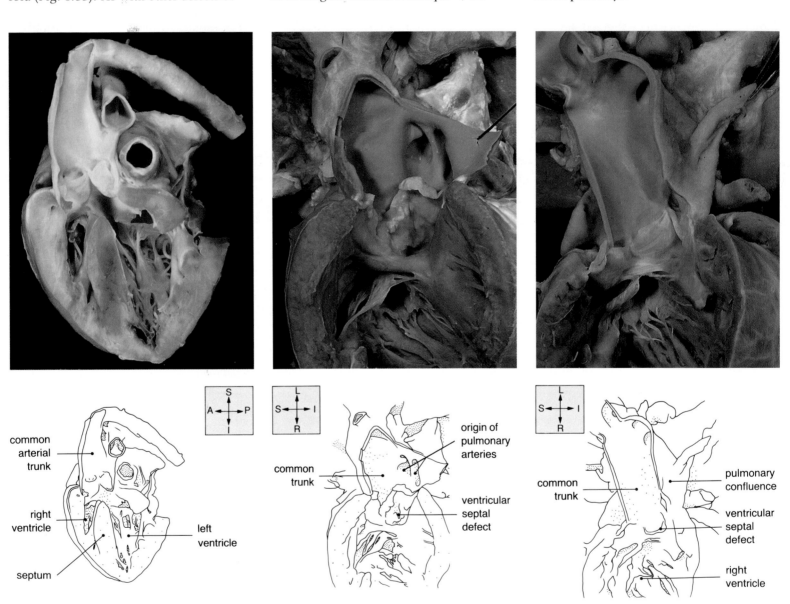

Fig. 8.52 *This long axis section shows a heart with a common arterial trunk overriding a juxtaarterial ventricular septal defect.*

Fig. 8.53 *This heart, shown in anatomic orientation from the right ventricle, has a common arterial trunk overriding a ventricular septal defect with a muscular postero-inferior rim. Note that the pulmonary arteries arise from a confluent channel (so-called type I).*

Fig. 8.54 *This heart with a common arterial trunk, again viewed in anatomic orientation, has a ventricular septal defect that is perimembranous, with fibrous continuity between the leaflets of the truncal and tricuspid valves.*

Origin of the Pulmonary Arteries
Following the classical studies of Collett and Edwards[63], common trunk is usually classified according to the mode of origin of the pulmonary arteries. The possibilities are for the arteries to arise from a short confluent channel ('type I'), to arise separately and directly from the left posterior aspect of the trunk ('type II'), or to arise separately from either side of the trunk ('type III'). Presence of a short pulmonary confluence would certainly facilitate banding but, in specialized centres, this procedure is now performed with far less frequency than once was the case. Either of the first two patterns facilitates connexion to a right ventricular conduit during complete repair (Fig. 8.55). The much rarer variant, in which each pulmonary artery arises from the side of the trunk ('type III'), makes complete repair more difficult though not impossible. As described above, we believe that the so-called 'type IV', where there is no evidence of intrapericardial pulmonary arteries, is best considered to be a solitary arterial trunk (Fig. 6.21, p.6.11) rather than a variant of common arterial trunk.

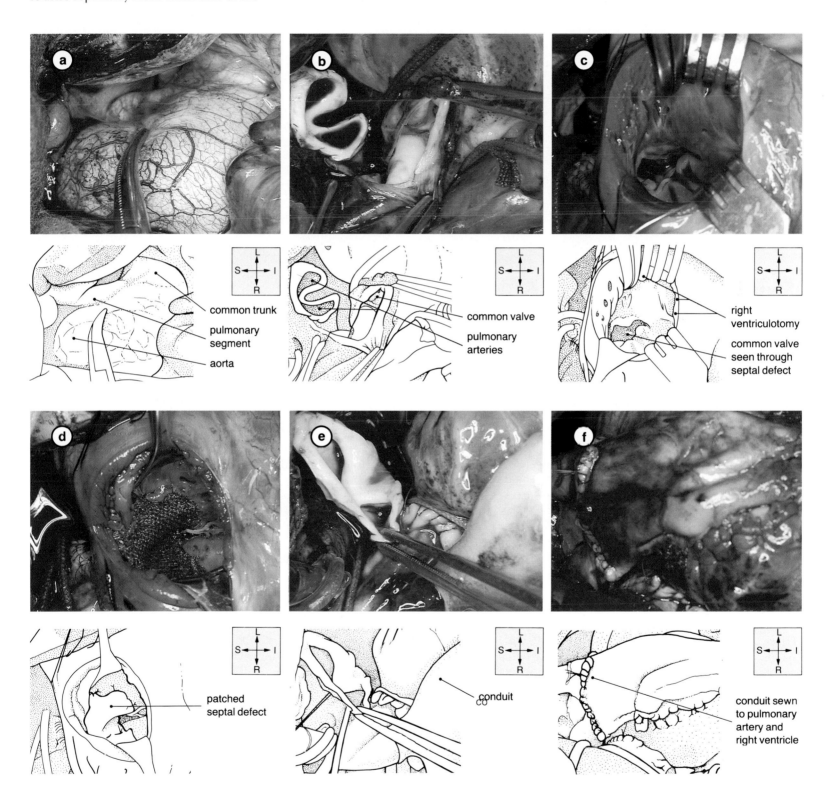

Fig. 8.55 *These panels illustrate the steps taken during surgical correction of a heart with common arterial trunk. Where (a) shows the origin of the common trunk from the base of the heart; (b) the pulmonary arteries have been removed from the trunk; while (c) shows the ventricular septal defect seen through a right ventriculotomy. (d) The defect has been patched while (e) shows sizing of the pulmonary arteries and (f) illustrates the completed repair.*

Pattern of the Aortic Arch
Categorization of a common arterial trunk has tended to concentrate on the patterns of the pulmonary arteries, but it is the pattern of the aortic arch which is of much more surgical significance. Usually the aorta arises in its anticipated position or, more rarely, anteriorly[64], but continues to supply the head, neck and arm arteries together with the descending aorta. The variant in which the aortic arch is interrupted is the pattern which will create problems for the surgeon. In this arrangement, the ascending aorta supplies all or only part of the arterial supply to the head, neck and arms[65]. The interruption is usually at the isthmus, but it can occur proximal to the origin of the left subclavian artery. In either case, the descending aorta is supplied by the arterial duct. If surgical repair is contemplated, therefore, it is imperative to recognize this arrangement and make appropriate modifications. Common trunks with interruption are not infrequent, being found in up to one-fifth of autopsy series[58,59,65,66]. Other rare variations in arterial pattern occur in association with common trunks, such as crossed pulmonary arteries[67].

References

1. Anderson, R.H., *et al.* (1983) Univentricular atrioventricular connection: the single ventricle trap unsprung. *Pediatric Cardiology*, **4**, 273–280.

2. Anderson, R.H., Becker, A.E., Tynan, M., Macartney, F.J., Rigby, M.L. & Wilkinson, J.L. (1984) The univentricular atrioventricular connection: getting to the root of a thorny problem. *American Journal of Cardiology*, **54**, 822–828.

3. Becker, A.E., Anderson, R.H., Penkoske, P.A. & Zuberbuhler, J.R. (1987) Morphology of double inlet ventricle. In *Double Inlet Ventricle. Anatomy, Diagnosis and Surgical Management*. Edited by R.H. Anderson, G. Crupi & L. Parenzan. Tunbridge Wells: Castle House Publications Ltd, pp. 36–71.

4. Gale, A.W., Danielson, G.K., McGoon, D.C., Wallace, R.B. & Mair, D.D. (1980) Fontan procedure for tricuspid atresia. *Circulation*, **62**, 91–96.

5. Laks, H., Williams, W.G., Hillenbrand, W.E., Freedom, R.M., Talner, N.S., Rowe, R.D. & Trusler, G.A. (1980) Results of right atrial to right ventricular and right atrial to pulmonary artery conduits for complex congenital heart disease. *Annals of Surgery*, **192**, 382–389.

6. Kirklin, J.K., Blackstone, E.H., Kirklin, J.W., Pacifico, A.D. & Bargeron, I.M. Jr. (1986) The Fontan operation. Ventricular hypertrophy, age, and date of operation as risk factors. *Journal of Thoracic and Cardiovascular Surgery*, **92**, 1049–1064.

7. Fontan, F., Fernandez, G., Costa, F., Naftel, D.C., Tritto, F., Blackstone, E.H. & Kirklin, J.W. (1989) The size of the pulmonary arteries and the results of the Fontan operation. *Journal of Thoracic and Cardiovascular Surgery*, **98**, 711–724.

8. Fontan, F., Kirklin, J.W., Fernandez, G., Costa, F., Naftel, D.C., Tritto, F. & Blackstone, E.H. (1990) Outcome after a "perfect" Fontan operation. *Circulation*, **81**, 1520–1536.

9. Kurosawa, H., Imai, Y., Fukuchi, S., Sawatari, K., Koy, Y., Nakazawa, M. & Takao, A. (1990) Septation and Fontan repair of univentricular atrioventricular connection. *Journal of Thoracic and Cardiovascular Surgery*, **99**, 314–319.

10. Stefanelli, G., Kirklin, J.W., Naftel, D.C., Blackstone, E.H., Pacifico, A.D., Kirklin, J.K., Soto, B. & Bargeron, I.M. (1984) Early and intermediate-term (10 year) results of surgery for univentricular atrioventricular connection ("single ventricle"). *Americal Journal of Cardiology*, **54**, 811–821.

11. McGoon, D.C., Wallace, R.B., Maloney, J.D. & Marcelleti, C. (1977) Correction of the univentricular heart having two atrioventricular valves. *Journal of Thoracic and Cardiovascular Surgery*, **74(2)**, 218–226.

12. Cheung, H.C., Lincoln, C., Anderson, R.H., Ho, S.Y., Sinebourne, E.A. & Rigby, M.L. Options for surgical repair in hearts with univentricular atrioventricular connexion and subaortic stenosis. Submitted for publication.

13. Abbott, M.E. (0000) Unique case of congenital malformation of the heart. *Museum Notes*. McGill University, pp. 522–525.

14. Mair, D.D., Rice, M.J., Hagler, D.J., Puga, F.J., McGoon, D.C. & Danielson, G.K. (1985) Outcome of the Fontan procedure in patients with tricuspid atresia. *Circulation*, **72(II)**, 88–92.

15. Fontan, F., Deville, C., Quaegebeur, J., Ottenkamp, J., Sourdille, N., Choussat, A. & Brom, G.A. (1983) Repair of tricuspid atresia in 100 patients. *Journal of Thoracic and Cardiovascular Surgery*, **85**, 647–660.

16. Yacoub, M.H. (1978) Fontan's operation — are caval valves necessary? In *Paediatric Cardiology*. Edited by R.H. Anderson & E.A. Shinebourne. Edinburgh: Churchill Livingstone, pp. 581–588.

17. Stellin, G., Mazzucco, A., Bortolotti, U., del Torso, S., Faggian, G., Fracasso, A., Livi, U., Milano, A., Rizzoli, G. & Gallucci, V. (1988) Tricuspid atresia versus other complex lesions: comparison of results with a modified Fontan procedure. *Journal of Thoracic and Cardiovascular Surgery*, **96**, 204–211.

18. Anderson, R.H., Arnold, R., Thaper, M.K., Jones, R.S. & Hamilton, D.I. (1974) Cardiac specialized tissues in hearts with an apparently single ventricular chamber. (Double inlet left ventricle.) *American Journal of Cardiology*, **33**, 95–106.

19. de Leval, M.R., Kilner, P., Gewillig, M. & Bull, C. (1988) Total cavopulmonary connection: a logical alternative to atriopulmonary connection for complex Fontan operations. *Journal of Thoracic and Cardiovascular Surgery*, **96**, 682–695.

20. Jonas, R.A., Mayer, J.E. & Castaneda, A.R. (1988) Invited letter concerning: Total cavopulmonary connection. *Journal of Thoracic and Cardiovascular Surgery*, **96**, 830–832.

21. Essed, C.E., Ho, S.Y., Hunter, S. & Anderson, R.H. (1980) Atrioventricular conduction system in univentricular heart of right ventricular type with right-sided rudimentary chamber. *Thorax*, **35**, 123–127.

22. Bull, C., de Leval, M., Stark, J. & Macartney, F. (1983) Use of a subpulmonary ventricular chamber in the Fontan circulation. *Journal of Thoracic and Cardiovascular Surgery*, **85**, 21–31.

23. Rao, P.S., Jue, K.L. Isabel-Jones, J. & Ruttenberg, H.D. (1973) Ebstein's malformation of the tricuspid valve with atresia. *American Journal of Cardiology*, **32**, 1004–1009.

24. Norwood, W.I., Kirklin, J.W. & Saunders, S.P. (1980) Hypoplastic left heart syndrome: experience with palliative surgery. *American Journal of Cardiology*, **45**, 87–91.

25. Norwood, W.I. & Stellin, G.J. (1981) Aortic atresia with interrupted aortic arch. Reparative operation. *Journal of Thoracic and Cardiovascular Surgery*, **81**, 239–244.

26. Norwood, W.I., Lang, P. & Hansen, D.D. (1983) Physiologic repair of the aortic atresia–hypoplastic left heart syndrome. *New England Journal of Medicine*, **308**, 23–26.

27. Van Praagh, R. (1971) Transposition of the Great Arteries. II. Transposition clarified. *American Journal of Cardiology*, **28**, 739–741.

28. Van Mierop, L.H.S. (1971) Transposition of the great arteries. Clarification or further confusion? Editorial. *American Journal of Cardiology*, **28**, 735–738.

29. Wilcox, B.R., Henry, G.W. & Anderson, R.H. (1983) The transmitral approach to left ventricular outflow tract obstruction. *Annals of Thoracic Surgery*, **35**, 288–293.

30. Buchler, J.R., Bembom, J.C. & Buchler, R.D. (1984) Transposition of the great arteries with posterior aorta and subaortic conus: anatomical and surgical correlation. *International Journal of Cardiology*, **5**, 13–18.

31. Aubert, J., Pannatier, A., Couvelly, J.P., Unal, D., Rouault, F. & Delarue, A. (1978) Transposition of the great arteries. New technique for anatomical correction: case report. *British Heart Journal*, **40**, 204–208.

32. Damus, P.S., Thomson, B.N. Jr. & McLoughlin, T.G. (1982) Arterial repair without coronary relocation for complete transposition of the great vessels with ventricular septal defect: report of case. *Journal of Thoracic and Cardiovascular Surgery*, **83**, 316–318.

33. Stansel, H.G. (1975) A new operation for d-loop transposition of the great vessels. *Annals of Thoracic Surgery*, **19**, 565–567.

34. Kaye, M.P. (1975) Anatomic correction of transposition of great arteries. *Mayo Clinic Proceedings*, **50**, 638–640.

35. Ceithaml, E.L., Puga, F.J., Danielson, G.K., McGoon, D.C. & Ritter, D.G. (1984) Results of the Damus–Stansel–Kaye procedure for transposition of the great arteries and for double outlet right ventricle with subpulmonary ventricular septal defect. *Annals of Thoracic Surgery*, **38**, 433–437.

36. Anderson, R.H., Henry, G.W. & Becker, A.E. (1991) Morphological aspects of complete transposition. *Cardiology Young*, **1**, 1–103.

37. Gittenberger-de-Groot, A.C., Sauer, U., Oppenheimer-Dekker, A. & Quaegebeur, J. (1983) Coronary arterial anatomy in transposition of the great arteries: a morphologic study. *Pediatric Cardiology*, **4(I)**, 15–24.

38. Gittenberger-de-Groot, A.C., Sauer, U. & Guaegebeur, J. (1986) Aortic intramural coronary artery in three hearts with transposition of the great arteries. *Journal of Thoracic and Cardiovascular Surgery*, **91**, 566–571.

39. Becker, A.E. & Anderson, R.H. (1977) Conditions with discordant atrioventricular connexions — anatomy and conducting tissues. In *Paediatric Cardiology*. Edited by R.H. Anderson & E.A. Shinebourne. Edinburgh: Churchill Livingstone, pp. 184–197.

40. Anderson, R.H., Becker, A.E., Arnold, R. & Wilkinson, J.L. (1974) The conducting tissues in congenitally corrected transposition. *Circulation*, **50**, 911–923.

41. Losekoot, T.G. (1978) Conditions with atrioventricular discordance — clinical investigation. In *Paediatric Cardiology*. Edited by R.H. Anderson & E.A. Shinebourne. Edinburgh: Churchill Livingstone, pp. 198–206.

42. Stewart, S., Manning, J. & Siegel, L. (1977) Automatic identification of cardiac conduction tissue in L-TGV and Ebstein's anomaly. *Annals of Thoracic Surgery*, **23**, 215–220.

43. de Leval, M., Bastos, P., Stark, J., Taylor, J.F.N., Macartney, F.J. & Anderson, R.H. (1979) Surgical technique to reduce the risks of heart block following closure of ventricular septal defect in atrioventricular discordance. *Journal of Thoracic and Cardiovascular Surgery*, **78**, 515–526.

44. Okamura, J. & Konno, S. (1973) Two types of ventricular septal defect in corrected transposition of the great arteries. Reference to surgical approaches. *American Heart Journal*, **85**, 483–490.

45. Anderson, R.H., Becker, A.E. & Gerlis, I.M. (1975) The pulmonary outflow tract in classically corrected transposition. *Journal of Thoracic and Cardiovascular Surgery*, **69**, 747–757.

46. Doty, D.B., Truesdell, S.C. & Marvin, W.J. Jr. (1983) Techniques to avoid injury of the conduction tissue during the surgical treatment of corrected transposition. *Circulation*, **68(II)**, 63–69.

47. Dick, M., Van Praagh, R., Rudd, M., Folkerth, T. & Castaneda, A.R. (1977) Electrophysiological delineation of the specialised atrioventricular conduction system in two patients with corrected transposition of the great arteries with situs inversus (I,D,D). *Circulation*, **55**, 896–900.

48. Kurosawa, H., Imai, Y. & Becker, A.E. (1990) Congenitally corrected transposition with normally positioned atria, straddling mitral valve, and isolated posterior atrioventricular node and bundle. *Journal of Thoracic and Cardiovascular Surgery*, **99**, 312–313.

49. McGoon, D.C., Danielson, G.K., Wallace, R.B. & Puga, F.J. (1981) Surgical implications of straddling atrioventricular valves. In *Paediatric Cardiology Volume 3*. Edited by A.E. Becker, T.G. Losekoot, C. Marcelletti & R.H. Anderson. Edinburgh: Churchill Livingstone, pp.431–440.

50. Wilcox, B.R., Ho, S.Y., Macartney, F.J., Becker, A.E., Gerlis, I.M. & Anderson, R.H. (1981) Surgical anatomy of double-outlet right ventricle with situs solitus and atrioventricular concordance. *Journal of Thoracic and Cardiovascular Surgery*, **82**, 405–417.

51. Van Praagh, R., Perez-Trevino, C., Reynolds, J., Moes, C.A.F., Keith, J.D., Roy, D.L., Belcourt, C., Weinberg, P.M. & Parisi, L.F. (1975) Double outlet right ventricle (S–D–L) with subaortic ventricular septal defect and pulmonary stenosis. *American Journal of Cardiology*, **35**, 42–53.

52. Lev, M., Bharati, S., Meng, C.C.L., Liberthson, R.R., Paul, M.H. & Idriss, F. (1972) A concept of double-outlet right ventricle. *Journal of Thoracic and Cardiovascular Surgery*, **64**, 271–281.

53. Stellin, G., Zuberbuhler, J.R., Anderson, R.H. & Siewers, R.D. (1987) The surgical anatomy of the Taussig–Bing malformation. *Journal of Thoracic and Cardiovascular Surgery*, **93**, 560–569.

54. Otero Coto, E., Quero Jimenez, M., Castaneda, A.R., Rufilanchas, J.J. & Deverall, P.B. (1979) Double outlet from chambers of left ventricular morphology. *British Heart Journal*, **42**, 15–21.

55. Milo, S., Ho, S.Y., Wilkinson, J.L. & Anderson, R.H. (1980) The surgical anatomy and atrioventricular conduction tissues of hearts with isolated ventricular septal defects. *Journal of Thoracic and Cardiovascular Surgery*, **79**, 244–255.

56. Anderson, R.H., Ho, S.Y. & Becker, A.E. (1983) The surgical anatomy of the conduction tissues. *Thorax*, **38**, 408–420.

57. Anderson, R.H. & Thiene, G. (1989) Editorial. Categorization and description of hearts with a common arterial trunk. *European Journal of Cardio-thoracic Surgery*, **3**, 481–487.

58. Van Praagh, R. & Van Praagh, S. (1965) The anatomy of common aortico-pulmonary trunk (truncus arteriosus communis) and its embryologic implications. *American Journal of Cardiology*, **16**, 406–426.

59. Calder, L., Van Praagh, R., Van Praagh, S., Sears, W.P., Corwin, R., Levy, A., Keith, D.J. & Paul, M.H. (1976) Truncus arteriosus communis. Clinical, angiographic, and pathologic findings in 100 patients. *American Heart Journal*, **92**, 23–38.

60. Thiene, G. & Anderson, R.H. (1983) Pulmonary atresia with ventricular septal defect. Anatomy. In *Paediatric Cardiology Volume 5*. Edited by R.H. Anderson, F.J. Macartney, E.A. Shinebourne & M.J. Tynan. Edinburgh: Churchill Livingstone, pp.80–101.

61. McGoon, D.C., Rastelli, G.C. & Ongley, P.A. (1968) An operation for the correction of truncus arteriosus. *JAMA*, **205**, 69–73.

62. Becker, A.E., Becker, M.J. & Edwards, J.E. (1971) Pathology of the semi-lunar valve in persistent truncus arteriosus. *Journal of Thoracic and Cardiovascular Surgery*, **62**, 16–26.

63. Collett, R.W. & Edwards, J.E. (1949) Persistent truncus arteriosus. A classification according to anatomic types. *Surgical Clinics of North America*, **29**, 1245–1270.

64. Angelini, P., Verdugo, A.L., Illera, J.P. & Leachman, R.D. (1977) Truncus arteriosus communis. An unusual case associated with transposition. *Circulation*, **56**, 1107.

65. Crupi, G., Macartney, F.J. & Anderson, R.H. (1977) Persistent truncus arteriosus. A study of 66 autopsy cases with special reference to definition and morphogenesis. *American Journal of Cardiology*, **40**, 569–578.

66. Bharati, S., McAllister, H.A. Jr., Rosenquist, G.C., Miller, R.A., Tatooles, C.J. & Lev, M. (1974) The surgical anatomy of truncus arteriosus communis. *Journal of Thoracic and Cardiovascular Surgery*, **67**, 501–510.

67. Becker, A.E., Becker, M.J. & Edwards, J.E. (1970) Malposition of pulmonary arteries (crossed pulmonary arteries) in persistent truncus arteriosus. *American Journal of Roentgenology*, **110**, 509–514.

ABNORMALITIES OF THE GREAT VESSELS 9

Anomalous Systemic Venous Drainage

Abnormal systemic venous connexions are usually of little surgical significance because their clinical consequences are limited. These anomalies are apt to be encountered as the surgeon pursues a more complex associated intracardiac anomaly. They may be grouped into the following categories: absence or abnormal drainage of the right caval vein(s); persistence or abnormal drainage of the left caval vein(s); and abnormal hepatic venous connexions. Abnormalities of the coronary sinus usually fall into one of these groups, except the 'unroofed' coronary sinus, which was discussed in Chapter 7.

Abnormal Drainage of the Right Caval Veins

Abnormalities of the right superior caval vein are extremely rare. It may be diminished in size. Alternatively, it may be completely absent and the venous return from the head, neck and arms passes through a persistent left superior caval vein to the right atrium via the coronary sinus or, rarely, directly into the left atrium. Only this last situation requires surgical intervention. The other conditions, if encountered during open-heart surgery, would require some adjustment from the usual technique used for cannulation. Though there is no definite evidence to this effect, we would not expect these abnormalities to affect the location of the sinus node.

The right inferior caval vein can be absent at its cavoatrial junction or in the abdomen, with its venous return being directed to the right atrium through the azygos or hemiazygos system. The azygos return can be to the left-sided atrium, producing right-to-left shunting. (Right-to-left shunting can also be an iatrogenic phenomenon occasionally observed when low-lying atrial septal defects are improperly closed; see Chapter 7. Such return via the azygos venous system is seen most frequently with isomerism of the left atrial appendages. The hepatic veins usually drain independently into the right-sided or left-sided atrium, although there can be a confluent suprahepatic channel. It can also occur in individuals with lateralized atrial chambers, and the hepatic veins then always connect to the right atrium through a suprahepatic segment of the inferior caval vein.

Persistent Left Caval Veins

A persistent left superior caval vein is joined to the right superior caval vein by an innominate vein in about 60% of reported cases[1]. When arranged in this fashion, the left caval vein can simply be clamped or ligated, so as to avoid flooding the field when the heart is opened. If connexions with the right vein are not apparent, a trial period of occlusion will usually indicate whether venous hypertension will give problems.

A left superior caval vein is found frequently in patients with cyanotic heart disease, being reported in as many as 20% of patients with tetralogy of Fallot and 8% of patients with Eisenmenger's syndrome[2]. This venous channel can be the route of partial anomalous pulmonary venous connexion, or it can empty through the left-sided pulmonary veins into the left atrium. It can also empty directly into the left atrium ('unroofed' coronary sinus). Much more frequently, it is encountered as an isolated lesion which usually receives the hemiazygos vein before penetrating the pericardium and passing between the left atrial appendage and the left pulmonary veins (Fig. 9.1). It then connects with the

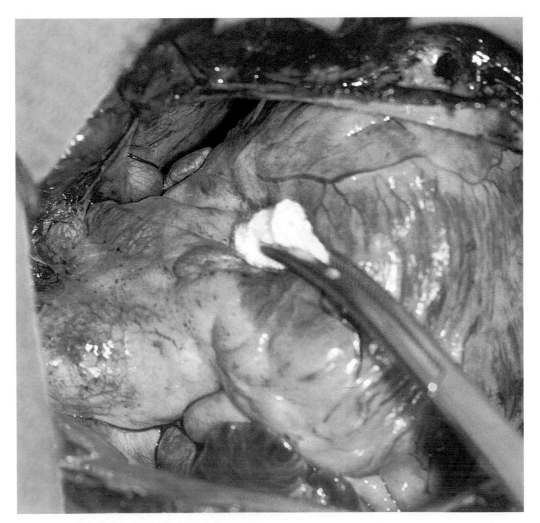

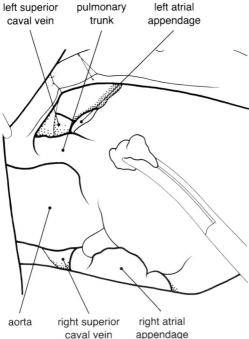

Fig. 9.1 *This operative view through a median sternotomy shows a left superior caval vein entering the pericardial cavity between the left atrial appendage and the pulmonary trunk.*

left superior caval vein   pulmonary trunk   left atrial appendage

aorta   right superior caval vein   right atrial appendage

coronary sinus behind the heart to empty into the right atrium through a larger than normal orifice. In such hearts, the Thebesian valve is often attenuated or absent.

Though relatively rare, there may be a persistent left-sided inferior caval vein[3], which may drain by way of the azygos system to the superior caval vein. As discussed above, this 'azygos continuation' of the inferior caval vein is commonly found with isomerism of the left atrial appendages[4]. Exceedingly rarely, the inferior caval vein may drain directly into the morphologically left atrium[5].

Another anomaly which, although rare, warrants consideration is the levoatrial cardinal vein[6]. This channel connects the left atrium to the systemic venous system. It is found with associated lesions such as mitral atresia, where it functions as the only route for pulmonary venous return. Then, although the pulmonary veins are normally connected to the morphologically left atrium, the pattern of venous return is comparable to the 'snowman' types of anomalous pulmonary venous connexion (see below).

Anomalous Pulmonary Venous Connexion

Very rarely, the pulmonary veins may be obstructed or totally atretic at their atrial junction[7,8]. Much more commonly, abnormalities of the pulmonary venous system take the form of an anomalous connexion. Because of the plethora of possibilities for abnormal pulmonary venous connexions[9–11], it is particularly important that they be described as specifically and as unambiguously as possible (Fig. 9.2).

The pulmonary veins connect anomalously when they are not joined to the morphologically left atrium. Consequently, if all the veins from one lung connect to a site other than the left atrium, the arrangement can be described as complete unilateral anomalous pulmonary venous connexion. If all the veins from both lungs connect to sites other than the morphologically left atrium, there is total anomalous pulmonary venous connexion. Obviously this implies bilateral complete anomalous connexion.

Describing Anomalous Connexion

Any combination can be readily described by treating each lung as an entity (that is, partial or complete unilateral anomalous connexion; Fig. 9.2). The unifying lesion in all of these combinations is the connexion of one or more pulmonary veins to the systemic venous system or to the right atrium (Fig. 9.3). It is equally important, therefore, that the site of drainage be identified. Historically, these have been described as supradiaphragmatic or infradiaphragmatic (Fig. 9.4).

Supradiaphragmatic Connexion

The supradiaphragmatic group can be subdivided into supracardiac and cardiac groups. Supracardiac connexion may be to a right or left superior caval vein, the innominate (brachiocephalic) vein or even the azygos vein. Connexion to the innominate vein is most frequent, and the combination of vertical vein and innominate vein (Fig. 9.5) draining to the superior caval vein produces the typical 'snowman' configuration seen on chest radiography.

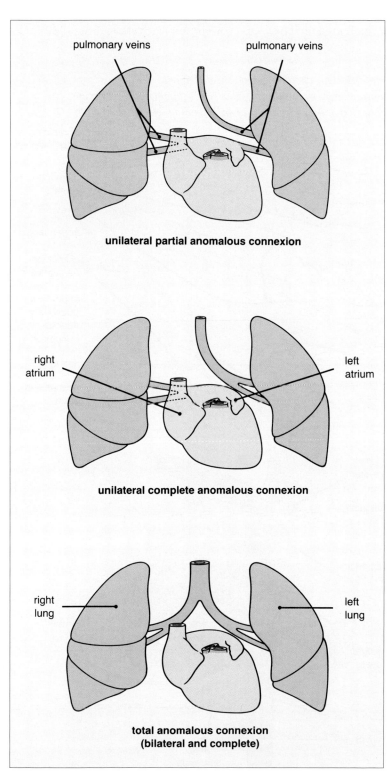

Fig. 9.2 *This diagram, in anatomic orientation, shows how anomalous connexion of the pulmonary veins can be described by specifying the connexion of the veins from each lung as separate entities.*

Cardiac drainage enters the right atrium directly or, more usually, through the coronary sinus (Fig. 9.6).

Infradiaphragmatic Connexion

Infradiaphragmatic connexion is usually total except when there is a partial right-sided connexion to the inferior caval vein. This produces the 'scimitar syndrome', a name taken from its likeness to a Turkish sword when seen roentgenographically[12]. In the usual infradiaphragmatic connexion, the common channel connecting both lungs lies outside the pericardium posterior to the left atrium. A vertical vein drains through the diaphragm as a single channel to enter the inferior caval vein, the portal vein or the venous duct (Fig. 9.7). Occasionally, however, the channel breaks up into a series of branches which connect to the gastric veins.

Surgical Anatomy of Anomalous Connexion

The salient anatomical features relating to the surgical repair of anomalous pulmonary connexions include the type of abnormal connexion (for example, total, unilateral or mixed), the site of anomalous connexion, and the proximity of the anomalous veins to the left atrium.

As pointed out in Chapter 7, an interatrial communication in the mouth of the superior caval vein is often accompanied by anomalous connexion of the right pulmonary veins to the superior caval vein. The need to safeguard the sinus node and its blood supply has already been emphasized.

Other sites of connexion, or potential sites of anastomosis, often require construction of an extensive atrial junction to guard postoperatively against pulmonary

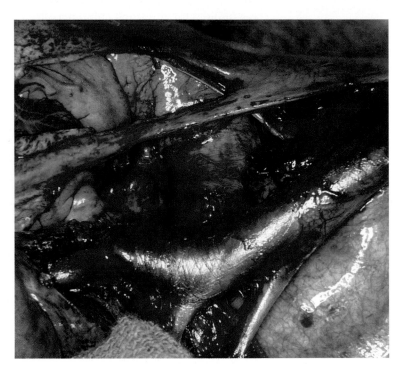

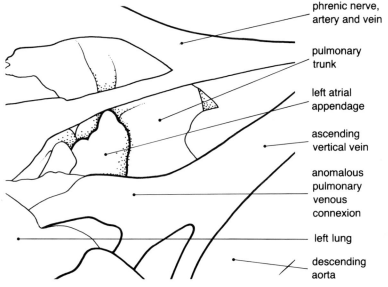

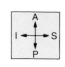

Fig. 9.3 *This operative view, through a left lateral thoracotomy, shows unilateral complete anomalous connexion of the left pulmonary veins to an ascending left vertical vein.*

phrenic nerve, artery and vein

pulmonary trunk

left atrial appendage

ascending vertical vein

anomalous pulmonary venous connexion

left lung

descending aorta

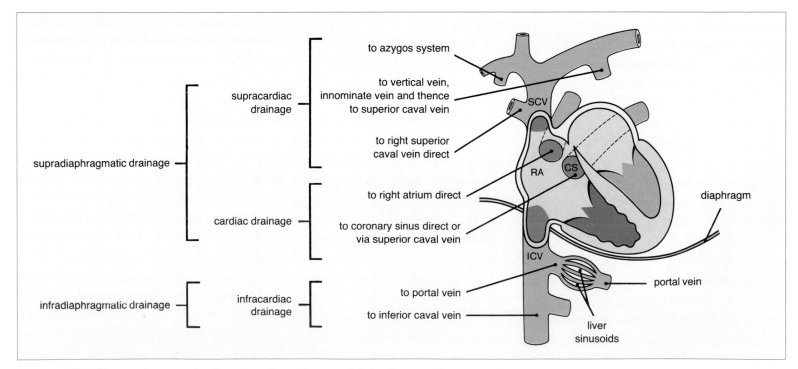

Fig. 9.4 *This diagram, in anatomic orientation, shows the potential sites for anomalous connexion of the pulmonary veins.*

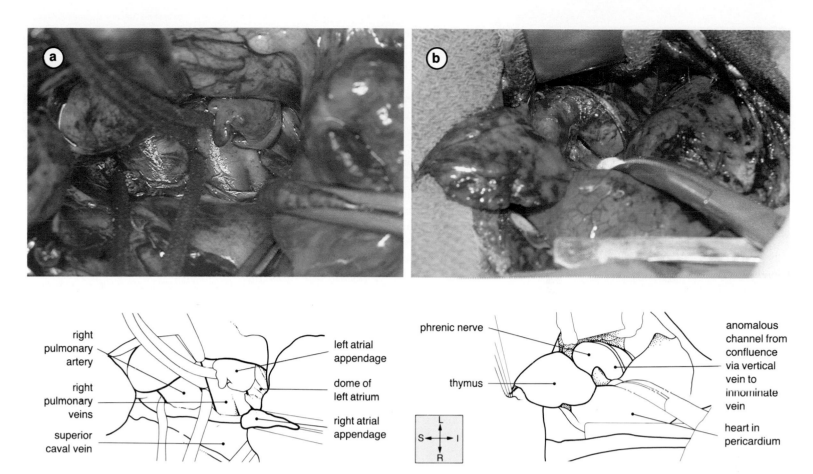

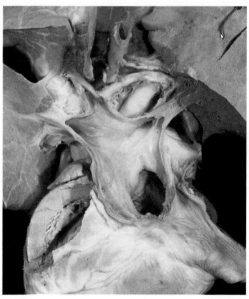

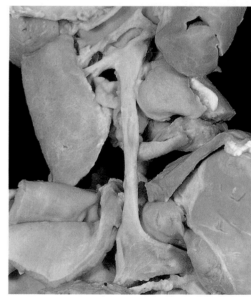

Fig. 9.5 *These operative views through a median sternotomy show total anomalous connexion of the pulmonary veins to the superior caval vein.* **(a)** *The course of the right pulmonary veins.* **(b)** *The vertical vein taking the pulmonary venous return to the innominate vein.*

Fig. 9.6 *This specimen, viewed from behind in anatomic orientation, has anomalous connexion of all four pulmonary veins to the coronary sinus.*

Fig. 9.7 *This specimen, viewed from behind in anatomic orientation, has anomalous connexion of all pulmonary veins to a descending channel that passes through the diaphragm to join the portal venous circulation.*

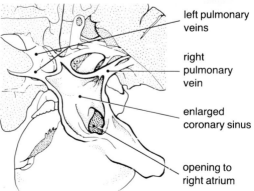

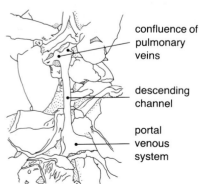

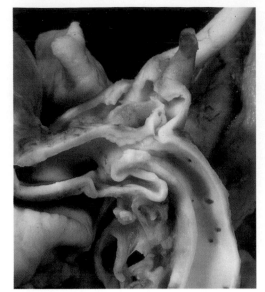

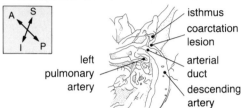

Fig. 9.8 *This specimen, viewed as it might be seen through a left thoracotomy, shows the ductal tissue that forms the shelf lesion of aortic coarctation. Note the co-existing hypopolasia of the aortic isthmus.*

venous obstruction. The appropriate landmarks must be borne in mind. Two types of anomalous connexion pose particular problems. The first is when the anomalous venous return is via the coronary sinus (Fig. 9.6), with a common 'party wall' between the coronary sinus and the left atrium. The logical repair is to incise this wall so as to unroof the sinus. At the same time, the orifice of the coronary sinus can be made confluent with the atrial septal defect, which is almost invariably within the oval fossa. It is important to remove enough of the party wall to ensure that the patch placed across the orifice of the coronary sinus and oval fossa does not produce an obstruction at the site of the incised sinus septum.

The second problematic type of connexion is the infradiaphragmatic variant. The extrapericardial common pulmonary venous trunk is farther from the posterior left atrial wall than might be expected. Because of this, the anastomosis effected between the trunk and left atrium is vulnerable to obstruction, particularly at its lateral extreme. This may become evident only when bypass is discontinued and the heart fills with blood.

Anomalies of the Aorta

The congenital anomalies of the thoracic aorta which are of interest to the surgeon include coarctation, the spectrum of partial to complete interruption of the aorta, and vascular 'rings'.

Coarctation of the Aorta

A coarctation is defined as a congenitally derived discrete shelf-like lesion within the aorta which causes obstruction to the flow of blood. It is most often found just distal to the left subclavian artery, but can occur proximally or more distally, and even in the abdominal aorta. It is usually accompanied by some degree of tubular hypoplasia of the aorta but is anatomically independent of the hypoplasia. Its presence may be linked with other lesions associated with diminished left-sided flow, but coarctation can and does occur independently. Tubular hypoplasia is considered as one extreme of a spectrum leading to atresia or interruption of the aortic arch[13].

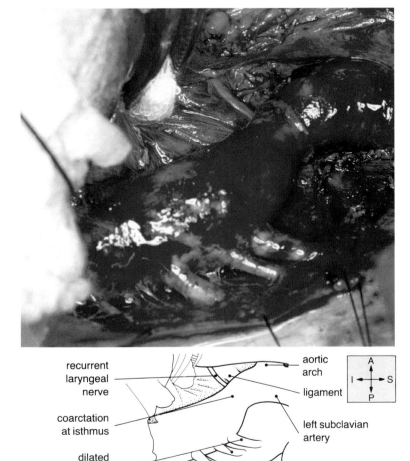

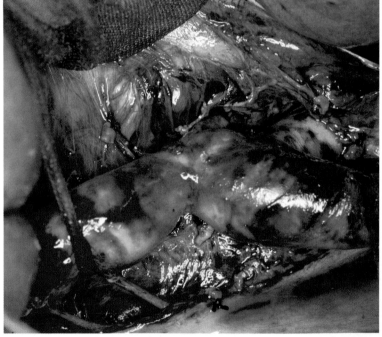

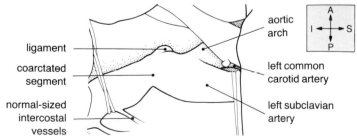

Fig. 9.9 *This operative view, through a left thoracotomy, shows aortic coarctation with enlarged intercostal arteries which are part of a well developed collateral circulation.*

Fig. 9.10 *In this operative view through a left thoracotomy, again from a patient with aortic coarctation (compare with Fig. 9.9), the collateral circulation is not well developed.*

The Role of Ductal Tissue

Much has been made of the role of ductal tissue in the etiology of coarctation. This subject has been extensively reviewed[14–16] and will not be discussed further, other than to stress the importance of removing ductal tissue during repair (Fig. 9.8). The significant features of the duct devolve upon its patency. If the duct is patent, almost invariably there is an associated congenital anomaly which promotes increased blood flow through the pulmonary trunk and diverts blood away from the proximal aorta. In these circumstances the associated anomaly tends to dominate the picture and to determine the most appropriate surgical therapy. On the other hand, coarctation with a closed duct is very likely to be an isolated lesion, except for the occasional association with a bicuspid aortic valve[17].

Surgical Anatomy of Coarctation

The chief concerns of the surgeon relate to the specific anatomy of the coarctation. The nature of the collateral circulation is of particular significance. With well developed collateral arteries (Fig. 9.9) there is little danger of cross-clamping the aorta during repair. If the collaterals are less well developed (Fig. 9.10), however, clamping the aorta may have several deleterious consequences. These include strain on the left ventricle due to proximal hypertension, which may also induce a cerebrovascular accident secondary to rupture of a 'berry' aneurysm. There may be distal aortic hypotension which endangers the splanchnic and spinal vascular beds. Irrespective of the nature of the collaterals, the spinal circulation is best preserved by interrupting none (or as few as possible) of the intercostal vessels. Temporary occlusion of the intercostal vessels adjacent to the operative field seems to be a reasonable compromise in this difficult situation.

Other noteworthy features include the position of the thoracic duct (Fig. 9.11a) and the occasional presence of an anomalous artery (Fig. 9.11b), sometimes referred to as 'Abbott's artery', which may arise from the posteromedial aspect of the proximal descending aorta. Whether this is an enlarged bronchial artery, or a 'persistence of the evanescent fifth arch', as suggested by Hamilton and Abbott[18], is irrelevant. What is important is that the surgeon be aware of the existence of this anomalous vessel which, if not properly managed, can lead to substantial bleeding during the repair[19].

Aortic Discontinuity

Discontinuity of the aorta, as opposed to coarctation, has been variously referred to as absence, atresia or interruption of the arch. Included in this group are those cases with a fibrous cord or bridge of tissue (Fig. 9.12) as well as those with a gap, or absolute discontinuity, at some point in the arch. Interruption can occur at one of three positions: at the isthmus; between the left subclavian and left common carotid

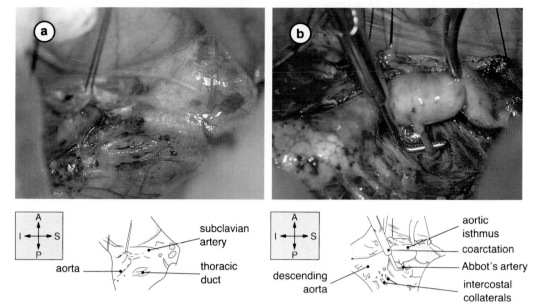

Fig. 9.11 **(a)** *This view through a left lateral thoracotomy shows the thoracic duct as it passes from the area of coarctation behind the left subclavian artery.* **(b)** *Through a left thoracotomy in a different patient, the proximal descending aorta and distal arch are rotated anteriorly. The large collateral referred to as 'Abbot's artery' is seen arising proximally to the area of coarctation.*

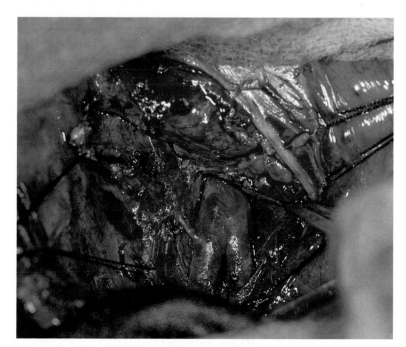

Fig. 9.12 *This operative view through a left lateral thoracotomy shows an aortic arch interrupted distal to the left subclavian artery. There is a thin fibrous cord connecting the interrupted arch to the distal descending aorta.*

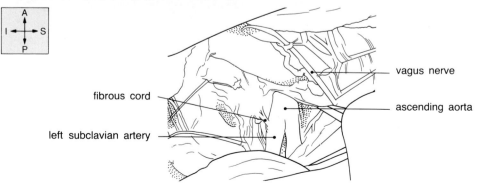

arteries; and between the left common carotid and brachiocephalic arteries (Fig. 9.13). Almost invariably, these lesions are associated with a unilateral left aortic arch but, rarely, a right arch can be similarly affected[20].

Associated Cardiovascular Malformations
Since patients with discontinuity of the aorta are unlikely to survive without surgical treatment, they are a particular challenge to the clinician. The associated cardiovascular malformations are of critical importance for they affect the operative outcome as much as the presence of the interrupted arch itself.

Almost always there is a patent connexion to the distal aorta through the duct (Fig. 9.14). A 'proximal' septal defect is also the rule. Frequently this is a ventricular septal defect but, occasionally, an aortopulmonary window is found (Fig. 9.15). The ventricular septal defect is usually peri-membranous in association with a posterior and leftward displacement of the outlet septum, resulting in sub-aortic stenosis (Fig. 9.16). Any type of defect can be found including, on rare occasions, those with anterior displacement which causes a Fallot-like obstruction to right ventricular outflow[21]. Abnormal ventriculo–arterial connexions are not unusual and present their own particular problems for operative reconstruction.

Aberrant right subclavian artery
A less lethal but fairly frequently associated arterial abnormality is an aberrant right subclavian artery which arises in a retro-esophageal position from the distal aorta. Since the arch is interrupted, symptoms of a vascular ring are unlikely unless a ring is created while reconstructing the arch. Conversely, if the aberrant artery is brought forward, it can be useful in repairing the aorta.

This emphasizes the critical importance of clearly defining the nature and effect of associated abnormalities. Successful anatomical correction is usually dependent

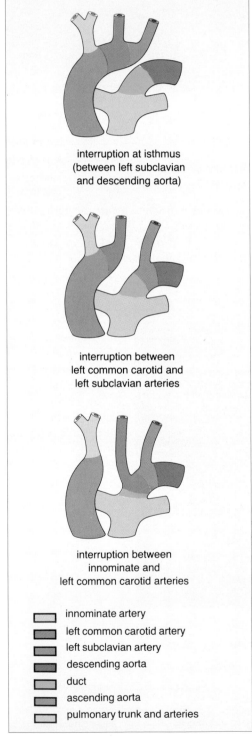

Fig. 9.13 *This diagram, in anatomic orientation, shows the different ways in which the aortic arch can be interrupted, the distal segment of the arch is then supplied through the arterial duct.*

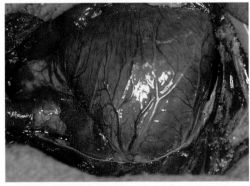
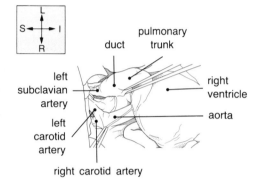

Fig. 9.14 *This operative view, seen through a median sternotomy, demonstrates an aortic arch interrupted distal to the left carotid artery. The ascending aorta gives rise to the left and right carotid arteries. The very large duct extends from the pulmonary artery to the distal aorta, which gives rise to the left subclavian and an aberrant right subclavian artery.*

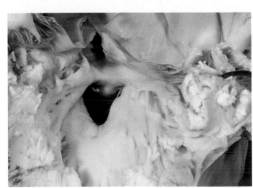
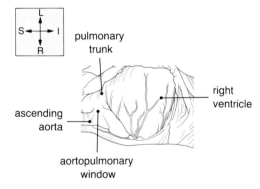

Fig. 9.15 *This operative view shows a patient with an interrupted aortic arch in association with an aortopulmonary window.*

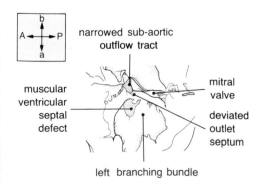

Fig. 9.16 *This anatomic orientation of the left ventricle with interrupted aortic arch shows the posterior deviation of the outlet septum that obstructs the sub-aortic outflow tract.*

on appropriate management of these accompanying lesions as it is on establishing aortic continuity

Aortic Rings

Aortic rings are malformations associated with an abnormal regression of part of a 'double aortic arch'. Knowledge of the development of aortic arches is a genuine aid to understanding the morphology of these anomalies, although it is undesirable to use embryological hypothesis as proven fact.

Of the six pairs of aortic arches connecting the anterior (ventral) and posterior (dorsal) aorta during development (Fig. 9.17), only the third, fourth and sixth arches remain recognizable in the postnatal heart. Most often, remnants of the third arch supply the head; the fourth becomes part of the definite aortic arch; and the left sixth arch becomes the duct (Fig. 9.18). The subclavian arteries, which are the seventh cervical intersegmental arteries, originate from the fourth arch between the third and sixth arches when the heart migrates inferiorly[22]. The hypothetical double aortic arch[23] consists of a midline anterior aorta which connects the bilateral fourth arches and bilateral posterior aortic segments to a midline descending aorta (Fig. 9.19). The fourth arches give rise to the remnants of the third arch and the bilateral sixth arches.

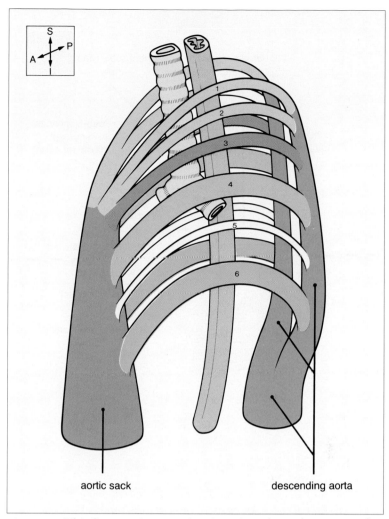

Fig. 9.17 *This diagram, in anatomic orientation, shows the patterns of formation of the aortic arches believed to exist during embryological development.*

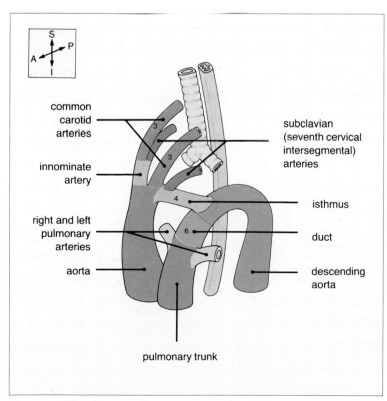

Fig. 9.18 *This diagram, drawn in comparable fashion to Fig. 9.17, shows how the definitive system of aortic arches is derived from the embryologic primordia.*

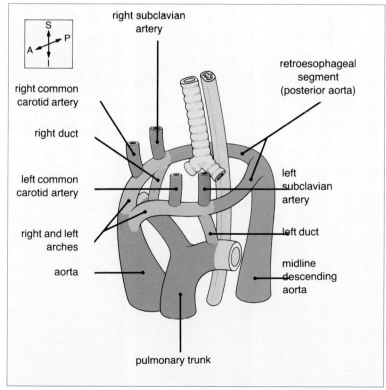

Fig. 9.19 *In this diagram, based on the series shown in Figs 9.17 and 9.18, the hypothetical perfect double arch is shown.*

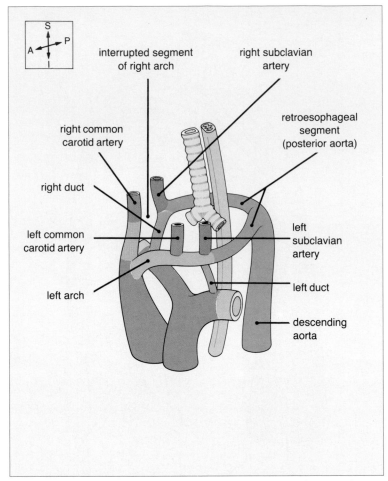

Fig. 9.20 *This diagram, continuing the series 9.16 through 9.18, shows how an abnormal arch with an aberrant subclavian artery and bilateral arterial ducts is explained on the basis of the hypothetical double arch.*

Initially, the arterial system is bilaterally symmetrical and the arches encircle the gut. Then, normally during early development, the entire distal right third arch regresses, leaving a left arch and a left-sided aorta (Fig. 9.18). Failure of this regression leads to various forms of a 'ring' around the trachea and the oesophagus. Most malformations of this nature are associated with a right aortic arch.

Persistent patency of an aortic ring can cause problems, and inappropriate interruption or atresia of part of the ring may result in abnormal anatomy. Such a situation is illustrated in Figure 9.20, which shows a left aortic arch with an aberrant right subclavian artery and bilateral ducts. In the scheme adopted by Stewart and co-workers[23], this anomaly would be placed in subgroup IIB3; however descriptive analysis rather than alphanumeric notation is preferable.

It should be noted that, as in the latter example of focal atresia, the atretic segment may not persist as a fibrous cord and may not necessarily cause compression of the trachea or oesophagus. Also, the size of the component parts of the ring is as least as important in producing symptoms as the particular anatomic arrangement. This accounts for the high incidence of symptoms associated with double aortic

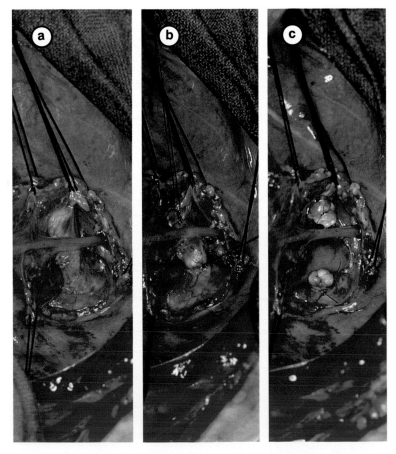

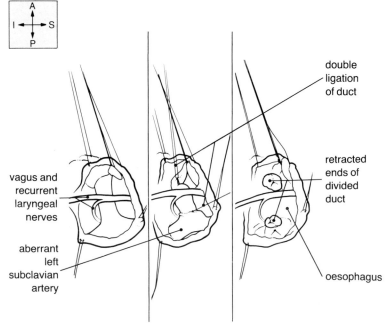

Fig. 9.21 *(a and b) These operative views, taken through a left thoracotomy, show an arterial duct that connects a right aortic arch to an aberrant left subclavian artery. Once the duct has been divided (c), the ends of the arch spring apart to free the oesophagus.*

arch. Indeed, when only a fibrous cord is found, compression is not always apparent. Figure 9.21a shows a duct attaching the left subclavian artery which arises from a right arch (Fig. 9.21b). The considerable tracheoesophageal compression is not obvious until the duct is divided and its ends allowed to retract (Fig. 9.21c). A detailed description of the various combinations of aortic rings can be found in the atlas by Stewart and his colleagues[23].

Right-sided Aortic Arch

A word must be said about the right-sided aortic arch apart from its association with vascular ring abnormalities. The definition of a right-sided aortic arch is one which crosses over the right main-stem bronchus. It may connect to a descending aorta on either the right or left side of the vertebral column. A right-sided aortic arch is considered abnormal with the usual atrial arrangement, but in patients with the mirror–image arrangement it is 'normal'. In either case it may or may not produce clinical problems. Its chief surgical significance lies in its association with about one-quarter of the cases of tetralogy of Fallot and approximately half of all patients with common arterial trunks.

When considering subclavian–pulmonary artery shunts in patients with a right aortic arch, it is important to recognize that one usually finds a mirror-image arrangement of the head, neck and arm arteries. The first branch of the aorta beyond the coronaries is a brachiocephalic trunk which gives rise to the left subclavian and common carotid arteries. Under such circumstances the surgeon may elect to perform a left-sided anastomosis so as to avoid kinking of the right subclavian artery as it is turned down into the mediastinum. The duct, however, is usually a left-sided structure connecting the brachiocephalic trunk to the left pulmonary artery (Fig. 9.22). Perhaps because of this mirror-image arrangement, it is unusual for the subclavian artery to have an aberrant origin and, thus, under these circumstances it is equally unusual to find a symptomatic vascular ring.

Pulmonary Arterial Anomalies

Aortic Origin of the Pulmonary Arteries

By far the most common malformation of the pulmonary arteries, excluding atresia or stenosis, is for either the right or left

pulmonary artery to have an aortic origin. Most frequently the anomalous artery arises from a duct. Although seen in the presence of pulmonary atresia, usually with the other lung supplied by major systemic-to-pulmonary collateral arteries, it can occur with the other pulmonary artery connected to the patent pulmonary trunk. In this arrangement, the duct will often close with time and consequently there will be apparent unilateral absence of that pulmonary artery which was initially fed through the duct. This is fairly common in tetralogy of Fallot or double outlet right ventricle, but about half of the patients thus afflicted have otherwise normal hearts[24]. It is rare to find true absence of the hilar pulmonary artery.

Less frequently, the anomalous pulmonary artery, usually the right, can arise directly from the ascending aorta (Fig. 9.23). This is sometimes called 'hemitruncus', but use of this term is not advocated because almost always there are two normally formed arterial valves, one of which is aortic and the other guards the pulmonary trunk supplying the normally connected pulmonary artery. Rarely, the right pulmonary artery may take an unusually high origin from the right side of the ascending portion of a common arterial trunk. It is preferable to use the descriptive title 'common trunk with anomalous origin of the right pulmonary artery' rather than 'hemitruncus'.

Surgical Repair of these Anomalies

When the anomalously connected pulmonary artery arises directly from the aorta, surgical repair consists simply of detachment from the aorta and reattachment to the pulmonary trunk. This is somewhat more difficult in the presence of a common trunk, but the same basic principle is followed for repair. When the anomalous pulmonary artery is fed through a duct or connected by a ligament, however, it will arise from the aortic arch or an innominate artery. Care must then be taken during surgical reconstruction to ensure that ductal tissue is not incorporated with the anastomosis, since it may subsequently constrict and produce stenosis at the site of repair. It should be remembered that, in cases with unilateral absence of a pulmonary artery, it is usual to find pulmonary hypertension and pulmonary hypertensive vascular disease in the normally connected lung, probably because it is disproportionately small and has to receive the entire right ventricular output[24].

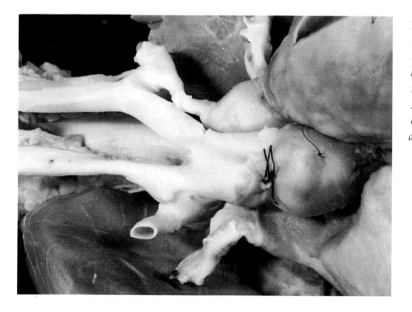

Fig. 9.22 *This view of a specimen, orientated as it might be seen through a median sternotomy, shows a right aortic arch with a left-sided arterial duct.*

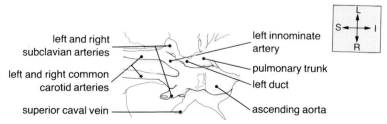

left and right subclavian arteries

left and right common carotid arteries

superior caval vein

left innominate artery

pulmonary trunk

left duct

ascending aorta

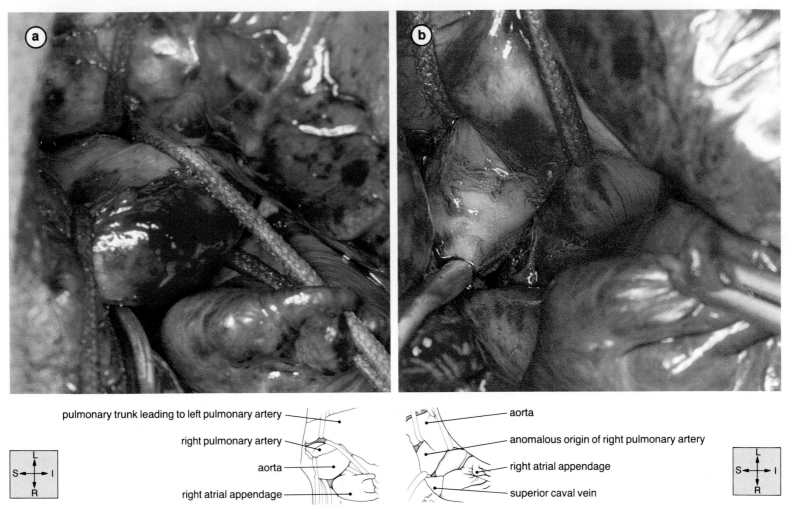

Fig. 9.23 *These operative views through a median sternotomy show the origin of the right pulmonary artery from the aorta. (a) Note the absence of its connexion to the pulmonary trunk, and (b) its course to the right lung.*

Origin of the Left from the Right Pulmonary Artery

A much rarer anomaly of the pulmonary arteries is when the left pulmonary artery arises from the right pulmonary artery. The abnormal left pulmonary vessel courses from the right chest and passes between the trachea and oesophagus to the left pulmonary hilum, creating a so-called 'vascular sling'[25] (Figs 9.24a and b). This may result in repeated respiratory problems requiring division and transplantation of the offending artery. As discussed above, the right pulmonary artery may arise anomalously from the aorta or innominate artery, but an abnormal right pulmonary vessel arising from the left pulmonary artery has not been reported. The reason for this is not clear.

Agenesis of the Right Lung

In the rare occurrence of agenesis of the right lung, displacement of the heart into the right chest may create a ring-like disposition which can obstruct the left

bronchus. The displaced heart, pulling on the left pulmonary artery, draws the ligament and descending aorta across the left bronchus, compressing the bronchus against the spinal column. Division of the ligament and grafting of the aorta may be necessary to allow the pulmonary trunk and aorta to spring apart and 'unroof' the constricting circle[26–28].

Persistent Duct and Aortopulmonary Window

Persistent Duct

Persistent duct occupies a special place in the study of cardiovascular disease because it was the first congenital cardiovascular malformation to be cured by operative intervention[29]. Though it has recently been subject to various medical manoeuvres[30,31], its interruption remains a paradigm of the best of surgical science. The anatomy is almost always predictable and the operative results uniformly excellent.

Because the arterial system develops with bilateral symmetry, a persistent duct may be either right- or left-sided, although the latter is overwhelmingly more common. Because the duct can persist on either side, or bilaterally, it may be important in vascular rings. Persistent patency may also play an important physiological role when it accompanies other complex congenital cardiovascular anomalies such as interruption of the aortic arch, aortic or pulmonary valvar atresia or complete transposition. This section is concerned with the primary congenital condition of isolated left-sided persistent patent duct.

Surgical Anatomy of Persistent Duct

Although an anterior approach to a patent duct is possible, and sometimes necessary (Fig. 9.25), the normal operative approach is through a left lateral thoracotomy (Fig. 9.26). The duct arises from the postero-superior aspect of the junction of the pulmonary trunk with the left pulmonary artery. It courses posteriorly and slightly leftward to join the junction of the aortic

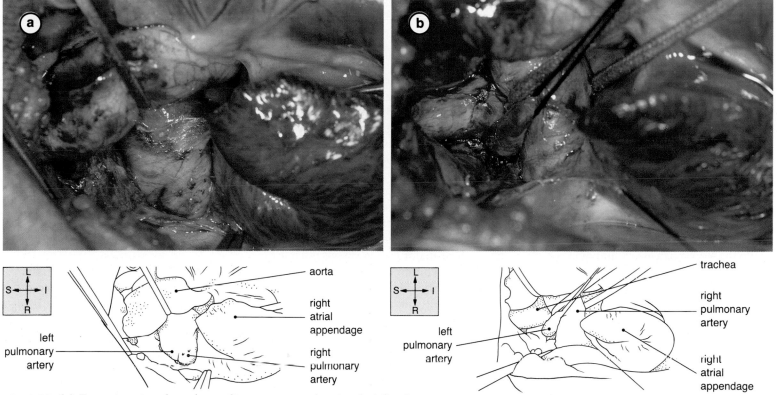

Fig. 9.24 *(a) Operative view through a median sternotomy showing the left pulmonary artery arising from the right pulmonary artery. (b) With the patient on bypass, the left artery can be seen to swing around the distal trachea.*

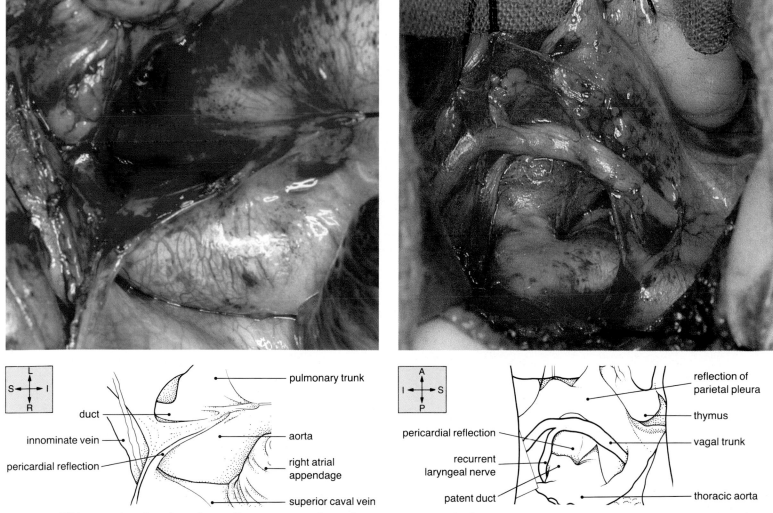

Fig. 9.25 *This operative view through a median sternotomy shows the appearance of a patent arterial duct arising from the distal pulmonary trunk.*

Fig. 9.26 *In this operative view, a patent arterial duct is seen through a left thoracotomy (compare with Fig. 9.25).*

arch and descending aorta just distal to, and opposite, the left subclavian orifice. Its pulmonary end is covered by a fold of pericardium and its aortic end by parietal pleura. It may be confused with the aortic isthmus, particularly in the infant, and the left pulmonary artery may also be erroneously identified as a patent duct. Even under the best conditions, these other structures may be mistakenly ligated in lieu of the duct. The caveats of this procedure have been elegantly reviewed by Pontius and co-workers[32]. Approached laterally, the best anatomical guide to the duct is the vagus nerve and its recurrent laryngeal branch. The vagus nerve passes along the subclavian artery and over the aortic arch before heading in a posterior direction to disappear behind the hilum. Just at the level of the duct, it gives rise to the recurrent nerve (Fig. 9.27), which then curves beneath the inferomedial wall of the duct before ascending along the posteromedial aspect of the aorta into the groove between the trachea and oesophagus.

Access to the duct may be achieved by incising the mediastinal parietal pleura, either between the phrenic and vagal nerves or more posteriorly over the aorta itself. With either approach, the recurrent nerve must be visualized to prevent direct trauma or injury by traction. The fold of pericardium extending over the pulmonary end of the duct may be lifted away by sharp dissection. The posteromedial wall

of the duct is firmly attached by another more fibrous band to the bronchus. It is this firm fibrous fold that prevents easy circumscription of the duct with a right-angle clamp. To minimize the risk of tearing the ductal wall, this tissue must be divided by sharp dissection. This can be done through a superior approach over the aortic end of the duct or by freeing the aorta and retracting it medially. In this latter case, small but potentially troublesome bronchial vessels may be encountered, arising from the posterior wall of the aorta. Another anatomical note of caution involves the thoracic duct and its tributaries at the origin of the subclavian artery. Division of any of these major lymph vessels is liable to lead to chylothorax and its attendant difficulties. Should the lymphatic trunks be inadvertently divided, they must be ligated to avoid chylothorax.

The duct in an infant or small child can measure 1–15mm in length and diameter. Rarely, one may encounter aneurysmal dilation of a duct. These may be aneurysms of a truly patent duct, or may simply be a dilated ductal diverticulum with a closed pulmonary end. In general, the short 'fat' duct should be cross-clamped, divided and oversewn to minimize the chances of incomplete ligation or tearing of the vessel wall. For the longer 'thin' duct, a triple ligation technique has proved to be safe and effective[34].

Aortopulmonary Window

The clinical presentation of aortopulmonary window is often similar to that of a common arterial trunk. The anatomical distinction lies in the mode of ventriculo–arterial connexion. Where, in a common trunk, there is a single valve, aortopulmonary window is always associated with separate aortic and pulmonary valves. Though the ventricular septum is usually intact, this defect is frequently associated with additional congenital cardiovascular anomalies[35].

Surgical Anatomy of Aortopulmonary Window

The defect itself is usually located in the right lateral wall of the pulmonary trunk anterior and opposite to the origin of the left pulmonary artery (Figs 9.15 and 9.28). This means that its opening into the left side of the ascending aorta is just distal to the sinutubular junction and coronary arteries. The defect may appear as a well demarcated short tubular structure or it may be more like a window.

The surgical repair of aortopulmonary window is best accomplished through an incision in the ascending aorta using standard cardiopulmonary bypass techniques. As a general rule, 'closed' methods are not advisable, not even for the more tubular defects. When the window supplies

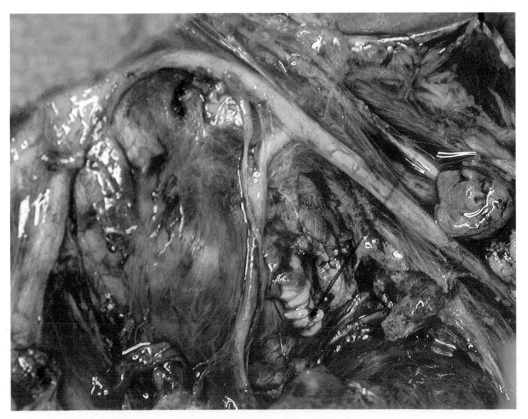

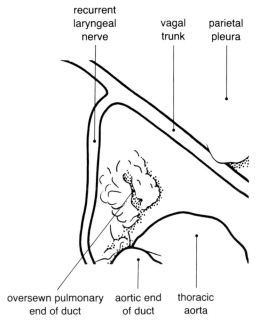

recurrent laryngeal nerve   vagal trunk   parietal pleura

oversewn pulmonary end of duct   aortic end of duct   thoracic aorta

Fig. 9.27 *In this operative view of the heart shown in Fig. 9.26, the recurrent laryngeal nerve is seen in relation to the duct.*

a vital part of the circulation, it cannot be closed without providing an alternate source of blood for the dependent segment of the circulation.

Anomalies of the Coronary Arteries

Congenital malformations of the coronary arteries in otherwise normally structured hearts have, traditionally, been categorized as major or minor. This approach was rooted in the belief that the so-called major anomalies were those that produced symptomatology, whereas the minor lesions were thought to be of no clinical relevance[36]. The potential danger of such a classification became evident when it was realized that some lesions categorized as minor could, in fact, underlie the occurrence of sudden death[37]. Because of this discrepancy between presumed anatomic and revealed clinical significance, it now seems preferable to account for these malformations on a descriptive basis. Within such a descriptive categorization, the anomalies can be grouped into those with anomalous origin of the coronary arteries from the arterial roots, those with an anomalous course of the epicardial coronary arteries, those with anomalous communications between the coronary arteries and other structures within the heart, or combinations of such findings (Fig. 9.29).

Anomalous Origin of the Coronary Arteries

The coronary arteries can arise anomalously either from the pulmonary trunk or, rarely, from a pulmonary artery, but can also take an anomalous origin from the aorta itself.

Anomalous Origin from the Pulmonary Trunk

It is the anomalous origin from the pulmonary trunk that is of the most clinical significance. Often described as the Bland–White–Garland syndrome, anomalous origin of the left coronary artery from the pulmonary trunk (Fig. 9.30) usually presents in infancy with ischaemia of the

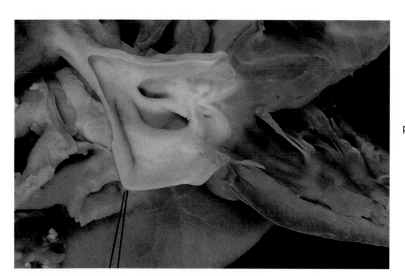

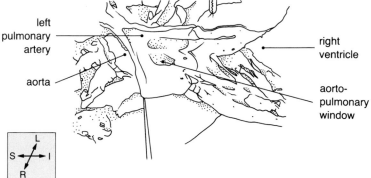

Fig. 9.28 *This specimen, viewed as it would be seen through a median sternotomy, shows an aortopulmonary window as seen from the pulmonary trunk.*

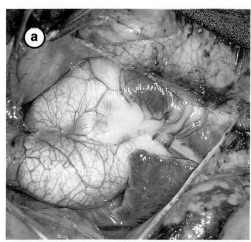
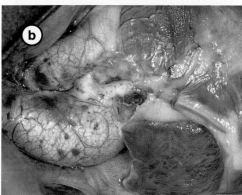

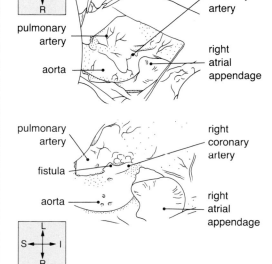

Fig. 9.29 *(a) This view through a median sternotomy shows a heart with the right coronary artery arising high on the ascending aorta. (b) With dissection the artery is seen to communicate as well with the pulmonary trunk. This resulted in a small left-to-right shunt and reverse flow in the right coronary artery.*

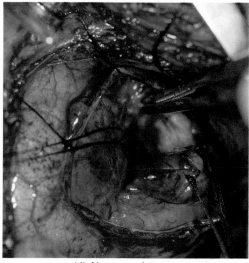
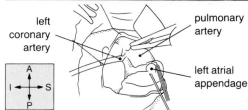

Fig. 9.30 *This view through a left lateral thoracotomy shows a silk ligature encircling the left coronary artery arising from the pulmonary trunk.*

left ventricle, although, if there is well-developed collateral circulation, presentation can be markedly delayed, some cases not presenting until childhood or even adolescence. The clinical problems are produced by the extent of ischaemia of the left ventricular myocardium, which can be extreme. It is important to reattach the artery to the aorta as soon as the diagnosis is made.

If the abnormal artery arises from the right-hand facing sinus of the pulmonary trunk[38], the arterial origin, together with a button of pulmonary sinus, may be transferred to the left-hand facing sinus of the aorta. Others have advocated creating an aortopulmonary tunnel to reconnect the artery to the aorta[39]. Either the creation of a tunnel, or direct transfer of the artery to the aortic root[40] is, if possible, usually preferable to simple ligation of the coronary artery. The pattern that may create problems in transfer is when the artery arises from a branch of the pulmonary trunk rather than the trunk itself.

Other patterns, such as anomalous origin of the right coronary artery from the pulmonary trunk, do not produce the same degree of symptomatology and often do not come to the attention of the surgeon. If necessary, the origin of the right coronary artery can readily be transferred back to the aortic root.

Anomalous Origin from the Aorta

The significance of anomalous origin of one coronary artery from the aorta has yet to be fully established. Usually the coronary arteries arise from the aortic sinuses that face the pulmonary trunk. In the normal heart, the left coronary artery arises from the left-hand facing sinus, while the right coronary artery arises from the right-hand facing sinus. Accessory orifices supplying either the infundibular artery, the artery to the sinus node, or an artery supplying the wall of the arterial trunks are by no means uncommon and should not be interpreted as representing anomalies. The circumflex and anterior descending branches of the left coronary artery can also, rarely, take a separate origin from the left-hand facing sinus in an otherwise normal heart. Usually the arteries arise within the sinuses, but origin at the sinutubular bar, or just above it, should not be considered abnormal. High origin, however, or an oblique course of a coronary artery through the wall, particularly when crossing a commissure (the so-called intramural course), should be considered anomalous, as should origin of the left coronary artery from the right-hand facing sinus or, as occurs very rarely[41], from the non-facing aortic sinus.

The finding of a single coronary artery also represents anomalous origin from the aortic root. This can be found in two patterns. In the first, all three coronary arteries arise from the same aortic sinus, with either one, two, or three orifices within the sinus. Usually it is the right-hand sinus that gives rise to the coronary arteries (Figs 9.31a and b). There is then an associated anomalous epicardial course of the branches of the left coronary artery as they reach their anticipated locations. Unlike the case shown in Fig. 9.31 this may involve the anterior interventricular branch tracking between the aorta and the pulmonary trunk, with the potential for its constriction. Another pattern is for the right coronary artery to take its normal origin from the right-hand facing sinus, but then to continue beyond the crux as the circumflex artery and to terminate at the obtuse margin as the anterior interventricular artery. This pattern probably has no clinical significance. Very rarely, a solitary coronary artery may originate from the non-facing aortic sinus (Fig. 9.32a). In the case illustrated, with tetralogy of Fallot, the abnormal course of the right coronary artery meant that repair was necessary through the right atrium, with only a limited incision being possible across the ventriculo–arterial junction (Fig. 9.32c). An alternative approach would have been to use a conduit.

In addition to anomalous origin, congenital malformations can also afflict

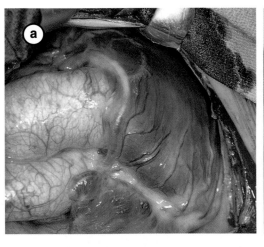
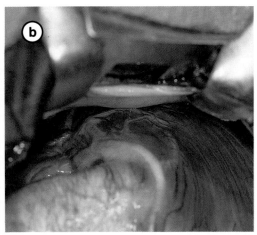
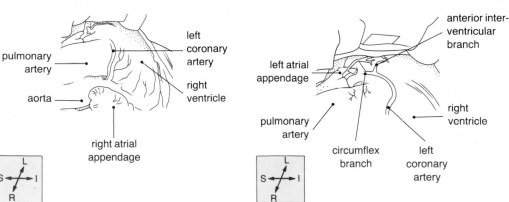

Fig. 9.31 *(a) This operative view through a median sternotomy demonstrates the coronary arteries arising from a single orifice in the right-hand facing sinus. (b) A close-up view shows the left coronary artery to cross the base of the pulmonary trunk. It divides into an anterior interventricular branch and a circumflex branch.*

normally attached arteries, producing the effect of anomalous origin. Particularly important in this respect is congenital atresia of the main stem of the left coronary artery (Fig. 9.33). This can be another condition for sudden death in an adolescent or young adult[42]. Unfortunately, this anomaly is unlikely to be diagnosed prior to the event, when it could readily be treated by surgical manoeuvres.

Anomalous Epicardial Course of the Coronary Arteries

Although an anomalous epicardial course can be found in otherwise normally structured hearts, it is seen more frequently in hearts that are themselves malformed, such as those with a complete transposition or a common arterial trunk. The clinical significance of these anomalies has yet to be fully determined. Some are found as chance observations at autopsy, such as the single case presenting with anomalous origin of the circumflex artery from the right-hand facing sinus with subsequent retroaortic course (Fig. 9.34), which was discovered in examination of 100 presumed normal hearts[43]. Others may be of signifi-

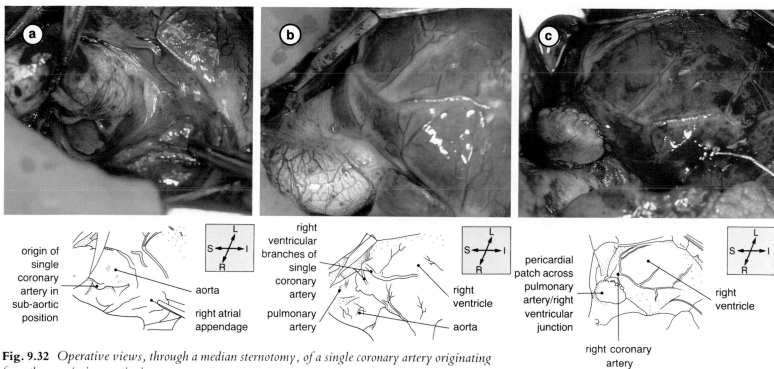

Fig. 9.32 *Operative views, through a median sternotomy, of a single coronary artery originating from the non-facing aortic sinus.*

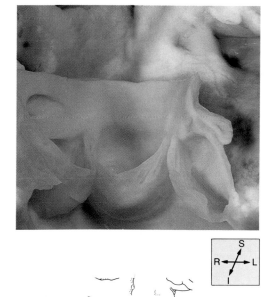

Fig. 9.33 *This specimen, in anatomic orientation, shows atresia of the left coronary artery.*

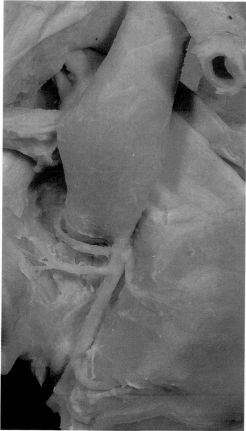

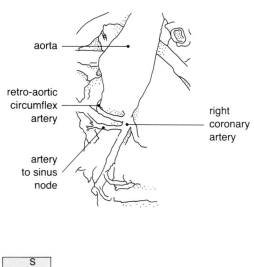

Fig. 9.34 *This specimen, in anatomic orientation, shows anomalous origin of the circumflex coronary artery from the right-hand facing sinus.*

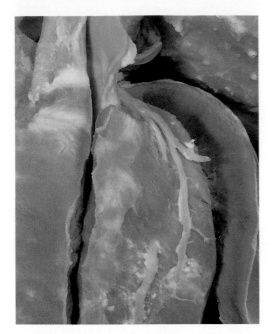

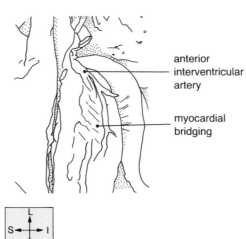

anterior interventricular artery

myocardial bridging

cance in sudden death, such as passage of the anterior interventricular artery between the aorta and the pulmonary trunk, sometimes coursing through the muscular ventricular septum, as discussed previously[44]. In this respect, muscular bridging of the epicardial coronary arteries may be of relevance, although this was seen in 34 of the series of normal hearts[43], with bridges being found over both the right and left coronary arteries in two of the specimens (Fig. 9.35).

Anomalous Communications of the Coronary Arteries

Fistulous communications between the coronary arteries and the ventricles are seen most frequently when atresia of an outflow tract is seen in the case of an intact ventricular septum, notably in pulmonary atresia with intact ventricular septum (see Chapter 7 p7.00). Such communications can also be found in otherwise normally structured hearts, and the anomalous artery can be joined to any other cardiac structure. The right coronary artery is most frequently involved, and it may connect to the right atrium (Figs 9.36a, b and c), the superior caval vein, the coronary sinus, the right ventricle (Fig. 9.37), the pulmonary trunk, a pulmonary vein, or the left ventricle. The communication itself can be a simple large orifice (Fig. 9.37b) or a complex worm-like aneurysmal cavity. When the communication is simple and large, shunting across it can be considerable and the artery itself can be markedly dilated. 'Steals' can also result, with consequent ischaemia in the area of myocardium from which the steal has occurred.

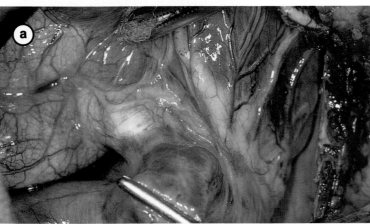

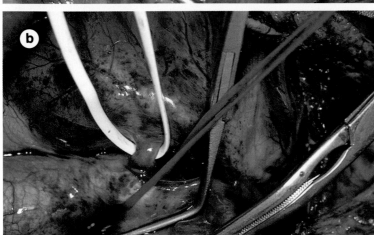

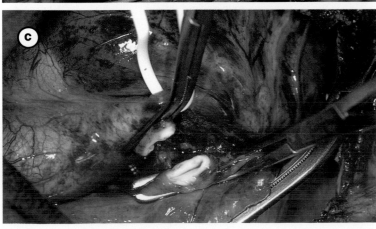

Fig. 9.36 *(a) This operative view with the right atrial appendage retracted demonstrates a fistula from the right coronary artery to the base of the appendage. (b) Here vessel loops are seen around the normal distal right coronary artery (white) and the fistula (red). (c) The broad fistula has been divided.*

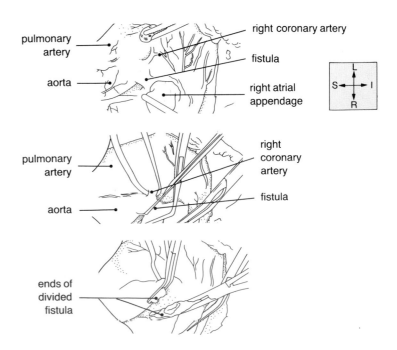

pulmonary artery

aorta

right coronary artery

fistula

right atrial appendage

pulmonary artery

aorta

right coronary artery

fistula

ends of divided fistula

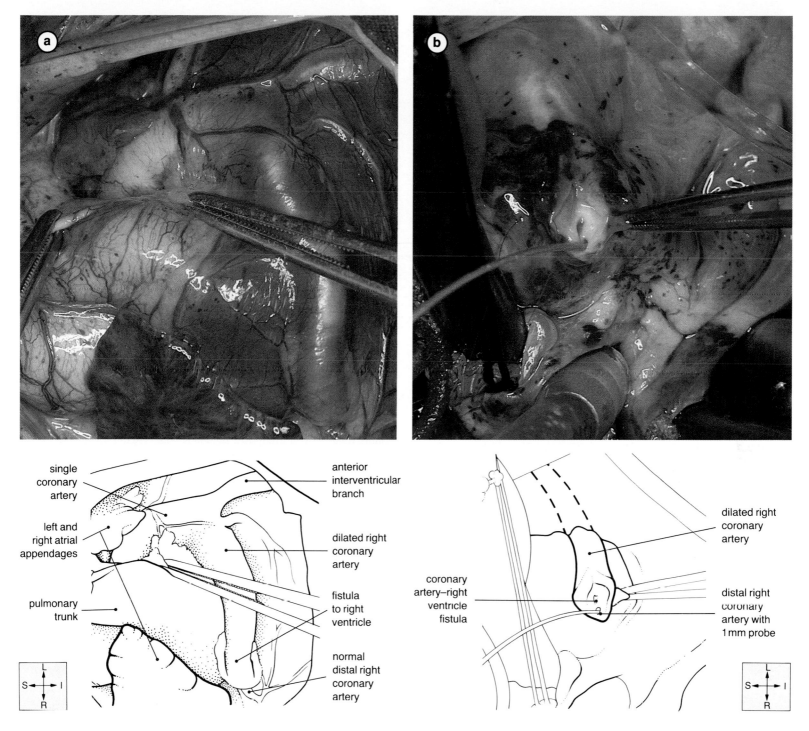

Fig. 9.37 *Operative views of a fistula between the right coronary artery and the right ventricle. The single coronary artery gives rise to (a) a grossly dilated right coronary artery (b) which becomes normal beyond the site of the fistulous communication.*

References

1. Winter, F.S. (1954) Persistent left superior vena cava: survey of world literature and report of 30 additional cases. *Angiology*, **5**, 90–132.

2. Bankl, H. (1977) In *Congenital Malformations of the Heart and Great Vessels*. Baltimore – Munich: Urban and Schwarzenberg, p. 194.

3. Anderson, R.C., Heilig, W., Novick, R. & Jarvis, C. (1955) Anomalous inferior vena cava with azygous drainage: so-called absence of the inferior vena cava. *American Heart Journal*, **49**, 318–322.

4. Moller, J.H., Nakib, A., Anderson, R.C. & Edwards, J.E. (1967) Congenital cardiac disease associated with polysplenia: A developmental complex of bilateral 'left-sidedness'. *Circulation*, **36**, 789–799.

5. Venables, A.W. (1963) Isolated drainage of the inferior vena cava to the left atrium. *British Heart Journal*, **25**, 545–548.

6. Edwards, J.E. & DuShane, J.W. (1950) Thoracic venous anomalies. I. Vascular connection between the left atrium and the left innominate vein (levoatriocardinal vein) associated with mitral atresia and premature closure of the foramen ovale (case 1). II. Pulmonary veins draining wholly to the ductus arteriosus (case 2). *Archives of Pathology*, **49**, 517–537.

7. Lucas, R.V. Jr., Woolfrey, B.F., Anderson, R.C., Lester, R.G. & Edwards, J.E. (1962) Atresia of the common pulmonary vein. *Pediatrics*, **29**, 729–739.

22. Barry, A. (1951) Aortic arch derivatives in the human adult. *Anatomical Record*, **111**, 221–238.

23. Stewart, J.R., Kincaid, O.W. & Edwards, J.E. (1964) *An Atlas of Vascular Rings and Related Malformations of the Aortic Arch System*. Springfield, Illinois: Charles C. Thomas.

24. Pool, P.E., Vogel, J.H.K. & Blount, S.G. Jr. (1962) Congenital unilateral absence of a pulmonary artery. The importance of flow in pulmonary hypertension. *American Journal of Cardiology*, **10**, 706–732.

25. Contro, S., Miller, R.A., White, H. & Potts, W.J. (1958) Bronchial obstruction due to pulmonary artery anomalies. I. Vascular sling. *Circulation*, **17**, 418–423.

26. Maier, H.C. & Gould, W.J. (1953) Agenesis of the lung with vascular compression of the tracheobronchial tree. *Journal of Pediatrics*, **43**, 38–42.

27. Harrison, M.R. & Hendren, W.H. (1975) Agenesis of the lung complicated by vascular compression and bronchomalacia. *Journal of Pediatric Surgery*, **10**, 813–817.

28. Harrison, M.R., Heldt, G.P., Brasch, R.C., de Lorimier, A.A. & Gregory, G.A. (1980) Resection of distal tracheal stenosis in a baby with agenesis of the lung. *Journal of Pediatric Surgery*, **15**, 938–943.

29. Gross, R.E. (1939) Surgical management of patent ductus arteriosus with summary of four surgically treated cases. *Annals of Surgery*, **110**, 321–356.

30. Starling, M.B. & Elliott, R.B. (1974) The effect of prostaglandins, prostaglandin inhibition, and oxygen on the closure of the ductus arteriosus, pulmonary arteries, and umbilical vessels *in vitro*. *Prostaglandins*, **8**, 187–203.

31. Heymann, M.A., Rudolph, A.M. & Silverman, N.H. (1976) Closure of the ductus arteriosus in premature infants by inhibition of prostaglandin synthesis. *New England Journal of Medicine*, **295**, 530–533.

32. Pontius, R.G., Danielson, G.K., Noonan, J.A. & Judson, J.P. (1981) Illusions leading to surgical closure of the distal left pulmonary artery instead of the ductus arteriosus. *Journal of Thoracic and Cardiovascular Surgery*, **82**, 107–113.

33. Mendel, V., Luhmer, J. & Oelert, H. (1980) Aneurysma des Ductus arteriosus bei einem Neugeborenen. *Herz*, **5**, 320–323.

34. Wilcox, B.R. & Peters, R.M. (1967) The surgery of patent ductus arteriosus: a clinical report of 14 years' experience without an operative death. *Annals of Thoracic Surgery*, **3**, 126–131.

35. Faulkner, S.L., Oldham, R.R., Atwood, G.F. & Graham, T.P. (1974) Aortopulmonary window, ventricular septal defect and membranous pulmonary atresia with a diagnosis of truncus arteriosus. *Chest*, **65**, 351–353.

36. Ogden, J.A. (1970) Congenital anomalies of the coronary arteries. *American Journal of Cardiology*, **25**, 474–479.

37. Becker, A.E. (1983) Variations of the main coronary arteries. In *Paediatric Cardiology Volume 3*. Edited by A.E. Becker, T.G. Losekoot, C. Marcelletti & R.H. Anderson. Edinburgh: Churchill Livingstone, pp. 263–277.

38. Smith, A., Arnold, R., Anderson, R.H., Wilkinson, J.L., Qureshi, S.A., Gerlis, L.M. & McKay, R. (1989) Anomalous origin of the left coronary artery from the pulmonary trunk. Anatomic findings in relation to pathophysiology and surgical repair. *Journal of Thoracic and Cardiovascular Surgery*, **98**, 16–24.

39. Takeuchi, S., Imamura, H., Katsumoto, K., Hayashi, I., Katohgi T., Yozu, R., Ohkura, M. & Inoue, T. (1979) New surgical method for repair of anomalous left coronary artery from the pulmonary artery. *Journal of Thoracic and Cardiovascular Surgery*, **78**, 7–11.

40. Neches, W.H., Matthews, R.A., Park, S.C., Lenox, C.C., Zuberbuhler, J.R., Siewers, R.D. & Bahnson, H.T. (1974) Anomalous origin of the left coronary artery from the pulmonary artery. *Circulation*, **50**, 582–587.

41. Ishikawa, T., Otsuka, T. & Suzuki, T. (1990) Anomalous origin of the left main coronary artery from the non-coronary sinus of Valsalva. (Letter). *Pediatric Cardiology*, **11**, 173–174.

42. Debich, D.E., Williams, K.E. & Anderson, R.H. (1989) Congenital atresia of the orifice of the left coronary artery and its main stem. *International Journal of Cardiology*, **22**, 398–404.

43. Debich, D.A., Devine, W.A. & Anderson, R.H. The pattern of origin of the coronary arteries and their epicardial course in the normal heart. Submitted for publication.

44. Kragel, A.H. & Roberts, W.C. (1988) Anomalous origin of either right or left main coronary artery from the aorta with subsequent coursing between aorta and pulmonary trunk: analysis of 32 necropsy cases. *American Journal of Cardiology*, **62**, 771–777.

8. Mortensson, W. & Lundstrom, N.R. (1974) Congenital obstruction of the pulmonary veins at their junctions. Review of the literature and a case report. *American Heart Journal*, **87**, 359–362.

9. Nakib, A., Moller, J.H., Kanjuh, V.I. & Edwards, J.E. (1967) Anomalies of the pulmonary veins. *American Journal of Cardiology*, **20**, 77–90.

10. Bharati, S. & Lev, M. (1973) Congenital anomalies of the pulmonary veins. *Cardiovascular Clinics*, **5**, 23–41.

11. DeLisle, G., Ando, M., Calder, A.L., Zuberbuhler, J.R., Rochenmacher, S., Alday, L.E., Mangino, O., Van Praagh, S. & Van Praagh, R. (1976) Total anomalous pulmonary venous connection: report of 93 autopsied cases with emphasis on diagnostic and surgical considerations. *American Heart Journal*, **91**, 99–122.

12. Neill, C.A., Ferencz, C., Sabiston, D.C. & Sheldon, H. (1960) The familial occurrence of hypoplastic right lung with systemic arterial supply and venous drainage 'scimitar syndrome'. *Johns Hopkins Medical Journal*, **107**, 1–15.

13. Becker, A.E. & Anderson, R.H. (1981) In *Pathology of Congenital Heart Disease*. London: Butterworths, pp. 319–338.

14. Brom, A.G. (1965) Narrowing of the aortic isthmus and enlargement of the mind. *Journal of Thoracic and Cardiovascular Surgery*, **50**, 166–180.

15. Ho, S.Y. & Anderson, R.H. (1979) Coarctation, tubular hypoplasia and the ductus arteriosus: a histological study of 35 specimens. *British Heart Journal*, **41**, 268–274.

16. Elzenga, N.J. & Gittenberger-de-Groot, A.C. (1983) Localised coarctation of the aorta. An age dependent spectrum. *British Heart Journal*, **49**, 317–323.

17. Becker, A.E., Becker, M.J. & Edwards, J.E. (1970) Anomalies associated with coarctation of the aorta. Particular reference to infancy. *Circulation*, **41**, 1067–1075.

18. Hamilton, W.F. & Abbott, M.E. (1928) Coarctation of the aorta of the adult type: Part I. Complete obliteration of the descending arch at insertion of the ductus in a boy of fourteen; bicuspid aortic valve; impending rupture of the aorta; cerebral death. Part II. A statistical study and historical retrospect of 200 recorded cases, with autopsy, of stenosis or obliteration of the descending arch in subjects above the age of two years. *American Heart Journal*, **3**, 381–421.

19. Lerberg, D.B. (1982) Abbott's artery. *Annals of Thoracic Surgery*, **33**, 415–416.

20. Pierpont, M.E.M., Zollikofer, C.L., Moller, J.H. & Edwards, J.E. (1982) Interruption of the aortic arch with right descending aorta. *Pediatric Cardiology*, **2**, 153–159.

21. Ho, S.Y., Wilcox, B.R., Anderson, R.H. & Lincoln, J.C.R. (1983) Interrupted aortic arch – anatomical features of surgical significance. *The Thoracic and Cardiovascular Surgeon*, **31**, 199–205.

POSITIONAL ANOMALIES OF THE HEART

10

Introduction

The surgical problems posed by cardiac malformations may be considerably increased when the heart is in an abnormal position. This is partly due to the unusual anatomical perspective presented to the surgeon because of the malposition, and also to the abnormal locations of the cardiac chambers which may necessitate approaches other than those already discussed. It is vital to stress that cardiac malposition is not itself a diagnosis. Any normal or abnormal segmental combination can be found in an abnormally located heart. The heart may be normal, despite the malposition, but extremely complex anomalies are frequently present. Consequently, the very presence of an abnormal cardiac position emphasizes the need for a full and detailed segmental analysis of the heart. All the rules enunciated in Chapter 6 apply when the heart is not in its anticipated position.

This chapter confines itself to a description of malpositioned hearts and a detailed discussion for specific types of malposition. It concludes with a brief review of the surgical significance of isomerism of the atrial appendages, which is generally held to be one of the major harbingers of abnormal cardiac position[1].

Describing the Abnormal Cardiac Position

When describing an abnormally located heart, it is necessary to take account of both its position within the chest and the direction of its apex. In the normal individual, the heart is positioned with its apex to the left and two-thirds of its bulk to the left of the midline. When a mirror-image atrial arrangement is the case it is usually accompanied by a mirror-image cardiac arrangement. The norm is then for the apex to point to the right with the greater part of the cardiac mass in the right hemithorax. With visceral heterotaxy and isomerism of the atrial appendages, however, there is no norm. Thus, for all patients with isomerism, and for those with the usual or mirror-image atrial arrangements as well as abnormally positioned hearts, it is necessary to have a system to describe the abnormal cardiac position.

In the past, formidable conventions have been constructed, using terms such as dextrocardia, dextroposition, dextrorotation and pivotal dextrocardia (for a review see Reference 2). In practice, the only requirement is a system which accounts for two major features: the position of the cardiac mass relative to the silhouette of the chest and the direction of the cardiac apex. This is because the position of the heart and the orientation of its apex, although usually congruent, are not invariably linked together. Some systems, such as that proposed by a group including one of the present authors[3], have defined dextrocardia as the heart in the right chest with the apex to the right (Fig. 10.1). But what happens on the rare occasion when the heart is in the right chest with its apex to the left? According to the convention recommended in Chapter 6, this is readily described as 'heart in right chest, apex to left'. The value of this approach is again emphasized. Those who wish to give nominative definitions to the arrangement are free to do so, but the descriptive terms will be found to be entirely adequate and less liable to misconstruction. Thus, the heart is described as being mostly in the left chest, in the right chest or symmetrical, and the apical orientation is to the left, to the right or to the middle.

Exteriorization of the Heart

The description given above does not account for the most severe cardiac malposition, namely exteriorization of the heart (ectopia cordis). It had been said that the heart can protrude from the thoracic cavity in cervical, thoracic, thoracoabdominal or abdominal positions. The review by Van Praagh and his colleagues[4] questions the cervical and abdominal variants, classifying all cases as effectively thoracic or thoracoabdominal. In the thoracic type, which is the most common, there is a sternal defect and the parietal pericardium is absent. The heart protrudes directly from the thorax as illustrated in the classical case of Byron[5]. Usually there is an associated omphalocele and a small thoracic cavity.

In the thoracoabdominal type, the sternal defect is usually confluent with defects of the abdominal wall and diaphragm, so the heart and various abdominal organs are displaced into an omphalocele. A variant of this abnormality is seen in patients with so-called Cantrell's syndrome[6]. These patients have a cleft lower sternum. The heart is beneath the skin in the upper epigastrium and is associated with an omphalocele (Fig. 10.2a). Opening the skin demonstrates the heart to be low in the midline (Fig. 10.2b) and extending toward the omphalocele through a diaphragmatic defect. These patients frequently have complex intracardiac defects, often including a diverticulum of the left ventricle. The heart illustrated here shows tetralogy of Fallot and right atrial isomerism (Fig. 10.2c) but no diverticulum.

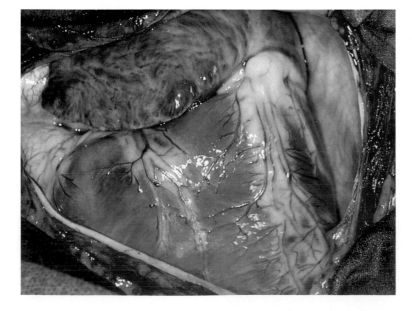

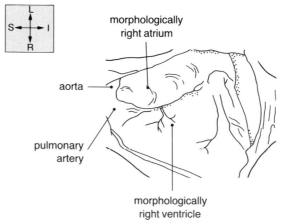

Fig. 10.1 *Operative view through a median sternotomy showing a patient with the heart in the right chest and the apex to the right.*

morphologically right atrium

aorta

pulmonary artery

morphologically right ventricle

Congenital Malformations

Our descriptive system provides no information as to whether the unusual situation is a result of congenital malformation. For example, the heart may be in the right chest secondary to a pulmonary defect or because of gross enlargement of its right-sided chambers. In each case, the problems of access presented to the surgeon are similar. Indeed, there is no reason why a patient with a lesion such as congenitally corrected transposition should not acquire a heart in the right chest because of pulmonary problems or right-sided hypertrophy.

There are certain lesions which readily spring to mind when the heart is located in the right chest with the usual atrial arrange-ment, and with hearts in the left chest and mirror-image atrial chambers. The most notable of these is congenitally corrected transposition[7]. An important point concerning patients with abnormally positioned hearts is that it is essential that the surgeon be aware of the locations of the chambers within the malpositioned organ so that the operation can be planned appropriately.

Diagnosing Difficult Cardiac Arrangements

With the sophistication of modern diagnostic techniques, it is unlikely that the surgeon will be presented with a patient with an abnormally located heart without a full preoperative diagnosis. There are, however, particular cardiac arrangements of the chambers which can still give major difficulties in diagnosis, notably the so-called 'criss-cross hearts' and 'supero-inferior ventricles'.

In these anomalies the ventricular relationships, or more rarely the ventricular topology (using the term 'topology' as defined in Chapter 6), are not as anticipated for a given atrioventricular connexion[8].

'Criss-cross Hearts'

In a patient with a congenitally corrected transposition and a 'criss-cross' arrangement, the morphologically right ventricle

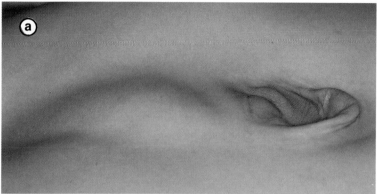

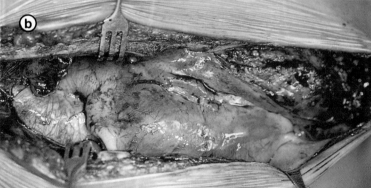

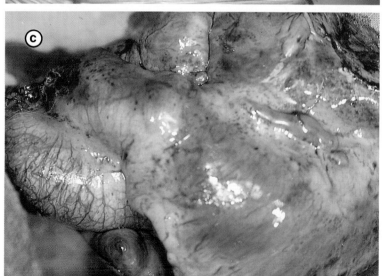

Fig. 10.2 *(a) View from the right side of a patient's epigastrium, as seen in the operating room with the patient supine. The bulging heart is seen through the skin because of the cleft lower sternum and diastasis of the rectus muscles. The associated abdominal hernia is collapsed.*

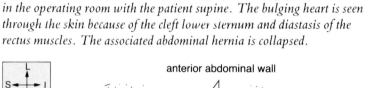

(b) The skin and upper sternum has been opened to show the heart in the midline with the apex in the midline.

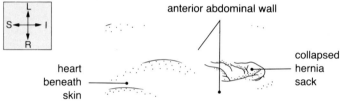

(c) The atrial appendages were both broad based, consistent with right isomerism.

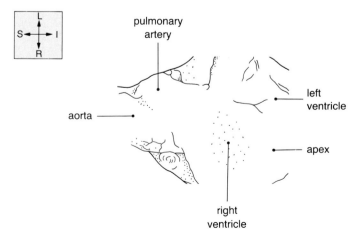

will be predominantly right-sided rather than in its anticipated left-sided position. This is a consequence of rotation of the ventricular mass in its long axis (Fig. 10.3).

In addition to these unusual relationships, there is the possibility that a catheter passed through the right atrioventricular valve, in a heart with discordant atrioventricular connexions and 'criss-cross' relationships, may slip through a ventricular septal defect and opacify the right-sided morphologically right ventricle. This will give the spurious appearance of concordant atrioventricular connexions[9].

Distribution of the Coronary Arteries

The distribution of the coronary arteries is of considerable help in determining the position of the ventricles since, in congenitally corrected transposition, the anterior interventricular coronary artery arises from the right-sided coronary artery. Thus, in a heart which at first sight appears to represent complete transposition, locating an anterior interventricular artery with such a disposition should alert the surgeon to the possible diagnosis of discordant atrioventricular connexions (congenitally corrected transposition).

Supero-inferior Ventricles

Hearts with supero-inferior ventricles present a similar situation to the 'criss-cross' arrangement except that the heart is tilted along its long axis (Fig. 10.4). In some cases it is rotated as well as tilted so that both 'criss-cross' and supero-inferior arrangements are present. Again, the interventricular coronary arteries are useful because they indicate the plane of the ventricular septum and are excellent guides to the position of the ventricular cavities.

A point of consideration is that the distribution of the conduction tissue in these bizarre hearts is governed by the connexions of the chambers and not by the position of the chambers. These hearts are often further complicated by straddling and overriding atrioventricular valves. It is important to be aware that these abnormal relationships can be found with any combination of atrioventricular and ventriculo–arterial connexions.

Isomerism of the Atrial Appendages

The problems of isomerism of the atrial appendages have already been mentioned. Hearts with this arrangement are not only found in unusual positions but are also almost invariably associated with an abnormal arrangement of the thoraco-abdominal organs, hence the popular rubric of 'visceral heterotaxy'.

Categorizing Atrial Morphology

It is still a widespread practice to classify these patients in terms of 'asplenia' and 'polysplenia'[10]. We believe it is of greater

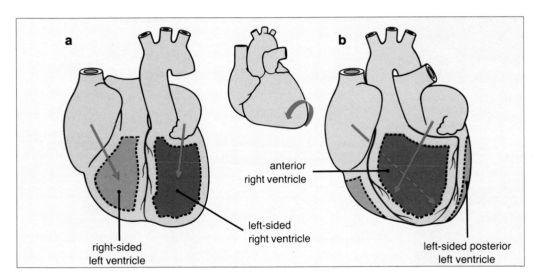

anterior right ventricle

left-sided right ventricle

right-sided left ventricle

left-sided posterior left ventricle

Fig. 10.3 *This diagram, in anatomic orientation, illustrates the abnormality around the long axis (inset) that produces the criss-cross relationship **(b)** in a heart with congenitally corrected transposition **(a)**.*

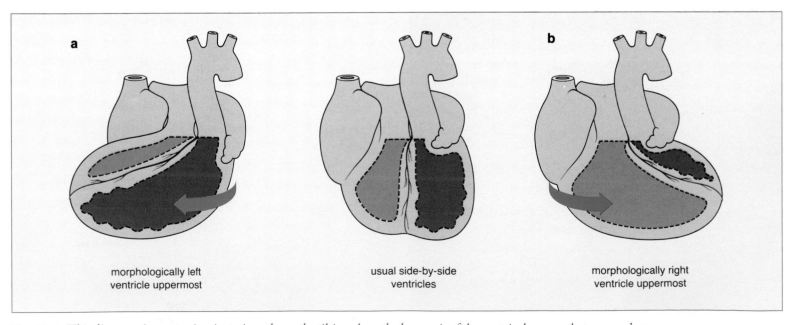

morphologically left ventricle uppermost

usual side-by-side ventricles

morphologically right ventricle uppermost

Fig. 10.4 *This diagram, in anatomic orientation, shows the tilting along the long axis of the ventricular mass that can produce supero-inferior ventricles with either **(a)** the morphologically left or **(b)** the morphologically right ventricle uppermost.*

value to base a system of categorization on atrial morphology. The first reason is that the splenic morphology does not always correspond to the atrial anatomy. There is a greater correspondence between the anatomy of the appendages and what is expected of the 'splenic syndrome' than between these syndromes and splenic morphology[11]. Second, and perhaps more important, it is of little consequence to the cardiac surgeon at the time of the operation whether his patient has one spleen, multiple spleens or no spleen at all. Using the morphology of the appendages to define these anomalies concentrates the attention upon the heart and enables the surgeon to diagnose isomerism at the time of surgery, even if this had not been predicted by the pre-operative studies.

The appendages are the best indicators of atrial morphology and can easily be distinguished as being morphologically right or left. The surgeon must always confirm that his patient possesses lateralized atrial appendages.

Intracardiac Anomalies

Isomerism of the left or right appendage should put the surgeon on immediate alert. In hearts with right isomerism, it is the rule to find complex intracardiac anomalies, usually with the absence of the spleen. There is a totally anomalous pulmonary venous connexion even if the pulmonary veins are connected to the heart. Almost always there are major anomalies of the systemic venous drainage. A common atrioventricular valve is usually present, often with a univentricular atrioventricular connexion. Pulmonary stenosis or atresia is frequently found and there are bilateral sinus nodes.

Although operative experience with these hearts is increasing, the various combinations of anomalies militate against successful outcomes. To be forewarned is of great value, so it should be remembered that the best preoperative guide to isomerism is either cross-sectional ultrasonography of the abdominal great vessels[11] or chest radiography to demonstrate bronchial morphology[12].

Although isomerism of the morphologically right appendages is usually accompanied by severe intracardiac malformations, it is not always so with isomerism of the left appendages. Thus, the surgeon is more likely to be confronted with an undiagnosed case. It then becomes important to know that the sinus node is in an anomalous position. It is usually hypoplastic and, if it can be found, will be located close to the atrioventricular junction[13]. Azygos return of the inferior caval vein is a frequent accompaniment. In the more severely affected cases, there may be a common atrioventricular valve. Pulmonary stenosis or atresia is not usually a feature, nor is the presence of a univentricular atrioventricular connexion.

Whatever the types of isomerism, in the presence of a common valve with each atrium connected to its own ventricle, a left hand pattern of ventricular topology is frequently found. In this setting the heart may well be diagnosed as a congenitally corrected transposition. The presence of isomeric appendages, however, makes it highly likely that there will be a sling of conduction tissue. This places the entire edge of the ventricular septum at risk should surgical correction be attempted.

When isomerism of the appendages is found with a biventricular atrioventricular connexion and a right-hand pattern of ventricular topology, an atrioventricular conduction axis in its usual posterior position is to be anticipated (Fig. 10.5). This entire discussion emphasizes the significance of full sequential segmental analysis of any patient presented for cardiac surgery.

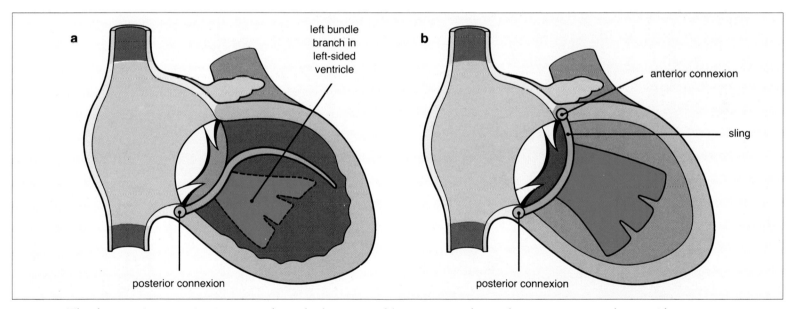

Fig. 10.5 *This diagram, in anatomic orientation, shows the disposition of the atrioventricular conduction tissue axis in hearts with isomerism of the atrial appendages and a biventricular atrioventricular connexion when there is (a) right hand ventricular topology or (b) left hand topology.*

References

1. Van Praagh, R., Van Praagh, S., Vlad, P. & Keith, J.D. (1964) Anatomic types of congenital dextrocardia. Diagnostic and embryologic implications. *American Journal of Cardiology*, **13**, 510–531.

2. Wilkinson, J.L. & Acerete, F. (1973) Terminological pitfalls in congenital heart disease. Reappraisal of some confusing terms, with an account of a simplified system of basic nomenclature. *British Heart Journal*, **35**, 1166–1177.

3. Calcaterra, G., Anderson, R.H., Lau, K.C. & Shinebourne, E.A. (1979) Dextrocardia – value of segmental analysis in its categorization. *British Heart Journal*, **42**, 497–507.

4. Van Praagh, R., Weinberg, P.M., Matsuoka, R. & Van Praagh, S. (1983) Malpositions of the heart. In *Moss's Heart Disease in Infants, Children and Adolescents*. Edited by F.H. Adams & G.C. Emmanouilides. Baltimore: Williams & Wilkins, pp. 422–458.

5. Byron, F.X. (1948) Ectopia cordis. Report of a case with attempted o correction. *Journal of Thoracic Surgery*, **17**, 717–722.

6. Cantrell, J.R., Haller, J.A. & Ravitch, M.M. (1958) A syndrome of congenital defects involving the abdominal wall, sternum, diaphragm, pericardium and heart. *Surgery, Gynecology & Obstetrics*, **107**, 602–614.

7. Anderson, R.H., Smith, A. & Wilkinson, J.L. (1987) Disharmony between atrioventricular connexions and segmental combinations – unusual variants of 'criss-cross' hearts. *Journal of the American College of Cardiology*, **10**, 1274–1277.

8. Symons, J.C., Shinebourne, E.A., Joseph, M.C., Lincoln, C., Ho, S.Y. & Anderson, R.H. (1977) Criss-cross heart with congenitally corrected transposition: report of a case with d-transposed aorta and ventricular preexcitation. *European Journal of Cardiology*, **5**, 493–505.

9. Stanger, P., Rudolph, A.M. & Edwards, J.E. (1977) Cardiac malpositions: an overview based on study of sixty-five necropsy specimens. *Circulation*, **56**, 159–172.

10. Sharma, S., Devine, W., Anderson, R.H. & Zuberbuhler, J.R. (1988) The determination of atrial arrangement by examination of appendage morphology in 1842 autopsied specimens. *British Heart Journal*, **60**, 227–231.

11. Deanfield, J., Leanage, R., Stroobant, J., Chrispin, A.R., Taylor, J.F.N. & Macartney, F.J. (1980) Use of high kilovoltage filtered beam radiographs for detection of bronchial situs in infants and young children. *British Heart Journal*, **44**, 577–583.

13. Dickinson, D.F., Wilkinson, J.L., Anderson, K.R., Smith, A., Ho, S.Y. & Anderson, R.H. (1979) The cardiac conduction system in situs ambiguus. *Circulation*, **59**, 879–885.

Index

A

Abbott's artery 9.7
aberrant right subclavian artery 9.8-9
accessory atrioventricular pathways 5.3-5
agenesis of right lung 9.12
aneurysm
  berry 9.7
  persistent duct 9.14
anomalous pulmonary venous connexion 9.3-6
ansa subclavia 1.8
anterior septum 5.6
aorta 2.17-19
  anomalies 9.6-11
  coarctation 9.6-7
    bronchial artery bleeding 2.19
aortic arch 2.18
  atresia 9.7-9
  in common arterial trunk 8.32
  double 9.9-10
  embryological development 9.9-10
  interruption (aortic discontinuity) 9.7-9
  right-sided 9.11
aortic bar 2.17, 4.2-3
aortic discontinuity 9.7-9
aortic leaflets of mitral valve 3.7
  clefts 7.30
aortic regurgitation 7.31
aortic rings 9.9-11
aortic root 2.3, 4.2
aortic sinuses 3.12, 4.2-3
  in complete transposition 8.19-20
aortic stenosis
  subvalvar 7.32-4
  supravalvar 7.35
aortic valve 2.17, 3.2-4
  anatomical features 3.12-14
  dysplasia 7.31
  endocarditis 7.36-7
  insufficiency, causes 7.36-7
  leaflets 3.12-14
    in tetralogy of Fallot 7.45
  stenosis 7.31-2
aortic-mitral curtain 3.4
aortopulmonary window 9.14-15
apical trabeculations 2.14-15
arcade lesions 7.30
arrhythmias 5.2-5
  after Mustard or Senning procedures 8.13
arterial duct 2.19
  aneurysm 9.14
  ductal tissue and coarctation of aorta 9.7
  persistent 9.12-14
arterial switch procedure 8.18-20
arterial valves 3.2-4
  imperforate 6.11
  leaflets 3.11
  malformations 7.31-49
  morphology 3.11-14, 6.11
  relationship with arterial trunks 6.12-13

arterial valves (cont.)
  sinuses 3.12
arteries
  Abbott's 9.7
  aberrant right subclavian 9.8-9
  bronchial 2.19
  circumflex 3.8, 4.6
  coronary *see* coronary arteries
  inferior thyroid 1.3
  intercostal 2.18-19
  internal thoracic 1.3, 1.5
  pulmonary *see* pulmonary arteries
  to sinus node *see* nodal artery
ascending aorta 2.17
asplenia 6.3, 10.4-5
atresia
  aortic arch (aortic discontinuity) 9.7-9
  left coronary artery 9.17
  mitral 6.5, 8.11-12
  pulmonary *see* pulmonary atresia
  tricuspid *see* tricuspid atresia
atrial appendages 2.4, 6.2-3
  isomerism 6.2-3, 10.4-5
  juxtaposition 2.4
  situs inversus 6.2-3
  situs solitus 6.2-3
atrial septal defects 7.4-8
atrial septum 7.2
  defects 7.4-8
  extent of 2.8-9
atrial shunting 7.4, 7.14-16
atrioventricular bundle 3.9, 3.14-15
  ablation 5.2
atrioventricular conduction system 5.2-6
  accessory pathways 5.3-5
  in atrioventricular septal defect 7.11
  and cardiac valves 3.14-15
  disposition in congenitally corrected transposition 8.20-22
  left bundle branch 2.17, 3.15
  pathways 2.10-11
  in perimembranous ventricular septal defect 7.20-21
  right bundle branch 3.15
  and ventricular relationship 6.10
atrioventricular connexions
  ablation 5.3-4
  biventricular and ambiguous 6.5
  concordant 6.4-5, 7.24
  discordant 6.4-5
  double inlet 6.5
  muscular, ablation 5.3-4
  univentricular 6.5-7, 6.10
atrioventricular groove 3.10
atrioventricular junction
  dilatation 7.29
  malformed heart 6.4-8
  overriding 6.8-9, 7.26
atrioventricular node 3.9
  artery, origin 4.7
  in complete transposition 8.13
  in congenitally corrected transposition 8.21-2